Step
Protoc...
Embryol...

System requirement:

- **Windows XP or above**
- **Power DVD player (Software)**
- **Windows media player 11.0 version or above (Software)**

Accompanying DVD ROM is playable only in Computer and not in DVD player.

Kindly wait for few seconds for DVD to autorun. If it does not autorun then please do the following:

- Click on my computer
- Click the **CD/DVD drive** and after opening the drive, kindly double click the file **Jaypee**

DVD Contents

Video number	Video folders	Folder contents	Chapter link
1.	Laboratory and operation theater	Ovum pickup procedure Laboratory protocols	Chapter 1
2.	Andrology and beyond	Denudation Insemination Oocyte cumulus complex Percutaneous epididymal sperm aspiration (PESA)	Chapter 10
3.	ICSI	ICSI plate preparation ICSI procedure	Chapter 11
4.	Gamete freezing	Cryobiology laboratory Oocyte vitrification Gamete freezing Semen freezing	Chapter 12
5.	Embryo transfer	Embryo transfer technique Postembryo transfer check	Chapter 6
6.	Embryo reduction	Embryo reduction procedure Postembryo reduction ultrasound	Chapter 16

Step by Step® Protocols in Clinical Embryology and ART

Editors

Lt Col Pankaj Talwar VSM
Assisted Reproductive Technology (ART) Center
Army Hospital (Research and Referral)
New Delhi, India

Surveen Ghumman Sindhu MD FICOG
Senior Specialist
Safdarjung Hospital

Assistant Professor
Vardhman Mahavir Medical College
Delhi, India

JAYPEE BROTHERS MEDICAL PUBLISHERS (P) LTD

New Delhi • Panama City • London

Jaypee Brothers Medical Publishers (P) Ltd.

Headquarter

Jaypee Brothers Medical Publishers (P) Ltd
4838/24, Ansari Road, Daryaganj
New Delhi 110 002, India
Phone: +91-11-43574357
Fax: +91-11-43574314
Email: jaypee@jaypeebrothers.com

Overseas Offices

J.P. Medical Ltd.,
83 Victoria Street London
SW1H 0HW (UK)
Phone: +44-2031708910
Fax: +02-03-0086180
Email: info@jpmedpub.com

Jaypee-Highlights Medical Publishers Inc.
City of Knowledge, Bld. 237, Clayton
Panama City, Panama
Phone: + 507-301-0496
Fax: + 507- 301-0499
Email: cservice@jphmedical.com

Website: www.jaypeebrothers.com
Website: www.jaypeedigital.com

© 2012, Jaypee Brothers Medical Publishers

All rights reserved. No part of this book and DVD ROM may be reproduced in any form or by any means without the prior permission of the publisher.

Inquiries for bulk sales may be solicited at: jaypee@jaypeebrothers.com

This book has been published in good faith that the contents provided by the contributors contained herein are original, and is intended for educational purposes only. While every effort is made to ensure accuracy of information, the publisher and the editors specifically disclaim any damage, liability, or loss incurred, directly or indirectly, from the use or application of any of the contents of this work. If not specifically stated, all figures and tables are courtesy of the editors. Where appropriate, the readers should consult with a specialist or contact the manufacturer of the drug or device.

Step by Step® Protocols in Clinical Embryology and ART

First Edition: **2012**

ISBN 978-93-5025-765-4

Printed at: Ajanta Offset & Packagings Ltd., New Delhi

Dedicated to

*Our Patients who in many ways
have been our best teachers*

CONTRIBUTORS

Ashok Khurana
Consultant in Reproductive Ultrasound
The Ultrasound Lab
New Delhi, India

Kuldeep Jain
Professor
Muzaffarnagar Medical College
Director
KJIVF and Laparoscopy Center
New Delhi, India

Lt Col Pankaj Talwar VSM
Assisted Reproductive Technology (ART) Center
Army Hospital (Research and Referral)
New Delhi, India

Preeti Chauhan
Assisted Reproductive Technology (ART) Specialist
Gurgaon, Haryana, India

Shashi Prateek
Professor and Head
Department of Obstetrics and Gynecology
Safdarjung Hospital and Vardhman Mahavir Medical College
Delhi, India

Surveen Ghumman Sindhu MD FICOG
Senior Specialist
Department of Obstetrics and Gynecology
Safdarjung Hospital
Assistant Professor
Vardhman Mahavir Medical College
Delhi, India

Ved Prakash BSc BAMS
Chief Embryologist
Southend Fertility and IVF Center
Delhi, India

PREFACE

Assisted reproductive technology (ART) has strengthened the hopes of the infertile population, thus increasing the demands of these services. ART has evolved as one of the fastest advancing science in medicine. Due to rapid advancement, protocols are fast changing and there is need for a comprehensive book which would get these protocols together in an easy-to-read manner. The book attempts to do this keeping in mind the recent advances.

The book begins with the chapter on setting up of an ART laboratory and selection of patients for IVF. It discusses the stimulation protocols with the pros and cons of each. The embryology section is extensively discussed with photographs and illustrations. It covers andrology, *in vitro* fertilization (IVF), intracytoplasmic sperm injection (ICSI) and cryopreservation. The chapters on oocyte retrieval and embryo transfer lay special emphasis on troubleshooting. Role of ultrasound and legal issues associated with ART are explicitly discussed. The growing attempt of providing therapy to all infertile patients is accompanied by efforts to forestall the complications that accompany these therapies. The chapter on ovarian hyperstimulation and multifetal embryo reduction throw light on these complications and methods to deal with them.

The book is an attempt to integrate information into a practical management protocol that is logical and easy-to-follow for the reader. We hope it is stimulating enough-to-help every practicing infertility and ART specialist to solve dilemmas in dealing with their patients.

Lt Col Pankaj Talwar vsm
Surveen Ghumman Sindhu

ACKNOWLEDGMENTS

I thank my father Mr Mohinder Pal Talwar and my mother Mrs Madhu Talwar for their guidance and constant support. Such monumental work would not have been possible without their blessings and encouragement. I give most sincere thanks to my wife Dr (Mrs) Neetu Talwar and sons Pratik and Arjun, for giving me unfailing support and encouragement during compilation of the book. It was their unflinching motivation and enthusiasm which gave me impetus to move ahead in trying times, which I faced during scripting of *Step by Step® Protocols in Clinical Embryology and ART*.

Lt Col Pankaj Talwar vsm

I would like to thank my husband, Sandeep, for his unconditional support in not only this, but all my ventures. His encouragement has been instrumental in making me focus on giving this academic project the face it has. My parents have given me the sound foundation of right values, which has helped me at each step including this one. I would like to thank them for their contribution. Jahnavi and Janya, my daughters are a source of constant inspiration and I would like to acknowledge their contributions through the patience and support they showed while the book took up my time.

Surveen Ghumman Sindhu

We would like to thank all the contributors for their valuable inputs and the team at M/s Jaypee Brothers Medical Publishers (P) Ltd, New Delhi, India, for bringing this book to its present form.

CONTENTS

1. **Setting up of an ART Center** 1
   Surveen Ghumman Sindhu

   *Location of the Laboratory 1 • Basic Infrastructure 1
   Floor Plan 7 • Laboratory Personnel 8
   Equipment 10 • Consumables 15 • Culture Media 15
   Protocols in the Laboratory—Do's and Dont's 16
   Quality Control 17 • Risk Management 18*

2. **Selection and Preparation of an IVF Patient** 21
   Surveen Ghumman Sindhu

   *Infection Screen 21 • Immunization Status 22 • Medical
   and Surgical Disease 22 • Assessment of BMI and Weight and
   Lifestyle Changes 22 • Role of Pelvic Ultrasonography in the
   Selection and Preparation of Patients for IVF 23 • Pretreatment
   Hormone Assessment to Optimize IVF Outcomes 24
   • Evaluation of the Ovarian Reserve 24 • Pre-IVF Laparoscopy/
   Hysteroscopy Assessment 27 • Assessment and Treatment
   of Specific Pathology Before an IVF Cycle 28 • Role of Oral
   Contraceptive Pills Before ART Cycle 34 • Assessment of the
   Male 34 • Patient Counseling and Education 35*

3. **Semen Analysis and Assessment of the
   Male Partner** 39
   Surveen Ghumman Sindhu

   *Sample Collection and Delivery 39 • Physical Parameters 42
   Initial Microscopic Examination 46 • Sperm Concentration 48
   Sperm Motility 50 • Sperm Morphology 53 • Cellular Elements
   other than Spermatozoa 59 • Tests for Sperm Membrane
   Integrity 60 • Sperm Membrane Binding, Capacitation
   and Penetration 61 • Acrosome Detection 62 • Biochemical
   Measurement of Sperm Function 62 • Antisperm Antibodies
   (ASA) 63 • Assessment of Sperm DNA Damage 65*

4. **Gonadotropins** 69
   Surveen Ghumman Sindhu

   *Gonadotropin Preparations 69 • Choice of Dosage 70
   Protocols 71 • Monitoring 76 • Side Effects and Risks 77
   Recombinant FSH 78 • Recombinant FSH-CTP in IVF 79
   Recombinant LH 80 • Human Chorionic Gonadotropin 80*

5. Role of GnRH Agonists and Antagonists in ART 85
Surveen Ghumman Sindhu

GnRH Agonist (GnRH-A) 85 • GnRH Antagonists 92
Gonadotropin Releasing Hormone 99

6. Embryo Transfer and Troubleshooting 103
Pankaj Talwar

Factors Affecting Embryo Transfer 103 • Relevant Issues to be
Addressed Before Embryo Transfer 103 • Relevant Issues to be
Addressed During Embryo Transfer 107 • Relevant Issues to be
Addressed Post Embryo Transfer 111
Embryo Transfer Step by Step 112

7. Ovum Pickup and Troubleshooting 127
Pankaj Talwar

Relevant Issues 127 • OPU Step by Step 137 • Common
Problems Encountered During Ovum Pickup 144
Complications 146 • Learning Curve 146

8. Embryo Selection 151
Ved Prakash, Pankaj Talwar

Embryo Assessment 153 • Fertilization Assessment 154
Pronuclei Scoring 155 • Evaluation of Embryo Quality 155
Blastocyst Scoring 161

9. Culture Media in IVF and Embryo Culture 167
Pankaj Talwar

Essential Concepts 168 • The Physiology of Sequential Culture
Media 171 • Use of Oil Overlay in ART 176
Quality Control Testing for the Culture Media 176
Essentials of Handling Media and Lab Equipment 179
Media Preparation and Pre-equilibration 188
Storage of the Media 189 • Shelf Life and Packaging 190
Disposables in ART 191 • Quality Control Tests 192
Types of Disposables 195

10. Andrology and Beyond 207
Pankaj Talwar, Kuldeep Jain

Semen Preparation for IVF 207 • Oocyte Assessment 230
Insemination Protocols in ART 233 • Denudation 238
Assessment of Fertilization 241

11. Intracytoplasm Sperm Injection and Troubleshooting 259

Pankaj Talwar

*Indications for ICSI 259 • ICSI Media 259 • Pipettes 260
Preparation of ICSI Dishes 263 • Denudation 268
Manipulation of Spermatozoa 272 • Manipulation of
Oocytes 272 • Microinjection of Oocytes with Mature
Spermatozoa 273 • Difficult ICSI Cases 280*

12. Gamete Cryopreservation 283

Pankaj Talwar

*Oocyte Freezing 283 • Oocyte Vitrification and Thawing 292
Sperm Cryopreservation 303*

13. Embryo Vitrification 329

Pankaj Talwar

*Principles of Vitrification 329 • Principles of Warming 330
Unique Vitrification Devices 331 • Superiority of Various
Vitrification Methods 333 • Vitrification Step by Step 334
Preventing Potential Contamination From Liquid Nitrogen 357*

14. Endometrial Receptivity and Luteal Support 361

Surveen Ghumman Sindhu

*Histological Changes 363 • Biochemical and Molecular
Changes 364 • Immunological Aspects of Endometrial
Implantation 365 • Endometrial Vascular Changes 366
Current Strategies to Assess Endometrial Receptivity 366
Endometrial Preparation for Frozen Embryo Transfer 370
Treatment of Poor Uterine Receptivity 370*

15. Ovarian Hyperstimulation Syndrome 385

Surveen Ghumman Sindhu

*Incidence 385 • Classification 385 • Pathophysiology of
OHSS 388 • Clinical Features 388 • Fatal Complications 390
Management of OHSS 390*

16. Multifetal Pregnancy Reduction 401

Preeti Chauhan

*Methods 403 • Complications of Pregnancy Reduction 412
Ethical Issues 413*

17. Ultrasound Assessment of Endometrial Receptivity and Oocyte and Embryo Quality............. 419

Ashok Khurana

Physiological and Biochemical Basis of Implantation 419
Lessons from IVF and Ovum Donation Cycles 421
Gray Scale, Power Doppler and 3D Ultrasound 422
Oocyte and Embryo Quality 430

18. Ethical and Legal Aspects in ART................................. 441

Shashi Prateek, Surveen Ghumman Sindhu

Legal Issues of ART in Marriage 447 • Rights of a Child Born by Donor Gamete 448 • Semen Banks 449 • Oocyte Donation 456 • Surrogacy 457

Index...461

Chapter 1

Setting up of an ART Center

Surveen Ghumman Sindhu

There are many factors that go into making a good IVF laboratory from a construction and facility standpoint, in addition to the people, that make it all work. Much depends on air quality, laboratory design and an ongoing quality control. An IVF program is only as good as the laboratory which supports it. The embryology laboratory must have adequate space to allow good laboratory practice and free movement. Attention should be given to the ergonomics of the operator like bench height, adjustable chairs, microscope eye height, efficient use of space and surfaces.

LOCATION OF THE LABORATORY

The laboratory should be away from traffic, dust and pollution, preferably on a higher floor (not ground floor). Moisture prone areas like basements must be avoided. It should be away from the hospital traffic.

Access to laboratory: Access should be large enough to allow bulky instruments to be moved in and out.

BASIC INFRASTRUCTURE

Electricity

Power points should be made at a regular distances over working benches above the estimated requirement.

Supply from different electric phases and provision for power backup in the form of uninterrupted power supply and/or a captive power generation system is important as there should be no interruption in power supply to the incubator.

Air Conditioning

The IVF laboratory has to have a separate air conditioning unit which is not common with the rest of the hospital air. This system should be attached to an air purifying unit.

Water Supply

Scrubbing and washing area will need adequate water supply and well concealed drainage.

Air Quality

For a successful IVF program it is important that the laboratory air is clean. Improved fertilization rates and embryo development were seen with superior air quality in an ART laboratory.[1] Volatile organic compounds (VOCs) are important air contaminants and include isopropanol (aka Isopropyl Alcohol) benzene, hexane, formaldehyde and, vinyl chloride and are found in fuel, solvents and adhesives are released by them. Air handling systems must keep the following facts in mind.

> *Note:*
> - VOCs may also be produced by instruments such as microscopes, television monitors, substances derived from building materials, flooring, paint and construction materials and all furniture from particle board, which is 10% formaldehyde resin by weight and off-gasses for over 20 years.
> - VOCs can increase in pulses when cleaning agents are used or be present continuously, like from those released from furniture made of particle board.

1. *Measurement of VOC:* When setting up an IVF laboratory, it is important to accurately measure VOCs in the building, in the laboratory, and in the incubators and should also be measured on an ongoing basis with a VOC meter. VOCs are typically measured in parts per million (ppm) or parts per billion (ppb). The air of the sterile area should not be mixed with unsterile area and the AC ducting should be such that there is no mixing of air.
2. *HEPA filters:* HEPA filtration removes 99.97% of airborne particles at 3 mm but do not remove VOC as they easily pass through these filters.
3. *Carbon filters:* Charcoal and potassium permanganate filters must be installed to remove VOCs and carbon-based contaminants.
4. An IVF laboratory must have a dedicated heating ventilation and air conditioning (HVAC) unit on the roof of the building directly above the laboratory. This separates the IVF laboratory environment from the rest of the building.

> For IVF a VOC count below 0.5 ppm, ideally below 0.2 ppm and preferably zero is required. VOCs levels at high levels (over 1 ppm) will be directly toxic to embryos and affect results.

5. *Pressure gradient:* Pressure gradient is maintained in such a manner that embryology laboratory air volume and pressure should be slightly higher than adjoining rooms forcing air out and keeping away any toxic fumes trying to come in. This is achieved by absorbing the circulating air outside the IVF laboratory and passing them through filters.
6. *Air exchanges:* HVAC system should have 10–15 air exchanges per hour with maximum air pressure so that air is going out of the room.

7. *Quality checks:* There must be regular quality checks to ensure that particles are removed to desired levels and number of air exchanges is adequate.
8. *Coda filters:* Coda filters remove VOCs and can also be installed within the laboratory or online for medical gasses which may contain VOCs to prevent these fumes from entering incubators.
9. *Ultraviolet light:* Photocatalytic oxidation units use ultraviolet light to breakdown VOCs into CO_2 and water. The disadvantage is that many times these units breakdown larger VOCs into smaller VOCs and they also generate high levels of free radicals which are not good for IVF. However, they are more economical than carbon media-based systems.
10. Certain basic protocols need to be followed to protect the laboratory environment like limited access to the laboratory, airlock systems, cleanliness of personnel and prohibition of use of perfumes and make-up.

> *Recommendation:* Air extracted from a brand new incubator shows a very high concentrations of VOC hence a new incubator must be off gassed for 3 to 5 months prior to putting it into use.

Temperature

The embryo grows in the body at a temperature of 37°C. Decreasing the temperature only 1°C will disrupt the spindle apparatus that helps the chromosomes separate. Ambient temperature should be 24 to 26°C.

Light

Sunlight and cool-white fluorescent office light, which is blue-white in appearance, were the most detrimental to the mice embryo development while warm-white light, which is typically used to illuminate homes and residential environments and has a yellow-white color, was significantly less damaging.[2] When exposed to light, the embryos produced increased levels of radical oxygen which is toxic to cellular development.

> *Recommendations:*
> - Lighting should be within sealed units
> - Harsh lighting should be replaced with warm-white light bulbs for illumination
> - Minimize light exposure as much as possible during each stage of embryo development
> - Filters are used in the microscopes and rheostats are used to control the amount of light.

Floors, Walls and Ceiling

The following points should be noted:
1. The floors should be scratch proof and non-slippery.
2. The edges and corners should be curved for easy cleaning.
3. The flooring can be a single sheet which wraps up the wall for 6 inches. This keeps the chance of dust or germs in the crevices between flooring tiles low and makes it easier to clean the flooring. Tiles should be as large as possible so that there are minimum joints which may accumulate dust particles.
4. Solvent free adhesives or vinyl glue used for floor covering with low VOC emissions are available.
5. Partition should be of non-porous inert material.
6. False ceilings are not recommended as it is inaccessible for maintenance. However, if they may be needed to conceal lights and filters the walls should go all the way up to the roof above the false ceiling so that laboratory is isolated. Additionally, the false ceiling should have solid panels.

7. Walls of IVF laboratory and OT should be dark, preferable black granite with minimum joints, smooth and non-porous.
8. Water based paint formulated with low VOC potential should be used. No paints containing formaldehyde, acetaldehyde, isocyanates, reactive amines, phenols and other water soluble volatile organics should be used.
9. Sinks and drains should be outside the laboratory. Ducts/pipes can be hidden between wall panels or covered.
10. Inert stainless steel tubing with medical gasses is now recommended and copper should be avoided.
11. Steps for vermin proofing should be planned at an early stage because no pesticide can be used in a fully functional IVF clinic, as it could be toxic to the gametes and embryos.

Doors

The entry should be restricted and preferably be with electric eye doors. The doors should be coated or of steel which can be cleaned with ethyl alcohol. In order to control the laboratory environment, it is best not to have windows or other surface that may not insulate the laboratory well.

Furniture

1. Stainless steel furniture is preferable as board releases VOCs and is less easy to clean.
2. Working benches, chairs and stools with adjustable height add to the comfort of the scientist and reduce fatigue.
3. Easily slidable drawers with adequate capacity for storage should be installed in the laboratory with working benches.

4. The surfaces should be non-porous and easily cleanable.
5. It is preferable not to put shelves on the wall as dust can collect on top and can go unnoticed.

FLOOR PLAN

An IVF clinic would require an area of 2500 sq feet. This would also take into consideration adding on instruments for ever expanding technology in this sector. The IVF clinic can be divided into sterile and nonsterile areas[3] (Fig. 1.1).

Nonsterile Area

1. A reception and waiting room for patients.
2. Office of the gynecologist and program director with a counseling room.
3. Conference room.
4. Examination room: An appropriate ultrasonographic machine with a transvaginal probe.[3]
5. Store room.
6. Record room.
7. Autoclave room.
8. Semen collection room: This must be a well-appointed room with privacy, an attached toilet and an appropriate environment located in a secluded area close to the laboratory.
9. Semen processing laboratory.
10. Room for for intrauterine insemination.
11. Recovery room.
12. Changing room.

Sterile Area

The sterile area shall house the operation theater, an adjoining embryology laboratory and a room to keep the cryocans for freezing. Entry to the sterile area must be

strictly controlled by an anteroom for changing footwear, area for changing into sterile garments and a scrub-station. The sterile area must be air-conditioned where fresh air filtered through an approved and appropriate filter system is circulated at an ambient temperature (22–25°C).
1. Scrub station.
2. The operation theater.
3. Room for intrauterine embryo transfer: It can be done in the same room as the operation theater.
4. The embryology laboratory complex: The embryology laboratory should be equipped with the following:
    - A laminar flow bench with a thermostatically controlled heating plate
    - A stereomicroscope
    - A routine high-powered binocular light microscope
    - A 'high resolution' inverted microscope with phase contrast or Hoffmann optics, preferably with facilities for video recording
    - A micromanipulator
    - Two CO_2 incubator with a back up
    - A laboratory centrifuge.

    The area for andrology should be separated by a door.
5. Room for storage of cryocans.

LABORATORY PERSONNEL

The practice of ART requires a well-orchestrated teamwork between many specialities.
1. Gynecologist and program coordinator.
2. Andrologist.
3. Ultrasonologist.
4. Clinical embryologist.

Setting up of an ART Center | 9

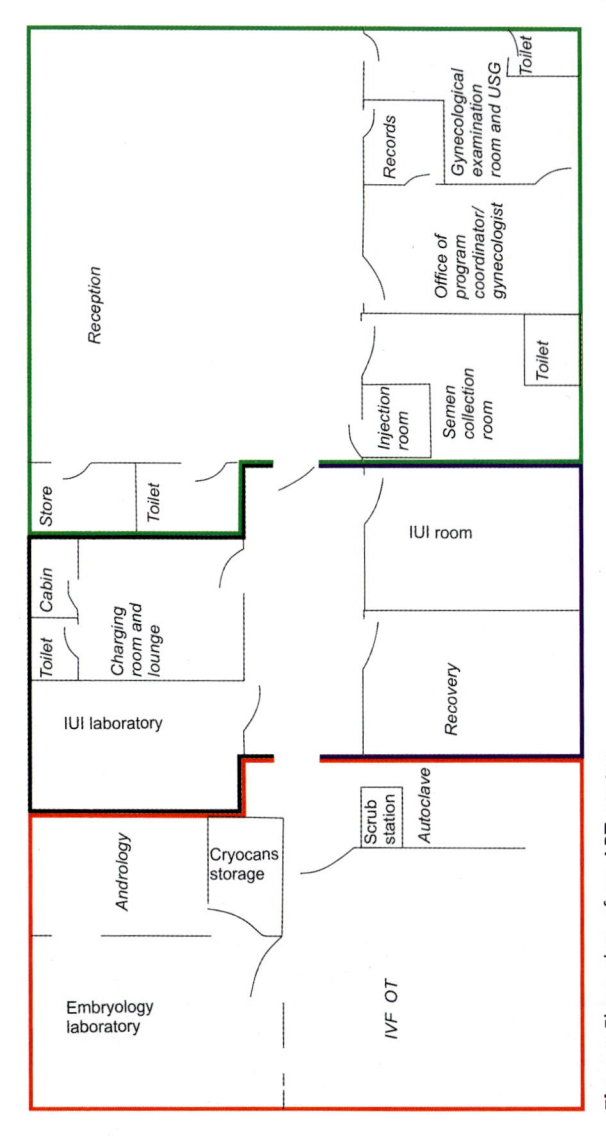

Fig. 1.1: Floor plan of an ART center

5. Counselors.
6. Trained OT nursing sisters.
7. Trained technicians.
8. Receptionist.

EQUIPMENT

1. Crucial equipment, like incubators and cryopreservation storage facilities must have appropriate monitors and alarms.
2. Gas cylinders should be placed outside with an automatic backup system.
3. Protocols for maintaining incubators and other equipment should be clearly defined on how frequently they must be sterilized and cleaned.
4. Records of maintenance on all the equipment must be documented.
5. All instruments must be calibrated periodically (weekly, monthly or yearly) and a record of such calibration maintained.
6. Besides, instruction manual for every instrument being available, written instructions should be available to all members of the staff for actions to be taken in the case of equipment failure.
7. New equipment should be "run in" to dissipate latent VOCs for a successful start.

Incubators

- The incubator which maintains the temperature accurately and has minimal CO_2 recovery preferred.
- Incubators may have either thermal conductivity or infrared sensors. Infrared are preferred.

- Between a water and air jacketed incubator, an air jacketed one is preferred.
- A minimum number of two incubators are recommended. This is for both, a backup facility, and to decrease the frequency of repeatedly opening the first, because samples are distributed.
- CO_2 supplied to the incubator should be of medical grade. Through a two stage regulator ideal pressure to minimize gas consumption without affecting CO_2 recovery time is maintained.
- There are alarm systems connected to mobile phones which notifiy the embryology staff if the incubators change temperature or CO_2 concentration.
- Metal gas tubing should be avoided.
- In line filter between CO_2 cylinder and incubator eliminates all contamination from the gas.
- Mini-incubators have shown better temperature and CO_2 recovery and embryo and blastocyst formation rate compared with the conventional incubator.[4]
- Triple gas incubators with lower oxygen concentration (5% O_2) environment consistently resulted in higher rates of live birth.[5]

Laminar Flow Hoods (Clean Air Work Station)

The size of the hood can be according to need. Accessories such as gas ports and humidifying systems can be added to the flow hood to control the pH and osmolarity. Temperature is controlled with a built-in heated area in the table plate. Microscopes are fixed. Usually there are 0.3 micron HEPA filters and 10 microns prefilters, i.e. a class 100 where 99.99% of airborne particles of 0.3 microns and above size are removable providing dust and bacteria free atmosphere.

Microscopes

Microscopes must deliver ample depth of field as well as clarity, detail, accurate color and the least possible distortion. Dependable, high-performance optics and good ergonomic features make even long-duration tasks easier and less demanding to perform.

A. *Stereozoom microscope:* Used for oocyte identification easy.
B. *Binocular microscope:* Binocular microscope is used for andrology. The standard microscope is provided with an objective of 10X, 20X, 40X and 100X. A trinocular microscope with CCD camera is also available and may be used for teaching purposes.
C. *Inverted microscope:* Inverted microscope is useful for studying the pronucleus stage and embryo morphology. Micromanipulation requires inverted microscope with Hoffmann modulation which can be adapted with a micromanipulator and PGD techniques in the future.

Micromanipulator

The specially selected adapter, a pair of positioners, joystick micromanipulators and universal joints are combined. Three-dimensional coarse movements are performed electrically and fine movements by an oil hydraulic mechanism can also be performed. This system enables exceptionally delicate manipulations.

Ovum Aspiration Pump

Ovum aspiration pump is used for oocyte retrieval. It ensures constant negative pressure for aspiration of follicular fluid.

Laboratory Purification System

Purification systems use a back-position Hospital Grade HEPA Filter with a 99.99% removal rating of 0.3 micron particles. There is also four different carbon types in activated charcoal granules, and UV chamber toxic compounds into benign constituents such as water and carbon dioxide. Purification system can be put in the room or online (Coda) for incubators.

Electric sensors with alarms may be installed which monitor air quality and automatically increase air purifier performance.

Heating Appliances

Maintaining temperature of the gametes all along the procedure in the laboratory is of prime importance and for this purpose warming blocks, petridish warmer and stage warmer are used.

a. *Warming blocks:* Warming block (Dry bath) is used for heating of test tubes used for follicular fluid and petri dishes in removable, autoclavable anodized aluminium blocks for maintenance of required temperature. Blocks are available in different shapes and for different applications.

b. *Petri dish warmer:* It maintains the temperature of the dishes before they are actually placed on the microscope stage.

c. *Stage warmer:* It maintains temperature of the culture dish during identification and manipulation of oocyte.

Programmable Biological Freezer with Cryocans

Programmable embryo freezer is used for slow freezing of embryos and gametes.

However, if the laboratory is doing vitrification this freezer is not needed.

Along with this cryocans of various sizes must be available for storage.

Laser System

Laser system for assisted hatching and embryo biopsy is attached to the micromanipulator.[6]

Spindle Imaging System

It is used in ICSI to bring into view the spindle before ICSI ensuring that the spindle is not harmed by the injection pipette. It also provides structural information closely related to the more invasive immunostaining method, and also enables study of the dynamic architecture of spindles.[7,8]

Sperm Counting Chamber

Makler sperm counting chamber is designed to produce 10 micron thick smear which avoids overlapping of sperms, and allows free movement of sperms in all directions.

Computer-assisted Semen Analyzer (CASA)

An automated analysis of semen is done on the screen and is used to asses sperm velocity and motion parameters.[9]

Centrifuge

A centrifuge with digital speed and time indicator is needed for semen preparation.

Ultrasound Machine

Ultrasound machine with a transvaginal probe is required for oocyte retrieval and embryo transfer.

Miscellaneous

- *Heat sealing machines:* Heat sealing machine is used for straws and polybags sealing.
- *Antivibration microscope table:* An antivibration table has vibration isolators with rolling diaphragm to give

isolation from surface borne vibrations in all directions. This helps in accurate manipulation of gametes and embryos.
- *Electronic thermometer.*
- *Fyrite kit:* Fyrite kit for measuring carbon dioxide concentration in incubators.
- *pH meter.*
- *Ultrapure water system:* A water filtration system should be installed to provide clean water for washing the laboratory.
- *Software for data entry:* The database systems are developed to manage patient and laboratory information and management of internal quality control and external quality assurance systems for andrology and embryology. There are many software programs for this purpose, which are commercially available today.

CONSUMABLES

Quality of consumables used in the laboratory: All disposable plasticware must be procured from reliable sources after ensuring that they are not toxic to the embryo. They are sterilized by gradiation and individually packed. Table 1.1 shows a list of consumables needed.

CULTURE MEDIA

When starting an IVF laboratory, it should be ensured that culture media be procured from reliable manufacturers. Each batch of culture medium needs to be tested for sterility, endotoxins, osmolality and pH to ensure that it is of tissue culture grade, preferably mouse embryo tested and with purity appropriate for the purpose. The media used are flushing medium, sperm preparation medium,

Table 1.1
Consumables for IVF laboratory

- Semen collecting containers
- Tissue culture grade plastic test tubes—6 ml and 14 ml
- Graduated conical tubes
- Plastic test tube stand
- 5 ml sterile serological pipettes
- Pasteur's pipette
- Pipette stands
- 1 ml syringe and 5 ml syringe with needle
- Glass slides
- Cover slip square 22 × 22 mm
- Nontoxic gloves
- Glass marking pencil
- Petri dishes, fourwell dishes, single well dish
- Oocyte retrieval set—single or double lumen
- Embryo transfer catheters
- Embryo reduction needle
- ICSI micropipettes

universal IVF medium, mineral oil and embryo freezing and thawing package (For details see Chapter 9).

PROTOCOLS IN THE LABORATORY—DO'S AND DONT'S

Protocols in the laboratory must be set-up before starting.
1. All consent forms should be in order for each procedure.
2. The detailed manuals for all procedures used should be available in the laboratory.
3. Written, signed and dated protocols and standard operating procedure should exist for every process performed in the laboratory.
4. Proper training of all the laboratory staff is mandatory.

5. All samples from the patients, like blood, follicular fluid and sperm samples, must bear identification of the treated couple.
6. Documentation of all critical steps in each patient's file is essential.
7. Strict observation of staff cleanliness is essential. Food, drinks and cigarettes are strictly forbidden. The use of make-up and perfumes should not be allowed.
8. Washing hands and change of clothes while entering the laboratory is important.
9. The handling of embryos, zygotes and gametes for ART should be performed in a laminar flow hood equipped with heating stages and prewarmed heating blocks with aseptic technique is a must.
10. Pipetting devices must be used only for one patient and must not be reused.
11. Treatment of more than one patient simultaneously should never be done in the same working place. Next sample should only be handled before the first is completely processed.
12. If the laboratory performs cryopreservation, a system should be in place for the detection of low levels of liquid nitrogen in the tanks and for high levels of nitrogen in the air.
13. Documentation of all records is a must.
14. An annual audit of stored gametes, zygotes and embryos must be carried out, cross-referencing contents with storage records.[10]

QUALITY CONTROL

Quality management system must be in place. A written record of adverse events, emergency situations and incorrect identification of specimens is maintained. Laminar flowhoods, laboratory tables, incubators and other areas where sterility is required must be periodically checked for microbial contamination using standard techniques, and a record of such checks must be kept. A logbook should be maintained which records the temperature, carbon dioxide content and humidity of the incubators and the manometer readings of the laminar air flow. All instruments must be calibrated periodically (weekly, monthly or yearly) and a record of such calibration maintained.

Internal quality assurance of laboratory performance is essential on a regular basis and indicators and their critical levels must be defined. The following indicators may be regularly assessed— fertilization and cleavage rates, rates of errors and adverse events, ratio of embryos of good quality, survival rate after thawing, implantation and clinical pregnancy rates, and multiple pregnancy rates.[11] Performance of laboratory staff should be recorded. External quality control (EQC) with commercial, or in collaboration with other laboratories, is recommended. Participation in EQC increases the degree of inter-laboratory agreement on embryo classification.

RISK MANAGEMENT

Before starting the laboratory each unit should establish procedures and policies for the safety of personnel and for preventing cross-contamination. All personnel must be vaccinated against hepatitis B or other viral disease. Screening patients and gamete donors for human immunodeficiency virus (HIV), hepatitis B/C should be the norm for the laboratory. The laboratory staff must be educated to treat each sample as potentially infectious and must be made aware about the risks of handling infected biological material. Care must be taken for the safe disposal of biological waste and other materials (syringes, glass slides, etc.).

The treatment of patients positive for HIV or hepatitis B/C should be only be performed in laboratories having dedicated areas, in which adequate safety measures are followed. Specimens known to be contaminated should be stored in high-security straws and, preferably, in dedicated tanks. A Class II laminar flow cabinet should be used when contaminated samples are handled for protection. Nontoxic (nonpowdered) gloves and masks are used for protection. Use of vertical laminar flow benches, mechanical pipetting devices and disposable material which can be discarded after usage are encouraged. Use of cryogloves if cryogenic materials are handled is recommended.

Setting up an IVF laboratory requires high-laboratory standards with extremely qualified personnel, as well as defined quality management program which, integrates quality control, quality assurance and quality improvement.

REFERENCES

1. Legro RS, Sauer MV, Mottla GL, Richter KS, Li X, Dodson WC, Liao D. Effect of air quality on assisted human reproduction. Hum Reprod. 2010;25(5):1317-24.
2. Oh SJ, Gong SP, Lee ST, Lee EJ, Lim JM. Light intensity and wavelength during embryo manipulation are important factors for maintaining viability of preimplantation embryos *in vitro*. Fertil Steril. 2007;88:1150-7.
3. National Guidelines for Accreditation, Supervision and Regulation of ART Clinics in India Ministry of Health and Family Welfare Government of India Indian Council of Medical Research National Academy of Medical Sciences (India), New Delhi-110029. 2008

4. Fujiwara M, Takahashi K, Izuno M, Duan YR, Kazono M, Kimura F, Noda Y. Effect of micro-environment maintenance on embryo culture after *in vitro* fertilization: comparison of top-load mini incubator and conventional front-load incubator. J Assist Reprod Genet. 2007;24(1): 5-9.
5. Meintjes M, Chantilis SJ, Douglas JD, Rodriguez AJ, Guerami AR, Bookout DM, Barnett BD, Madden JD. A controlled randomized trial evaluating the effect of lowered incubator oxygen tension on live births in a predominantly blastocyst transfer program. Hum Reprod. 2009;24(2):300-7.
6. Hammadeh ME, Fischer-Hammadeh C, Ali KR. Assisted hatching in assisted reproduction: a state of the art. J Assist Reprod Genet. 2011; 28(2):119-28.
7. Keefe D, Liu L, Wang W, Silva C. Imaging meiotic spindles by polarization light microscopy: principles and applications to IVF. Reprod Biomed Online. 2003;7(1):24-9.
8. Montag M, Schimming T, van der Ven H. Spindle imaging in human oocytes: the impact of the meiotic cell cycle. Reprod Biomed Online. 2006;12(4):442-6.
9. Krause W. The significance of computer-assisted semen analysis (CASA) for diagnosis in andrology and fertility prognosis. Int J Androl. 1995;18:32-5
10. Magli MC, Abbeel EV, Lundin K, Royere D, Elst JV, Gianaroli L. Revised ESHRE guidelines for good practice in IVF laboratories. Hum Reprod. 2008;23:1253-62.
11. Balaban B, Urman B. Embryo culture as a diagnostic tool. Reprod Biomed Online. 2003;7(6):671-82.

Chapter 2

Selection and Preparation of an IVF Patient

Surveen Ghumman Sindhu

Selection and preparation of an IVF patient is part of the quality management of the whole procedure and can contribute significantly to the success of the program. As IVF involves high cost and is stressful to the patient, optimizing its results is mandatory. In order to explain what is the indication and why IVF is required to the couple, accurate evaluation has to be relied on (Table 2.1). Most patients have been extensively investigated before they reach an ART specialist. All these investigations are reviewed and updated if necessary.

INFECTION SCREEN

Pelvic examination with an infection screen is a must. Screening is done for *Chlamydia* and *Gonococcus*. Couples are screened for HIV, hepatitis B and C, and syphilis. In India, where there is a high prevalence of tuberculosis screening for this disease is a must and is done by sending an endometrial sample for AFB culture, histopathology or PCR. Tuberculosis is known to affect implantation and often remains undetected due to its latent nature. Nonspecific chronic endometritis is an important cause of IVF failure and is a histopathological finding. These conditions must be treated if found positive before patient is taken up for IVF, as they affect results.

Table 2.1
Indications of IVF

1. Male factor infertility
   a. Azospermia—Obstructive and nonobstructive
   b. Retrograde ejaculation
   c. Severe oligoasthenoteratospermia
   d. Immunological infertility
2. Age-related infertility—Premature menopause: oocyte donation
3. Absent or damaged fallopian tubes
4. Severe endometriosis
5. Unexplained infertility
6. Recurrent intrauterine insemination failure
7. Tubal and pelvic adhesions (pelvic inflammatory disease, tuberculosis, previous pelvic surgery)
8. Genetic disease requiring preimplantation genetic diagnosis (PGD)
9. Severe intrauterine adhesions—surrogacy
10. Medical disease in mother not permitting pregnancy—surrogacy

IMMUNIZATION STATUS

Immunization status for rubella is checked in case, the woman conceives.

MEDICAL AND SURGICAL DISEASE

A review of history of medical or surgical conditions, which can affect the treatment options is done.

ASSESSMENT OF BMI AND WEIGHT AND LIFESTYLE CHANGES

BMI is assessed. Increased weight is associated with reduced fertility, and increased treatment costs as higher doses of gonadotropins are required, the follicular response is poorer and the miscarriage rate is 30–50%. Hence, weight reduction forms an important goal in preparation. Lifestyle practices like smoking, excessive alcohol or caffeine intake, excessive exercise, inadequate micronutrient intake, and increased psychological stress contribute to IVF failure and pregnancy complications. Hence they should be rectified.

Assessment of Nutritional Status and Role of Supplements

Her hemoglobin level must be checked and any anemia corrected. Folate supplements must be started. With important role of reactive oxidation species emerging in infertility, antioxidants can be started in both partners if indicated.

ROLE OF PELVIC ULTRASONOGRAPHY IN THE SELECTION AND PREPARATION OF PATIENTS FOR IVF

It an essential tool in selection, preparation and monitoring of IVF patients. It helps in the following ways:
1. Assessment of endometrial receptivity by assessing endometrial thickness, morphology and vascularity.
2. Diagnosing uterine conditions, baseline ovarian cysts, endometriosis and hydrosalpinx which may need to be dealt with before starting IVF.
3. Ovarian reserve assessment to decide prognosis and protocol of ovarian stimulation.
4. Diagnosing PCOS and prediction of OHSS.
5. Judging location, mobility and accessibility of ovaries for planning oocyte retrieval.
6. A trial embryo transfer may be performed in previous cycle to assess the cervical os, length and curvature of cervical canal and length of endometrial cavity.

PRETREATMENT HORMONE ASSESSMENT TO OPTIMIZE IVF OUTCOMES

Baseline hormonal test must be done. Thyroid, testosterone and prolactin levels are to be assessed. Besides this day 2 LH and FSH is a must. Raised LH levels must be brought down before stimulation. In these cases an agonist protocol with recombinant FSH is preferred to keep LH levels down. Raised androgens and a abnormal thyroid profile also must be treated before starting IVF cycle.

EVALUATION OF THE OVARIAN RESERVE

A woman's advancing age is directly related to poor ovarian response to simulation. This situation arises from the natural process of aging and the depletion of the primordial follicular pool and consequent failure in recruitment of follicles. Ovarian reserve assessment is essential as it helps us to categorize patients into poor responders or hyper-responders. This helps in counseling patients about prognosis and deciding which ovarian stimulation protocol is to be used. Women with low ovarian reserve require protocols with higher initial FSH dose and GnRH antagonist cycles are preferred to agonist. The assessment of ovarian reserve (OR) is based on a series of clinical, biological, and ultrasound criteria. No single test for assessment of ovarian reserve is adequate, so a combination of following tests is recommended (Table 2.2).

Basal follicle stimulating hormone levels: Raised early follicular FSH level is one of the earliest indications of reproductive aging (Table 2.3). It has been shown that women with elevated FSH levels have a higher minimum threshold level of FSH required to initiate sustained follicular development. Cycling women with a history of elevated FSH should be offered treatment without further delay.[1]

Early follicular phase estradiol levels: Early elevation of serum estradiol level reflects advanced follicular development and early selection of dominant follicle seen in older women due to rising FSH levels. A premature elevation of estradiol may suppress FSH causing masking of an elevated day 3 FSH. Hence, it is better if both FSH and estradiol are measured, to eliminate false negative results.

Table 2.2
Ovarian reserve tests

1. Basal FSH (day 2)
2. Day 2 or 3 serum estradiol
3. Basal inhibin B
4. Mullarian inhibiting substance
5. Antral follicle count and ovarian volume
6. Clomiphene citrate challenge test
7. Dynamic assay of estradiol and inhibin B after GnRH-a (GAST)
8. Exogenous FSH ovarian reserve test (EFORT)

Table 2.3
Basal follicle stimulating hormone levels

FSH levels IU/L	
<9	Reassure
9–10	Suboptimal
10–12	Decreased ovarian reserve
12–17	Markedly reduced ovarian reserve
17–20	Poor prognosis
>20	No pregnancy

Basal E2 level of more than 80 pg/ml is associated with poor follicular response and development.

Early follicular phase inhibin B levels: Inhibin B levels decline with increasing age due to decreased number of follicles and decreased secretion by the granulosa cells. Since, inhibin is decreased there is poor negative feedback and FSH level is increased. Low levels of inhibin B on day 3 are associated with a poor outcome of IVF. Its role is limited due to less reliability and difficult serum estimation. A value of more than 45 pg/ml is taken as normal.

Anti-Mullerian hormone: Like inhibin, levels of anti-mullerian hormone reflect the health of the granulosa cell. Circulating AMH has the ability to predict excessive and poor response to stimulation with exogenous gonadotropins. This biomarker is superior to basal FSH and AFC, and has the potential to be incorporated into workup protocols to predict patient's ovarian response to treatment and to individualize strategies aiming at reducing the cancellation rate and the iatrogenic complications of controlled ovarian hyperstimulation like ovarian hyperstimulation.[2,3]

Ovarian volume and antral follicle count: Decreased ovarian volume and antral follicle count are useful indicators of ovarian reserve and response to superovulation and may be observed earlier than rise in FSH level in older women (Table 2.4).

Table 2.4

Antral follicle count

<4	Poor
4–7	Low count—High dose of FSH needs to given
8–12	Slightly reduced
>12	Normal

Clomiphene challenge test: In women with a decreased ovarian reserve FSH increases much more because a smaller follicle cohort in aging women produce less inhibin resulting in decreased negative feedback. FSH and LH levels are evaluated on day 2 and day 10 after giving clomiphene citrate from day 5 to day 9 in a dose of 100 mg/day. A value more than 26 IU on day 10 is suggestive of a decreased reserve. Positive predictive value is 90% for both day 3 FSH and clomiphene challenge test.[4]

Dynamic assessment following GnRH-a administration (GAST): GnRH-a produces an initial rise in LH, FSH, inhibin B and estradiol. The test evaluates the change in serum E2 levels between cycle day 2 and 3 after administering 1 mg of subcutaneous leuprolide acetate. Patients with E2 elevations by day 2 and decline by day 3 had better implantation and pregnancy rates than those with either no rise in E2, or persistently elevated E2 levels. This initial increase in estradiol is a better predictor than basal FSH, and FSH: LH ratio.[5]

Exogenous FSH ovarian reserve test (EFORT): This is a dynamic test. A increase in E2 of more than 30 pg/ml 24 hours after administration of 300 IU of purified FSH would be predictive of a good response in a subsequent IVF cycle.

In the recent years, these tests are occupying an increasingly important place in the workup of infertile women and usually basal FSH, antral follicle count and AMH are relied upon. Although they are reliable, rigid interpretation is discouraged as each treatment cycle may be different from the next.

PRE-IVF LAPAROSCOPY/HYSTEROSCOPY ASSESSMENT

Regarding endoscopic assessment practices differ widely from one center to the other. In some centers commencing

IVF would not be accepted until thorough investigations, including systematic evaluation of the uterine cavity (hysteroscopy) and the pelvis (laparoscopy), have been performed.[6] 40% women revealed an unsuspected intrauterine abnormality like polyp, submucus fibroid, intrauterine adhesions or septum when hysteroscopy was routinely performed prior to *in vitro* fertilization. A significant percentage of patients have uterine pathology that may impair the success of fertility treatment by affecting implantation or causing spontaneous abortion.[7] Hence, ruling out evidence of any intrauterine pathology becomes an important step before subjecting the patient to assisted reproductive techniques. It is seen that a pre-IVF hysteroscopy increased success rate of ART treatment.[8]

ASSESSMENT AND TREATMENT OF SPECIFIC PATHOLOGY BEFORE AN IVF CYCLE

Uterine Abnormality: Should it be Treated Before IVF?

Evidence suggests that pathology which distorts the endometrial cavity like fibroids, polyps, septa or adhesions may impact implantation and the success of fertility treatments. A balanced decision has to be taken on whether treatment of these conditions will improve fertility versus risk of development of postoperative morbidity such as endometrial scarring and myometrial damage which may further contribute to infertility.

Fibroids and polyps: It was seen that clinical pregnancy rates improved from 31 to 77% postmyomectomy in women with submucus myoma.[9] Hysteroscopic Polypectomy improved pregnancy rates from to 28 to 63%.[10]

Subseptate uterus: Pregnancy rates improved from 9.6 to 43% in patients undergoing IVF who were treated by hysteroscopic resection of septum.[11]

Intrauterine adhesions: They are known to negatively impact implantation. Flimsy adhesions must be lysed hysteroscopically. If there are dense adhesions prognosis is poor and surrogacy should be suggested as an alternative.

Hydrosalpinx

Tubal disease is an important indication for IVF and may be present in 10–30% of these patients. The clinical pregnancy and implantation rate was approximately 50% lower in patients who had hydrosalpinx. Appropriate management of hydrosalpinges is an important key in improving IVF success rates. Hydrosalpinges might have a negative effect on the oocytes, the transferred embryo, and on the implantation process due to toxic factors, in the hydrosalpinx fluid. The fluid may hinder implantation mechanically by a wash out effect on the newly implanted embryo.[12] Patients with hydrosalpiges who underwent proximal tubal occlusion before IVF demonstrated significantly increased implantation, clinical pregnancy, and ongoing pregnancy rates compared with those with no surgical intervention.[13] A recent Cochrane review (2010) stated that surgical treatment should be considered for all women with hydrosalpinges prior to IVF treatment. Laparoscopic tubal occlusion is an alternative to laparoscopic salpingectomy for improving IVF pregnancy rates in women with hydrosalpinges.[14]

Endometriosis

Endometriosis can cause distortion of pelvic anatomy, ovulatory and endocrine abnormalities, and impair implantation. Optimizing fertility in women with endometriosis can be challenging. The reduced oocyte yield in such patients is because of impaired folliculogenesis and difficulties in monitoring and oocyte retrieval. Fertilization and implantation rates are impaired.[15] There is a lower cleavage rate and aberrant nuclear and cytoplasmic morphology is higher in these embryos.[16]

Surgical treatment would be justified in these cases before taking them up for IVF, with the view that endometriosis causes adverse effects on embryo and oocyte quality. Endometriotic cysts less than 3 cms can be left as such and do not effect success rates in IVF. Surgery on the ovary may result in a decreased ovarian reserve which may lead to unpredictable response to gonadotropins.[17] Large cysts should be removed or cyst wall destroyed keeping in mind preservation of maximum ovarian tissue.

In patients with small endometriomas or peritubal adhesions a baseline transvaginal sonography is done to evaluate periovarian pouches, and the site and size of endometrioma in order to avoid confusion with follicles at a later stage. In patients with symptoms of pain ovum pickup should not be done under local anesthesia.

Ovarian Cyst

Functional ovarian cyst is seen in 9.3% of IVF cycles. Functional cysts can secrete estrogen and progesterone and interfere with ovarian stimulation. Patients with cyst showed a statistically significant decrease in the quality and number of oocytes retrieved, fertilization rate, number and quality of embryos, implantation and pregnancy rates, with a significant increase in cancellation and abortion rates.[18] Most clinicians aspirate these cysts. However, recent studies show that aspiration does not improve pregnancy rate.[19]

Polycystic Ovary Patients—Is there a Role for Metformin in Women Undergoing IVF?

Polycystic ovarian syndrome (PCOS) is a heterogeneous collection of signs and symptoms which form a spectrum of mild to severe disturbance of reproductive, endocrine and metabolic functions. Presence of two out of the following three criteria are essential for diagnosis.

1. Oligo and/or anovulation.
2. Hyperandrogenism (clinical and/or biochemical).
3. Polycystic ovaries with exclusion of other etiologies.

PCOS is characterized by insulin resistance which causes increased insulin levels that inhibit hepatic synthesis of sex hormone binding globulin (SHBG), leading to increased testosterone and estradiol levels. High levels of estradiol cause increased LH secretion and suppress FSH secretion. As FSH secretion is not totally suppressed follicular growth is continuously stimulated but not to the point of full maturation and ovulation. Small follicles 2 to 10 mm in diameter are present which may last for months. These are surrounded by hyperplastic theca cells which under the influence of LH get luteinized. The tissue derived from follicular atresia contributes to stromal compartment which secretes androstenedione and testosterone. High androgens prevent normal follicular development and premature atresia of follicles. They also affect endometrial receptivity. Serum prolactin levels may be high in 30 to 40% of PCOS women because of increased estrogen levels. All anovulatory women who are androgenic should be assessed for glucose tolerance and insulin resistance.

Goals of Treatment

1. Reducing insulin.

2. Treating anovulation—assessing for hyperstimulation and deciding dose for ovarian stimulation.
3. Antagonizing androgens.
4. Maintaining a normal endometrium.

Problems of Controlled Ovarian Stimulation in PCOS

1. Disturbed folliculogenesis leading to poor response to induction.
2. Large number of antral follicles sensitive to FSH leading to multiple follicular development, OHSS and multiple pregnancy.
3. Tonically elevated serum LH levels leading to premature luteinization, low pregnancy rates and high miscarriage rates.

Several Modes of Inducing Ovulation are Used (Flow chart 2.1)

Weight loss: Weight loss improves ovarian function and hormonal abnormality by decreasing insulin and androgens and increasing sex hormone binding globulin (SHBG) thus restoring ovulation and improving response to ovulation inducing drugs. Five to ten percent of weight loss is enough to decrease the visceral fat by 30% and restore reproductive function.

Insulin sensitizer: Metformin, an insulin sensitizer acts by reducing hyperinsulinemia which decreases in intraovarian androgens. This in turn leads to a reduction in E2 levels and favors orderly follicular growth in response to exogenous gonadotropins. There is a decrease in testosterone, free testosterone, DHEAS, androstenedione and LH, normalization of LH: FSH ratio and an increase in SHBG. It is indicated in documented hyperinsulinemia. The drug is usually started in the follicular phase in a dose of 500 mg/day for 5 to 7 days. This is increased in weekly increments of 500 mg up to 1500 to 2000 mg/day. Metformin treatment for 12 weeks before and during IVF or ICSI in nonobese women with PCOS significantly increased pregnancy and live birth rates.[20] A Cochrane review stated that metformin does not improve the success rates of IVF but does prevent hyperstimulation.[21]

Glucocorticoids: Fifty percent of patients of PCOS show involvement of an adrenal component with raised DHEAS. The desired effect should be to normalize without suppressing adrenal component, with dexamethasone (0.25–0.5 mg/day).

Flow chart 2.1: Modes of ovulation induction in PCOS

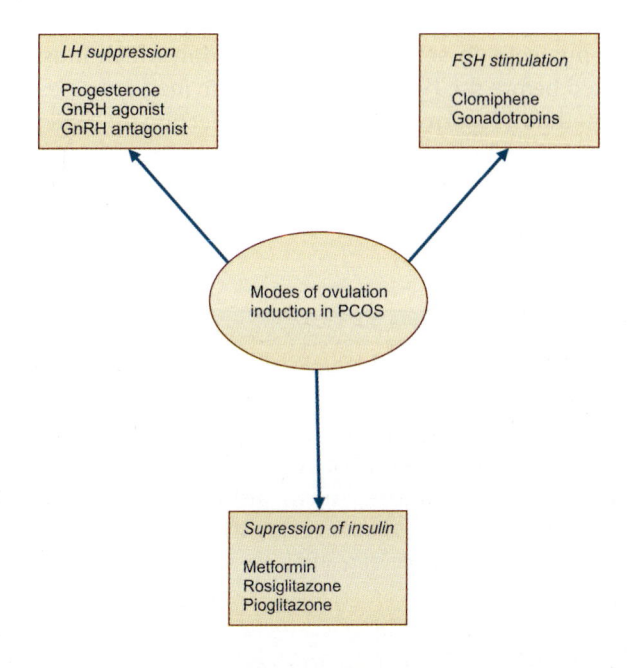

LH suppression

Progesterone
GnRH agonist
GnRH antagonist

FSH stimulation

Clomiphene
Gonadotropins

Modes of ovulation induction in PCOS

Supression of insulin

Metformin
Rosiglitazone
Pioglitazone

ROLE OF ORAL CONTRACEPTIVE PILLS BEFORE ART CYCLE

The combined oral contraceptive pill (OCP) given prior to the hormone therapy in an IVF cycle may result in better pregnancy outcomes of ART. There was evidence of improved pregnancy outcomes with progestogen pretreatment.[22] It is helpful where basal LH levels are raised specially in stimulation protocols which do not down regulate with GnRH agonist, like when a GnRH antagonist protocol is used.

ASSESSMENT OF THE MALE

A recent semenanalysis and post wash count should be done to decide the ART procedure of choice (Table 2.5). Any pus cells in semen indicate infection which must be treated before the IVF cycle. Azospermic men are assessed for method of sperm collection. The collection for testicular or epidydimal sperms is done before starting stimulation protocols and the sample is cryopreserved. In case of retrograde ejaculation urinary alkalizers are given before collection.

Table 2.5

Indications for ICSI

- Total motile inseminate count—less than 1 million
- Motility—less than 40%
- Normal morphology—less than 4%
- Hypo-osmotic swelling—less than 40%
- Immunobead test—positive in more than 80%
- Testicular or epidydimal sperms

PATIENT COUNSELING AND EDUCATION

Facts about IVF have to be clearly explained and instruction given (Table 2.6). Both emotional and financial counseling is a must. Individual assessment of prognosis is done and explained. The results, stimulation and monitoring protocols, adverse effects and alternatives in case of failure are to be spelled out. There could be a problem with understanding these facts due to stress, fatigue or selective hearing. Repetition and visual aids may help. A patient information booklet is useful. Stress assessment and psychological support is essential.

Table 2.6

Instruction to couple before IVF

Female
- Avoid drugs, alcohol and smoking for three months before treatment and during the IVF cycle
- Loose weight if obese
- Have no more than two caffeinated beverages a day
- Avoid dietary changes or weight fluctuation during the IVF cycle.

Male
- Any fever 1–2 months prior to IVF procedure should be informed as sperm quality can be affected by fever
- Avoid hot tubs or saunas
- Avoid wearing tight-fitting underwear
- No intercourse for at least 3 days but not more than 7 days before giving a semen sample
- Avoid drugs, alcohol and smoking for three months before treatment and during the IVF cycle
- Avoid excessive exercise.

IVF assessment is an opportunity to summarize infertility investigations, past treatment, current prognosis and plan a stimulation protocol individualized to patient. Couple must be seen together and all difficult decisions require involvement of both. There is no substitute for through understanding of the procedure as it helps patients to deal with failure and reduces medication errors by them.

REFERENCES

1. Abdalla H, Thum MY. Repeated testing of basal FSH levels has no predictive value for IVF outcome in women with elevated basal FSH. Hum Reprod. 2006;21(1):171-4.
2. Nardo LG, Gelbaya TA, Wilkinson H, Roberts SA, Yates A, Pemberton P, Laing I. Circulating basal anti-Müllerian hormone levels as predictor of ovarian response in women undergoing ovarian stimulation for *in vitro* fertilization. Fertil Steril. 2009;92(5):1586-93.
3. Broer SL, Dólleman M, Opmeer BC, Fauser BC, Mol BW, Broekmans FJ. AMH and AFC as predictors of excessive response in controlled ovarianhyperstimulation: a meta-analysis. Hum Reprod Update. 2011;17(1):46-54.
4. Jain T, Soules MR, Collins JA. Comparison of basal follicle stimulating hormone versus clomiphene citrate challenge test for ovarian reserve screening. Fertil Steril. 2004;82:180-6.
5. Amir R, Stuart L, Sappho M, Mandy D, Raul M, Geoff T, et al. Dynamic assays of inhibin B and oestradiol following buserelin acetate administration as predictors of ovarian response in IVF. Hum Reprod. 2000;15:2297-301.
6. El-Mazny A, Abou-Salem N, El-Sherbiny W, Saber W. Outpatient hysteroscopy: a routine investigation before assisted reproductive techniques? Fertil Steril. 2011;95(1):272-6.
7. Doldi N, Persico P, Di Sebastiano F, Marsiglio E, De Santis L, Rabellotti E, Fusi F, Brigante C, Ferrari A. Pathologic findings in hysteroscopy before *in vitro* fertilization-embryo transfer (IVF-ET). Gynecol Endocrinol. 2005;21(4):235-7

8. El-Toukhy T, Sunkara SK, Coomarasamy A, Grace J, Khalaf Y. Outpatient hysteroscopy and subsequent IVF cycle outcome: a systematic review and meta-analysis. Reprod Biomed Online. 2008;16(5):712-9.
9. Pritts EA. Fibroids and infertility: a systematic review of the evidence. Obstet Gynecol Surv. 2001;56(8):483-91.
10. Pérez-Medina T, Bajo-Arenas J, Salazar F, Redondo T, Sanfrutos L, Alvarez P, Engels V. Endometrial polyps and their implication in the pregnancy rates of patients undergoing intrauterine insemination: a prospective, randomized study. Hum Reprod. 2005;20(6):1632-5.
11. Tomaževič T, Ban-Frangež H, Virant-Klun I, Verdenik I, Požlep B, Vrtačnik-Bokal E. Septate, subseptate and arcuate uterus decrease pregnancy and live birth rates in IVF/ICSI. Reprod Biomed Online. 2010;21(5):700-5.
12. Zeyneloglu HB, Arici A, Olive DL. Adverse effects of hydrosalpinx on pregnancy rates after *in vitro* fertilization-embryo transfer. Fertil Steril. 1998;70(3):492-9.
13. Kontoravdis A, Makrakis E, Pantos K, Botsis D, Deligeoroglou E, Creatsas G. Proximal tubal occlusion and salpingectomy result in similar improvement in *in vitro* fertilization outcome in patients with hydrosalpinx. Fertil Steril. 2006;86(6): 1642-9.
14. Johnson N, van Voorst S, Sowter MC, Strandell A, Mol BW. Surgical treatment for tubal disease in women due to undergo *in vitro* fertilisation. Cochrane Database Syst Rev. 2010 Jan 20;(1):CD002125.
15. Coccia ME, Rizzello F, Mariani G, Bulletti C, Palagiano A, Scarselli G. Impact of endometriosis on *in vitro* fertilization and embryo transfer cycles in young women: a stage- vc dependent interference. Acta Obstet Gynecol Scand. 2011;90(11):1232-8.
16. Pellicon A, Oliviera N, Ruiz A, et al. Exploring the mechanism of endometriosis related infertility: an analysis of embryo development and implantation in assisted reproduction. Hum Reprod. 1995;10:91-7.
17. Donnez J, Wynes C, Nisolle M. Does ovarian surgery for endometriomas impair the ovarian response to gonadotropins? Fertil Steril. 2001;76: 662-5.

18. Qublan HS, Amarin Z, Tahat YA, Smadi AZ, Kilani M. Ovarian cyst formation following GnRH agonist administration in IVF cycles: incidence and impact. Hum Reprod. 2006;21(3):640-4.
19. Firouzabadi RD, Sekhavat L, Javedani M. The effect of ovarian cyst aspiration on IVF treatment with GnRH. Arch Gynecol Obstet. 2010; 281(3):545-9.
20. Kjøtrød SB, et al. Use of metformin before and during assisted reproductive technology in non-obese young infertile women with polycystic ovary syndrome: a prospective, randomized, double-blind, multi-centre study. Hum Reprod. 2011;26(8):2045-53.
21. Tso LO, Costello MF, Albuquerque LE, Andriolo RB, Freitas V. Metformin treatment before and during IVF or ICSI in women with polycystic ovary syndrome. Cochrane Database Syst Rev. 2009 Apr 15;(2):CD006105.
22. Smulders B, van Oirschot SM, Farquhar C, Rombauts L, Kremer JA. Oral contraceptive pill, progestogen or estrogen pre-treatment for ovarian stimulation protocols for women undergoing assisted reproductive techniques. Cochrane Database Syst Rev. 2010 Jan 20;(1):CD006109.

Chapter 3

Semen Analysis and Assessment of the Male Partner

Surveen Ghumman Sindhu

Semen analysis is a part of the initial diagnostic workup of the infertile couple and may provide the first indication that male factor is contributing to infertility. The clinical usefulness of semen evaluation is improving rapidly as more objective, standardized, methodology is introduced into practice. Semen analysis is not only essential for diagnosis of male infertility but is useful for determining the line of therapy and prognosis.

SAMPLE COLLECTION AND DELIVERY

Normal semen can be reported as abnormal if not correctly collected and handled.

1. *Abstinence:* Sample should be collected after abstinence of at least 48 hours but not more than 7 days. Less than 2 days of abstinence leads to decrease of sperm concentration and more than 7 days leads to decrease in sperm motility. The following should be recorded:
   - Period of abstinence
   - Date and time of collection
   - Completeness of collection
   - Difficulties in producing sample
   - Interval between collection and analysis.
2. *Number of samples:* Two samples must be evaluated initially. The collection of the second sample should not

be before 7 days or beyond 3 weeks. Day-to-day and seasonal variations are seen, with decreased sperms in the summer. Transient semen abnormalities may also be induced by infection trauma, environmental stress or medication. With history of such events, a repeat analysis should be done after 2-3 months.

3. *Transportation of semen:* Sample should be delivered within half an hour to one hour of collection.[1] The semen sample should be completed and should be transported at optimal temperature between 20 to 37°C.

> If tests of sperm function are performed, it is critical that the spermatozoa be separated from the seminal plasma within one hour of ejaculate.

4. *Container for collection:* The glass container should be wide mouthed, at 20 to 40°C, and checked for toxic effects. Ideally it should be 60 to 100 ml in capacity to avoid spillage.

5. *Method of collection:*
   - Masturbation
   - *Nontoxic condom:* If sample cannot be collected by masturbation special nontoxic condoms are used
   - *Coitus interruptus:* Coitus interruptus is not used since first part of ejaculate, which is sperm rich, is often spilled. If vaginal cells are found in the semen, this method of collection is suspected.

Postejaculatory urine sample: If no semen is produced despite ejaculation or volume is low, suspect retrograde ejaculation. Post-ejaculatory urine samples should be examined microscopically. It may be centrifuged at 300 gm for 10 minutes.

Note:
- Any sample for microbiological assessment should be recovered after urine has been passed.
- The time between collection and microbiological examination should not exceed 3 hours.

Semen analysis consists of a number of parameters to be assessed (Table 3.1).

Table 3.1
Parameters for semen analysis

Physical parameters
- Coagulation
- Liquefaction
- Viscosity
- Volume
- Color
- Odor
- pH.

Wet preparation examination
- General appearance
- Agglutination and cells.

Basic parameters
- Concentration
- Motility
- Morphology.

Functional tests for sperms
- Hypo-osmotic swelling tests
- Acrosome reaction
- Study of hyperactivated motility.

Biochemical tests
- Sperm fertilizing capability—Nuclear chromatin decondensation test, aniline blue, reactive oxygen species.
- Male genital tract inflammation—Elastase

Contd...

Contd...

- Accessory sex gland epidydimal dysfunction— Fructose, glucosidase, acid phosphatase, prostatic specific antigen.

Bioassay
- Hemizona assay—Study of zona binding and penetration defects
- Sperm penetration assay—Study of acrosome reaction, fusion and condensation.

Others
- Supravital staining
- Antisperm antibody tests
- Semen culture
- Kremer test.

Note: Substantial number of sperms must be observed in urine as, even with antegrade ejaculation, some spermatozoa will normally be present in the urine because of urethral contamination.

WHO (2010) has recommended a normal range of values (Table 3.2). The normal reference range does not represent an absolute minimum value needed for conception. Similarly, a normal value does not ensure fertility. The odds of male infertility increase with the number of semen parameters (motility, morphology, concentration) in subfertile range.[2]

PHYSICAL PARAMETERS

Before examination, the semen is thoroughly mixed with a pipette.

Coagulation

Coagulation is because of protein kinase enzyme secreted by seminal vesicle. It is absent in congenital absence of vas deference, ejaculatory duct or seminal vesicles. A normal semen sample liquefies within 60 minutes at room temperature.

Table 3.2
Normal values for semen analysis (WHO)

Semen analysis values (WHO	Normal reference Manual 2010)[3]
Volume	>1.5 ml
pH	≥ 7.2
Viscosity	< 3 (Scale 0-4)
Sperm concentration	> 15 million/ml
Total sperm number	> 39 million
Total motility (PR+NP)%	> 40%
Progressive motility %	> 32
Normal morphology	> 4% normal
WBC	< 1 million/ml
MAR test	< 50%
Immunobead test	< 50% motile sperms with boundbeads
Vitality %	> 58%
Seminal zinc (µmol/ejaculate)	≥2.4
Seminal fructose (µmol/ejaculate)	≥13
Seminal neutral glucosidase (µU/ ejaculate)	≥ 20

Liquefaction

Liquefaction is the natural change in consistency of semen from a semiliquid to a liquid.

Incomplete liquefaction may adversely affect the semen analysis. Liquefaction is completed within 15 to 30 minutes and is because of fibrinolysin enzyme secreted by the prostate gland. Delayed liquefaction (> 60 minutes) is due to prostatic dysfunction.

If semen does not liquefy at 60 minutes: Additional treatment like mechanical mixing or enzymatic digestion may be necessary as follows:

1. An equal volume of physiological solution is added followed by repeated pipetting
2. Repeatedly passing through gauge 18 needle
3. Digestion by bromelain, a proteolytic enzyme, dilute semen 1:1 with 10 IU/ml of bromelain. This treatment can effect motility morphology and biochemistry and must be taken into account when calculating sperm concentration.

Appearance

A normal sample has a homogenous, gray opalescent appearance. It can become yellow with increased abstinence. A translucent appearance is associated with low sperm counts.

Odor

The odor is due to spermine from prostate gland.

Volume

Normal volume is 1.5 to 6 ml. Less than 1.5 ml is considered abnormal. Calculation of volume can also be done by weighing the sample collected in a preweighed container, the density being taken as 1 gm/ml.

Cause of Low Volume

- Faulty collection
- Failed emission
- Short abstinence interval
- Obstruction in the male genital tract due to previous infections
- Ejaculatory duct obstruction
- Hypogonadism—Secretion of seminal vesicles and prostate are stimulated by androgens which are low in hypogonadism

- Congenital absence of vas deferens and seminal vesicles
- Retrograde ejaculation
- Previous surgery of bladder neck or prostate.

Cause of High Volume
- Active exudation in case of acute inflammation.

> A postejaculatory urinalysis is indicated when ejaculate volume is less than 1 ml except when hypogonadism, congenital bilateral absence of vas deferens, collection problems or short abstinence intervals offer an obvious explanation.

Viscosity

Viscosity refers to liquefied specimens tendency to form drops from the tip of the pipette. If drops form freely, the specimen has normal viscosity. If drops do not form or the semen cannot be easily drawn up into the pipette, viscosity is high (Table 3.3).

Increased viscosity can cause difficulties in assessing sperm concentration, motility and antibody coating. Mix with saline or culture medium before assessing.

Causes of Increased Viscosity
- Abnormal prostate function due to infection
- Artifact due to unsuitable plastic container

Table 3.3
Viscosity of semen
- Normal: If semen is released as a single drop within a distance of 2 cm from the tip of the pipette
- Minimally Increased: If strands of 2 to 4 cm are formed
- Increased: Strands of 4 to 8 cm
- Grossly Increased: Strands of > 8 cm.

- Antisperm antibody
- Frequent ejaculation
- Psychological state of patient.

If semen viscosity is high, it may be necessary to reduce the viscosity before the semen can be analyzed. Viscosity reduction can be achieved by aspirating the semen in and out of a hypodermic syringe fitted with a 18 gauge blunt needle. Treatment with an enzyme such as chymotrypsin may also decrease the viscosity improving distribution of sperms.

pH

The pH should be measured within one hour of ejaculation. The pH strip should be of range 6 to 10 and is read after 30 seconds. Normal pH should be between 7.2 to 7.8 (Table 3.4).

For viscous sample, a small aliquot of the semen sample is measured by a pH meter.

Semen pH increases with time as natural buffering decreases and has little significance.

INITIAL MICROSCOPIC EXAMINATION

A wet preparation is made and phase contrast microscope is recommended for all examinations of unstained fresh or washed semen (Flow chart 3.1).

Table 3.4
pH values

pH	Cause
7.2-7.8	Normal
> 7.8	Acute infection
< 6.8	Ejaculatory duct obstruction, congenital absence of vas, Chronic infectio

Semen Analysis and Assessment of the Male Partner | **47**

Flow chart 3.1: Initial basic microscopic examination

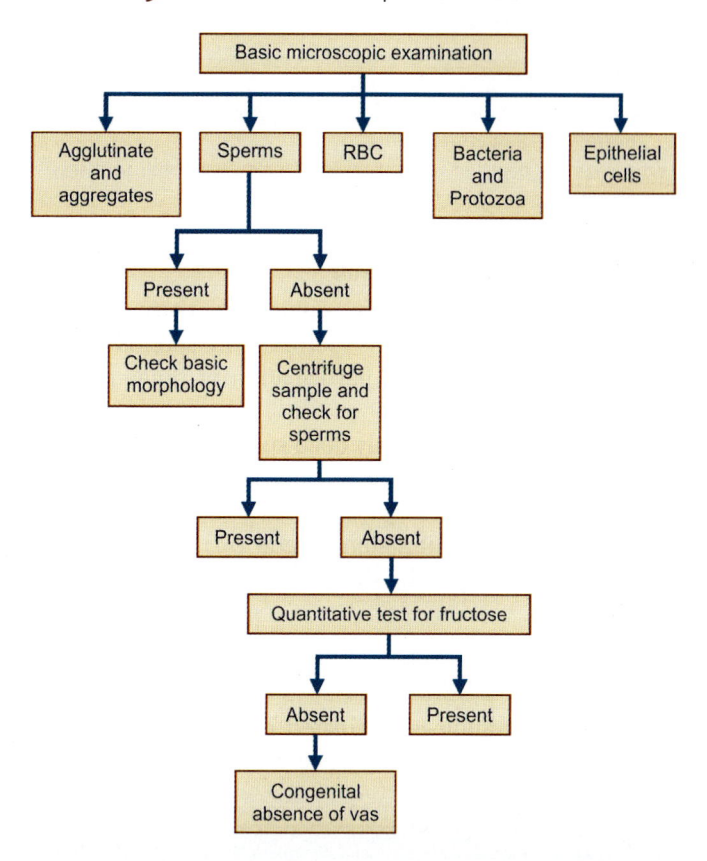

```
                    Basic microscopic examination
        ┌──────────┬──────────┬──────────┬──────────┐
   Agglutinate   Sperms     RBC      Bacteria    Epithelial
      and                              and          cells
   aggregates                        Protozoa
                    ┌────────┴────────┐
                 Present           Absent
                    │                 │
              Check basic        Centrifuge
              morphology         sample and
                                 check for
                                   sperms
                              ┌──────┴──────┐
                          Present        Absent
                                            │
                               Quantitative test for fructose
                                    ┌───────┴───────┐
                                 Absent          Present
                                    │
                               Congenital
                              absence of vas
```

> Before examination, mix the semen properly by aspirating 10 times into a wide bore (1.5 mm) pipette without creating air bubbles.

Making a wet preparation: Mix sample well. Volume of aliquot and size of cover slip should be standardized to create a depth of 20 µl.

- 10 µl with 22 × 22 mm coverslip
- 6.5 µl with 18 × 18 mm coverslip.

> *Note:*
> - A chamber depth of less than 20 µl constrains the rotational movement of spermatozoa
> - A chamber depth of more than 20 µl makes it difficult to assess spermatozoa as they move in and out of focus.

Agglutination and Aggregation

- Agglutination is caused by multivalent sperm antibody and usually involves live sperms. Only sperms adhere to each other without participation of other cells or debris (Table 3.5)
- Aggregation involves only dead sperms, other cells and debris and its presence is considered abnormal and should be noted.

The grade of agglutination (Grade 1-4) and the site of attachment (Grade A –E) should be classified (Tables 3.5 and 3.6).[4]

SPERM CONCENTRATION

Sperm concentration is calculated as number of sperms per ml. Oligospermia would be termed as count less than

Table 3.5

Scoring of agglutinates

Grade	No of sperms per agglutinate	No of free sperms
1 Isolated	<10	Many
2 Moderate	10-50	Some
3 Large	>50	Some
4 Gross	All	None

	Table 3.6
	Site of attachment of agglutinated spermatozoa
A	: Head to head
B	: Tail to tail
C	: Tail tip to tail tip
D	: Mixed—Clear head to head and tail to tail
C	: Tangled—Head and tail are entangled and no pattern made out

15 million/ml. Total sperm count is the product obtained by multiplying semen volume and sperm concentration. Normal is considered to be 39 million.

Note:
- The probability of conception increases with increasing sperm concentration up to approximately 40-50 million/ml but does not rise further with higher sperm densities.
- Endocrine and genetic evaluation is indicated in men with severe oligospermia.

Azoospermia

Azoospermia is present in 1 percent of all men and 10-15 percent infertile men.

Obstructive (40%): Blockage anywhere in the ductal system from efferent ductules to ejaculatory ducts as a consequence of:
- Severe infection
- Iatrogenic injury during scrotal or inguinal surgery
- Congenital absence of vas.

Nonobstructive: It may be due to:
- Intrinsic testicular disease (Primary testicular failure)
- Endocrinopathies or other conditions that suppress spermatogenesis (Secondary testicular failure).

To establish diagnosis of azoospermia: Semen specimen is centrifuged at high speed (3000 gm for 15 minutes) and pellet is examined at magnification of 400 X. If no spermatozoa are found recorded, check fructose in the sample which, if absent, signifies congenital absence of vas (Flow chart 3.2)

> Note:
> - Absence of sperms should be documented on two occasions to diagnose azoospermia.
> - Men with nonobstructive azoospermia should have a careful examination of centrifuged sample as in one-third of these men a very low sperm production, insufficient to drive epididymal transport and entry to ejaculate is present. These sperms can be recovered by TESE for ICSI.

Method of Assessment of Sperm Concentration

The semen is mixed thoroughly. Concentration can be determined by hemocytometer method which requires dilution of semen sample, or Makler's chamber where no dilution is required. Ten μl of raw semen is put on the chamber covered with a cover slip and seen under 20 X magnification. Although computer assisted semen analysis (CASA) system can also be used to automatically measure sperm concentration, errors are encountered when there are high and low concentrations, significant agglutinates or large amount of debris.

SPERM MOTILITY

Sperm motility is assessed as a percentage of total sperm population exhibiting any motion. It should be assessed within 30-60 minutes to limit effect of pH changes, dehydration and temperature on motility. Procedure must be performed at room temperature or at 37°C.

Semen Analysis and Assessment of the Male Partner | **51**

Flow chart 3.2: Protocol for examination of sperm morphology

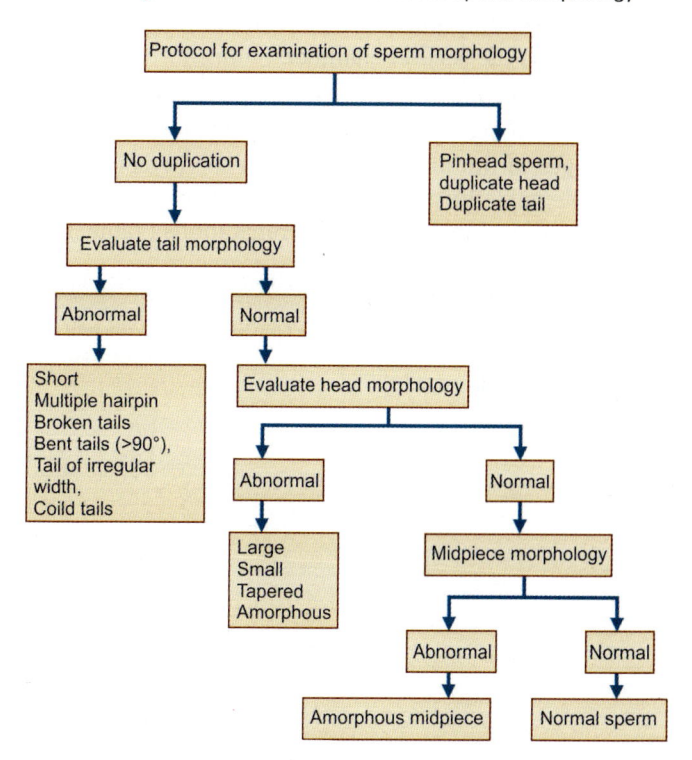

```
                    Protocol for examination of sperm morphology
                                        |
                    ┌───────────────────┴───────────────────┐
                No duplication                      Pinhead sperm,
                        |                           duplicate head
                        |                           Duplicate tail
            Evaluate tail morphology
                        |
            ┌───────────┴───────────┐
         Abnormal                 Normal
            |                       |
    Short                  Evaluate head morphology
    Multiple hairpin               |
    Broken tails           ┌───────┴───────┐
    Bent tails (>90°),   Abnormal        Normal
    Tail of irregular      |               |
    width,              Large       Midpiece morphology
    Coild tails         Small              |
                        Tapered    ┌───────┴───────┐
                        Amorphous Abnormal      Normal
                                    |             |
                            Amorphous midpiece  Normal sperm
```

Motility assessment can be done in two ways:
1. A wet preparation.
2. Computer aided sperm analysis (CASA). CASA provides numbers that quantitate the vigour and pattern of movement on per sperm basis.

Number of fields to be examined: At least 5 randomly selected fields are sampled.

Number of sperms to be counted: 200 spermatozoa are counted for motility and classified. The counting procedure is repeated in the second chamber.

Difference in counts between two chambers

Calculate average percentage and difference in two percentages. If the difference between the percentages is acceptable, take the average, if not take two new aliquots from sample and make two new preparations (Table 3.7).

Table 3.7
Acceptable difference for two percentages in a given average determined from replicate count of 200 spermatozoa (WHO Manual 2010)[3]

Average%	Acceptable difference
0	1
1	2
2	3
3-4	4
5-7	5
8-11	6
12-16	7
17-23	8
24-34	9
35-65	10
66-76	9
77-83	8
84-88	7
89-92	6
93-95	5
96-97	4
98	3
99	2
100	1

Grading of Motility

1. *Progressive motility (PR):* Sperms moving actively either linear or in large circles regardless of speed. Earlier this movement was graded according to speed </> 25 µm/sec. However, in the WHO manual 2010 this grading has been removed. The lower reference standard for PR is 32 percent.[3]
2. *Nonprogressive (NP):* All other patterns of motility with absence of progression, e.g. swimming in small circles with flagellar force hardly displacing the head or if flagellar beat can be observed
3. *Nonmotile:* No movement.

Total motility: Sum of PR + NP. The lower reference standard for total motility is 40 percent as per the WHO manual 2010.

Total progressive motility: Percentage of sperms exhibiting purposeful forward motion (Grade 2-4). The probability of conception increases with increasing motility up to 60 percent.[3]

Poor sperm motility may be due to:
- Testicular dysfunction
- Antisperm antibody
- Genital tract infection
- Partial obstruction of ejaculatory duct
- Varicocele
- Prolonged abstinence
- Immotile cilia syndrome.

SPERM MORPHOLOGY

Normal sperm morphology has been related to fertilizing potential of sperm. Sperm morphology usually is assessed from seminal smears that are prepared at the time of semen evaluation and subsequently stained. It can be assessed in several ways, the most common classification system being, the WHO standard and the Kruger strict criterion.[5] According to the WHO manual 2010, the cut off is 4 percent for normal sperm morphology.

Method of Preparation

Rapid addition of fixative to semen does not permit adequate visualization of the sperms as they are obscured by denatured seminal protein. For morphological analysis smears which are air dried before fixing and staining are used. Air dying leads to shrinkage in dimension of spermatozoa, expansion of immature sperm head and loss of osmotically sensitive cytoplasmic droplets.[3] Smears are made with fresh sample on a slide by 'feathering' method where the semen drop spreads along the back edge of the slide and is pulled forward over the slide to make a smear.

Quality of the smear depends on the:
1. Volume of the semen and the sperm concentration
2. Angle of the dragging slide smaller the angle the thinner the smear
3. *Speed of smear:* The more rapid the movement the thicker the smear

WHO manual recommends to start with a 10 µl volume, a 45° angle and one second for making. These are altered accordingly.

Samples with low sperm count (2 milliom/ml): Centrifuge, remove most of supernatant and resuspend in remainder of supernatant to obtain a concentration of not more than 50 million.

Viscous samples result in uneven smears: Treatment with mixing with equal quantities of media and repeated pipetting before making a smear.

Debris laden or viscous sample and for CASA analysis: Wash, centrifuge and resuspend. This helps in reducing background for computer aided analysis.

The greatest accuracy and precision in morphometric measurement are obtained when sperms are washed, and resuspended to standard concentration, before slide preparation.

- If sperm concentration is > 20×10^6/ml 5 µl, semen is used
- If concentration is < 20×10^6/ml 10-20 µl, semen is used.

They are fixed and stored for staining.

Staining

They may be stained by Shorr stain, Papanicolaou stain or Diff Quik method. With all three stains the head is stained pale blue in acrosomal region, and dark blue in postacrosomal region. The midpiece may show some red staining and the tail is stained blue or reddish. Excess residual cytoplasm is stained reddish.

Examining the Slide

Examination is done in oil immersion at 100 X field magnification. Defects are expressed per 100 sperms for that region.

Number of sperms to be assessed: 200 sperms are assessed. Only recognizable spermatozoa with tails are considered in the count. Immature cells upto the stage of round spermatids are not counted. 100 consecutive sperms are counted in two randomly selected areas.

If percentage difference between the two is:
- Less than 15 percent then the mean of the two is recorded as percentage morphology

- More than 15 percent, a third reading is taken and average of all three is taken.

Protocol for evaluation: Criterion for further evaluation is a single head and tail. Sperms with more than one head or tail are scored as duplicate sperms and are not evaluated further. So, also those without head, classified as headless or pinhead sperms. Sperms with any tail abnormality are classified as 'amorphous tail' regardless of head or midpiece morphology. The rationale for primacy of tail morphology is that such sperms can be considered dysfunctional because absent or severely abnormal flagellar activity will result in failure of sperm transport to site of fertilization or penetration of oocyte. If sperm tails are normal in size and shape, the head of the sperm is considered. Midpiece morphology is assessed last only if head and tail are normal. To be classified as normal the sperm must be normal in all three—head, tail and midpiece (Flow chart 3.2).

There may be sperms with more than one abnormality.

Teratospermic index: Average number of sperm defects per sperm.

WHO Criterion for Sperm Morphology

WHO criterion for assessing sperm morphology includes the following (Fig. 3.1):

Head
- Oval, smooth regularly contoured head is normal
- Round, pyriform, pin, double, and amorphous head is abnormal.

Midpiece
Straight, slightly thicker than the tail.

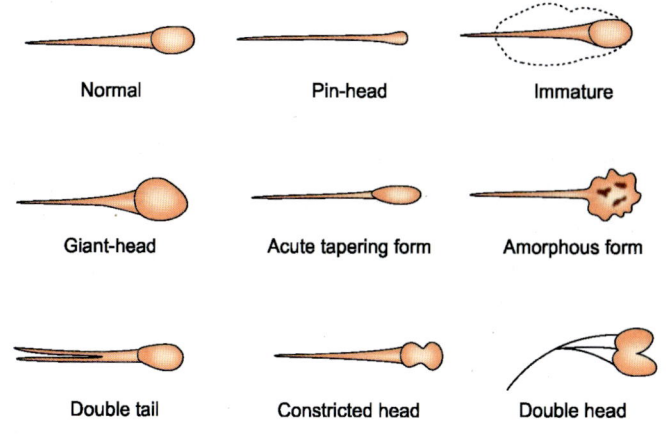

Fig. 3.1: Abnormal sperms

Tail
Single, unbroken straight without kinks or coils.

Abnormal Spermatozoa
The defect could be in the head, midpiece or tail (Fig. 3.1).

Head defects: These are:
- Large
- Small
- Tapered (length to width ratio is >2)
- Round
- Amorphous heads
- Vacuolated heads (>20% of head area occupied by unstained vacuolar area)
- Head with small acrosomal area (< 40% of head area)
- Double heads
- Combination of these

- Pin-head (absent head) or microhead sperm are not counted.

Neck and midpiece defects:
- Bent neck (The neck and tail form an angle of greater than 90° to the long axis of the head)
- Asymmetrical insertion of the midpiece into head
- Thick and irregular midpiece
- Abnormally thin midpiece (no mitochondrial sheath)
- Combination of these.

Principal Piece or Tail defects: The defect seen are:
- Short
- Multiple
- Hairpin
- Broken tails
- Bent tails (> 90°)
- Tails of irregular width
- Coiled tails
- Combination of these.

A high number of coiled tails indicate that the sperms have been subjected to hypo-osmotic stress. It may also be due to sperm ageing. If > 20 percent, it must be noted. Sperms with any tail abnormality are classified as 'amorphous tail', regardless of head or midpiece morphology.

Cytoplasmic droplets: Cytoplasmic droplets are more than one-third the area of normal head sperm. They are usually located in the midpiece.

> *Note:*
> - Pin-heads and free tails are not counted as spermatozoa, hence they are not counted as abnormal
> - Overlapping spermatozoa and those lying on the edge should not be assessed.

CELLULAR ELEMENTS OTHER THAN SPERMATOZOA

The ejaculate contains cells, other than spermatozoa, referred to as round cells. These include germinal line cells sloughed from seminiferous tubules, epithelial cells from genitourinary tract, prostate cells, spermatogenic cells and leukocytes.

Leukocytes

Leukocytes are predominantly neutrophils, and indicate infection in male genital tract which generates free radicals This has a detrimental effect on sperm function.

Although leukospermia has been implicated as a cause of poor sperm motility and function, more recent studies have failed to demonstrate an association between the two.[6]

The number of leukocytes should not exceed 1×10^6. The concentration of granulocytes in semen can be determined using peroxidase staining and hemocytometer counts Leukocytes are counted in five fields. The concentration is then calculated using the following formula.

$$\text{Concentration} = \frac{\text{Total leukocytes in five fields} \times \text{Sperm concentration in semen}}{\text{Total sperms in five fields}}$$

Immature Germ Cells

Round cells that lack polymorphonuclear morphology may be immature germinal cells (spermatocytes, spermatids) or exfoliated epithelial cells.

Differentiation of leukocytes from immature germ cells
1. They can be differentiated with papanicolaou staining based on staining color and nuclear size and shape. Polymorphonuclear leukocytes stain blue in contrast to spermatids which stain pink.

2. Leukocytes are peroxidase positive giving a brown color with peroxidase
3. *Immunocytochemical assay:* Leukocyte specific antigens are present.

TESTS FOR SPERM MEMBRANE INTEGRITY

Sperm vitality test is indicated if percentage of motile sperms is less than 40 percent. These tests determine the sperm membrane structure and function. The presence of large number of vital, but immotile sperms may be indicative of structural defect in flagellum. Assessment should be done preferably within 30 minutes to maximum of one hour after ejaculation before deleterious effects due to temperature and pH changes occur.

Sperm Viability by Dye Exclusion

The functionally intact sperm membrane excludes eosin dye from nuclear component of spermatozoa. Dead cells retain dye while normal cells remain uncolored. If the stain is retained in the neck region and not the head it is a ' Leaky membrane' and these sperms are alive. The vital stains used are eosin Y, trypan blue, and nigrosin. Nigrosin is used to increase contrast. Lower reference limit for sperm vitality is 58 percent.

> *Reverse stain ratio:* Particular attention should be paid to a reverse stain ratio where more sperms stain dead than are nonmotile in the sample, thus indicating a sperm membrane problem.

Hypo-osmotic Swelling Test

When live spermatozoa are exposed to a solution of low osmolarity they demonstrate tail swelling. The percentage of sperms, with curled tails in the treated sample, should be subtracted from the percentage of those that reacted from hypo-osmotic solution. A normal value is taken as more than 58% reacted sperms per sample.

> *Clinical significance:*
> - The test may play a significant role in selecting appropriate sperms for ICSI when only immotile sperms are present
> - Supravital staining indicates structural integrity of membrane while hypo-osmotic swelling test tells us about the functional integrity of sperm membrane.

Sperm Longevity Test

The capacity of motility of the sperm to survive incubation under optimal conditions for an extended period, correlates with fertilizing potential. After incubation for 24 hours the decline in motility should not be more than 30-40 percent.

SPERM MEMBRANE BINDING, CAPACITATION AND PENETRATION

Hemizona Assay

Hemizona assay uses matched zona halves from a human egg to compare the binding of the patient's sperm with that of a comparable fertile control after 4 hours of incubation. It has been shown to correlate with success rates of IVF and IUI.[7]

Hamster Egg Human Sperm Penetration Assay (SPA)

Zona free hamster eggs allow penetration of human sperms. Percentage of eggs which are penetrated and contain decondensed sperm heads are determined.[8]

ACROSOME DETECTION

The presence of acrosome cannot be verified easily with normal sperm morphology stains and light microscopy. Several techniques like triple staining and fluorescence techniques allows laboratories to count sperms with an intact acrosome.

BIOCHEMICAL MEASUREMENT OF SPERM FUNCTION

Various substances may be measured to assess the sperm function like acrosin, adenosine triphosphate, creatinine phosphokinase, zinc, acid phosphotase, hyaluronidase activity and alpha glucosidase.

Reactive Oxygen Species

Oxidative stress is one of the major causes of male infertility because it damages spermatogenic cells, the spermatogenic process and sperm function. Reactive oxygen species (ROS) are metabolites of oxygen and include superoxides, hydrogen peroxide, hydroxyl, and nitric oxide. When present in excess they can produce oxidative damage to cellular lipids, proteins and DNA impairing sperm function. ROS is produced by spermatozoa and leukocytes. A single leukocyte can generate 100 times more ROS than spermatozoa. Seminal plasma has antioxidative enzymes and removal of seminal plasma in semen preparation can damage sperms. A chemiluminescent procedure employing probes such as luminal or lucigenin may be used to measure ROS. Men treated with antioxidants have shown an improvement in semen parameters.[9]

ANTISPERM ANTIBODIES (ASA)

Because the spermatozoa are formed after puberty, they are recognized as foreign protein by man's immune system. If there is a breach in the blood testis barrier an immune response may be initiated, as occurs with vasectomy, varicocele repair, testicular biopsy or trauma.

Sperm antibodies in semen belong exclusively to two immunoglobulin classes IgA and IgG.[10] Clinical manifestations of significant antisperm antibody in males include:

- Sperm agglutination (differentiated from sperm clumping) in a definitive pattern
- Poor sperm motility
- Poor sperm function as evidenced by poor viability and low HOS score.

Mixed Antiglobulin Reaction Test

This test involves mixing fresh untreated semen with latex particles or RBC coated with human IgG and IgA. To this is added nonspecific anti human IgG antiserum. Mixed agglutinates between particles and motile sperms indicates presence of IgG and IgA antibodies on sperms. Immunological infertility is kept as a possibility when more than 50% or more motile sperms have adherent particles.

Immunobead Test (IBT)

A passive transfer of antisperm antibody from test sample (seminal plasma, serum or solubilized cervical mucus) to the surface of washed donor spermatozoa is done. These treated spermatozoa are then examined.

The WHO considers a level of binding of more than 20 percent to be significant. Clinically significant binding is considered to be a level more than 50 percent.

Clinical Significance of Positive Test (Flow chart 3.3)

- Immunobead binding restricted to the tail tip is not associated with impaired fertility and can be present in fertile men
- 50–80% IBT midpiece or tail—Try IUI or can go straight for IVF (Flow chart 3.3)
- 50–80% IBT head—Increase motile sperm numbers to compensate.
- More than 80 percent IBT midpiece/tail—Try IVF or can go directly for ICSI
- More than 80 percent IBT head—ICSI.

In a study four (57.1%) of seven patients who had IB-bound sperm of more than or equal to 80 percent,

Flow chart 3.3: Clinical significance of positive IBT

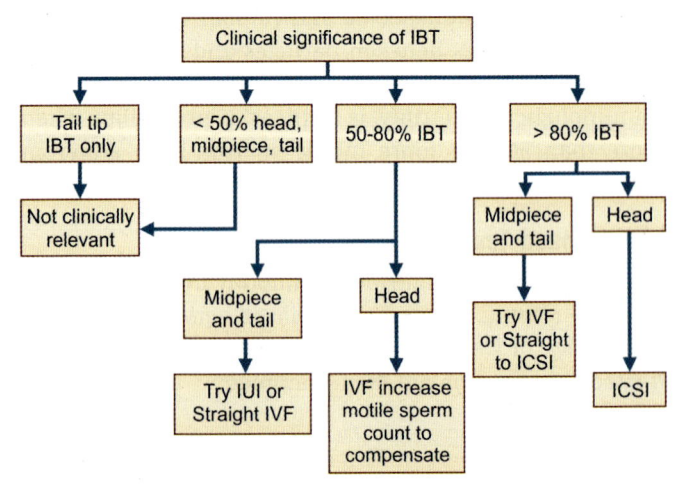

fertilizing ability was inhibited, while none of the eight patients who had less than 80% IB-bound sperm had an inhibitory effect on fertilization.[11]

ASSESSMENT OF SPERM DNA DAMAGE

In recent year it has been seen sperm DNA integrity is a prerequisite for normal spermatozoal function. DNA fragmentation index (DFI) in sperm of infertile men was found to be significantly higher as compared to controls. Sperm count, forward motility, and normal morphology were found to be negatively associated with DFI. Higher sperm DNA fragmentation may be the underlying cause for poor semen quality in idiopathic infertile men.[12]

Assessment of sperm chromatin can be made by dyes that bind to histone (aniline blue) or nucleic acid (acridine orange, chromomycin) and are assessed by flow cytometry. They could also measure DNA strand breaks like Tunnel assay, Comet assay or sperm chromatin dispersion. Many feel that these test should be included in workup of an infertile male since sperm DNA damage has shown an association with fertilization, embryo quality, implantation, spontaneous abortion.[13]

Semen analysis is the basic and most important test for male factor infertility. The basis of each parameter and its clinical implications need to be well understood to place patients into appropriate categories.

REFERENCES

1. Yavas Y, Selub M. Intrauterine insemination (IUI) pregnancy outcome is enhanced by shorter intervals from semen collection to sperm wash, from sperm wash to IUI time, and from semen collection to IUI time. Fertil Steril. 2004;82(6):1638-47.

2. Gluick DS, Overstreet JW, Factor Litwick P, Brazil CK, Nakajima ST, Coutiaris C, et al. Sperm morphology, motility and concentration in fertile and infertile men. New Engl J Med. 2001;345:1388.
3. World Health Organization Manual for Examination and Processing of Human Semen, 5th edn, Switzerland, 2010.
4. Rose et al. Techniques for detection of iso and auto antibodies to human spermatozoa Clin Exper Immunol. 1976;23:175-199.
5. Kruger TF, Acosta AA, Simmons KF, Swanson RJ, Matta JF, Oehninger S. Predictive value of abnormal sperm morphology in in vitro fertilization. Fertil Steril. 1988;49:112.
6. Ludwig M, Vidal A, Huwe P, Diemer T, Pabst W, Weidner W. Significance of inflammation on standard semenalysis in chronic prostatitis/chronic pelvic pain syndrome. Andrologia. 2003;35:152.
7. Arslan M, Morshedi M, Arslan EO, Taylor S, Kanik A, Duran HE, et al. Predictive value of the hemizona assay for pregnancy outcome in patients undergoing controlled ovarian hyperstimulation with intrauterine insemination. Fertil Steril. 2006;85(6):1697-707.
8. Ho LM, Lim AS, Lim TH, Hum SC, Yu SL, Kruger TF. Correlation between semen parameters and the Hamster Egg Penetration Test (HEPT) among fertile and subfertile men in Singapore. J Androl. 2007;28(1):158-63.
9. Agarwal A, Sekhon LH. Oxidative stress and antioxidants for idiopathic oligoasthenoteratospermia: Is it justified? Asian J Androl. 2011;13(3):420-3.
10. Bohring C, Krause W. The role of antisperm antibodies during fertilization and for immunological infertility. infertility Chem Immunol Allergy. 2005;88:15-26.
11. Shibahara H, Shiraishi Y, Hirano Y, Suzuki T, Takamizawa S, Suzuki M. Diversity of the inhibitory effects on fertilization by anti-sperm antibodies bound to the surface of ejaculated human sperm. Hum Reprod. 2003;18(7):1469-73.
12. Venkatesh S, Singh A, Shamsi MB, Thilagavathi J, Kumar R, K Mitra D, Dada R. Clinical significance of sperm DNA damage threshold value in the assessment of male infertility. Reprod Sci. 2011 18(10):1005-13.

13. Sadeghi MR, Lakpour N, Heidari-Vala H, Hodjat M, Amirjannati N, Hossaini Jadda H, Binaafar S, Akhondi MM. Relationship between sperm chromatin status and ICSI outcome in men with obstructive azoospermia and unexplained infertile normozoospermia. Rom J Morphol Embryol. 2011;52(2):645-51.

Chapter 4

Gonadotropins

Surveen Ghumman Sindhu

The first birth after gonadotropin stimulation was reported by Alan Trounson in 1981. Since then it has become the cornerstone of ART stimulation protocols. FSH with LH separated by polyvalent antibodies was commercially available by 1987, but these still contained urinary proteins. A highly purified FSH was obtained on removing LH by monoclonal antibodies.[1] Finally, the recombinant technology was used for a FSH preparation with absolutely no LH activity.

GONADOTROPIN PREPARATIONS

1. Human pituitary gonadotropin.
2. Human menopausal gonadotropins (75 IU of FSH, 75 IU LH).
3. Highly purified hMG (75 IU of FSH and 75 IU of LH with < 5% of urinary protein).
4. Purified urinary FSH (75 IU of FSH and < 0.7 IU of LH).
5. Highly purified urinary FSH (75 IU of FSH and <0.1 IU of LH and <5% urinary protein).
6. Recombinant FSH (75 IU of FSH and no LH).
7. Recombinant LH.
8. Human chorionic gonadotropin (hCG)
9. Recombinant hCG

Effective daily dose: It is the dose of gonadotropins which can elicit an ovarian response.

There are 2 phases of stimulation:
1. *The latent phase:* An initial period of 3 to 7 days where there is no measurable ovarian response in spite of follicular growth.
2. *Active phase:* After latent phase, a 4 to 7 days period where there is an exponential rise of estrogen with follicular growth.

CHOICE OF DOSAGE

The dose and duration of gonadotropin required may vary with the patient and also from cycle to cycle in the same patient. There is a relationship with body weight and dose requirement but the response threshold with all individuals is unpredictable.

The choice of gonadotropin also depends on indication of controlled ovarian stimulation. In women with hypogonadotropic hypogonadism, the drug of choice is menotropin because it contains both FSH and LH. LH is essential for ovulation and luteinization and in these cases LH levels are low. These patients respond to low doses of gonadotropin stimulation. Luteal phase support may be vital where endogenous LH levels are low (less than 3IU/L) These patients are prone to hyperstimulation and must be monitored carefully if hCG is given as luteal support (Table 4.1).

In patients with PCOS, LH levels are high. Recombinant FSH is given after down regulation (E2 < 30 pg/ml, LH < 4IU/L). There is a very narrow margin between doses which induce successful ovulation and those which cause hyperstimulation (Table 4.1). Patients with unexplained infertility are older

Table 4.1

Choice and dose of gonadotropin

	Type of gonadotropin	Dose of gonadotropin
Hypogonadotropic hypogonadism (LH low)	FSH and LH (menotropin)	Adequate dose
Clomiphene dose resistance/PCOS (LH high)	Recombinant FSH	Low
Unexplained infertility	Any preparation	High dose

subfertile women and the aim is multifollicular ovulation. Hence, higher doses of gonadotropins are used. In these, normally ovulating women where endocrinopathies have been ruled out, any available gonadotropin preparation can be used. Patients who are obese, above 35 years of age, poor responders, those with a baseline FSH of more than 10 IU/L or those down regulated with GnRH agonists, should be started on a higher dose of 225 IU of FSH. A day 8 LH assay of more than 10 IU/L predicts failure or increased risk of miscarriage if pregnancy occurs (Table 4.2).[2]

PROTOCOLS

The treatment is started within the first 2 days of the menstrual cycle.

Step up High Dose Protocol

This conventional protocol is started with 150 IU of FSH per day. Serum estradiol is measured on day 8 and transvaginal ultrasonography is done. The dose of gonadotropin is

Table 4.2

Factors influencing the dose of gonadotropin

1. Weight
2. Baseline FSH If > 10 IU/l—give higher dose.
3. Age beyond 35 years—a higher dose is required.
4. Higher effective daily dose in previous cycle.
5. Poor responders.
6. PCOS patients are usually started on a lower dose to avoid hyperstimulation.
7. Prior down regulation with GnRH agonists—a higher dose is required.
8. Hypogonadotropic hypogonadism.
9. Unexplained infertility.

maintained or increased accordingly as indicated. Once the serum estradiol begins to rise, the size and number of the developing follicles is determined every 1 to 2 days along with serum estradiol. If estradiol levels are not increasing then the dose of gonadotropins needs to be increased. A maximum of 300 to 375 IU of FSH can be used. There are studies where doses have gone up to 600 IU. Injection hCG is given once follicle is more than 16 to 17 mm. Patients will ovulate 36 hours after the hCG. This regime is useful for poor responders but has a high rate of multiple pregnancy and ovarian hyperstimulation syndrome. The effective daily dose of gonadotropins must be noted for each cycle. In subsequent stimulation cycles while determining the dose of gonadotropins, the response threshold and pattern of follicular development observed in previous cycles should be considered.

Step up Low Dose Protocol

It is started with an initial dose of 37.5 to 75 IU/day. If no response is seen in terms of estradiol level or follicle, it is increased in increments of 37.5 IU every week. This protocol though safe has an extended duration. Lesser ampules of gonadotropin are used and preovulatory estradiol levels are lower. Age, obesity and raised serum LH levels can adversely affect the outcome of treatment.[3] It is useful in patients of PCOS who are prone to hyperstimulation as they have a large number of antral follicles ready to respond to FSH stimulation. Administration of FSH converts already present androgens to estrogens producing very high levels of estrogens and overstimulation of ovary. This is avoided by this protocol as small doses of FSH provide the right amount of stimulation needed to make the process occur in a controlled manner. Homberg et al found in their study comparing conventional vs low dose regimen that patients treated with low dose regimen had a greater pregnancy rate and no hyperstimulation or multiple pregnancy. Patients on conventional treatment had an 11% incidence of OHSS and 33% incidence of multiple pregnancy.[4]

Step Down Protocol

Since many anovulatory women are very sensitive to low doses of exogenous gonadotropin stimulus the initiating dose of this protocol is determined in one or more pervious stimulation cycles before starting the regime. Total amount of gonadotropins are reduced in this regimen. The treatment is usually started with 225 IU hMG/FSH (or 300 IU in some cases) until follicles of 10 mm is seen. The dose is then reduced to 112.5 IU and 3 days later decreased to 75 IU and this is continued till administration of hCG. This is an effort to promote continued development of the more sensitive dominant follicle while withdrawing support from less sensitive smaller follicles in the cohort. It is indicated in oligo-amenorrheic women with PCOS or in high responders in IVF. FSH promotes follicular growth because of 2 events, the 'FSH threshold' and the 'FSH window'. FSH threshold is the level of FSH below which no follicular growth can be initiated.[5] Usually this level in normal women is 7.8 IU/l. The FSH window is the number of days that serum FSH levels are above the threshold and determines the number of follicles which are activated. Since sensitivity of the follicle increases with development, the required FSH for a follicle will decrease. The balance between the decreasing FSH levels and increasing FSH sensitivity is responsible for the growth of the follicle. Using this concept FSH levels are raised by exogenous FSH to reach the threshold and prolong the window in order to obtain specific number of follicles to be growing. The decreased dose would switch off the recruiting phase and limit the number of dominant follicles. A multiple pregnancy rate of 8% and OHSS rate of 2% is seen. This regimen mimics the physiological normal menstrual cycle.[6] It is a second line protocol in PCOS patients where other regimens do not achieve success.

Sequential Step up, Step Down Regimen

It is started similar to the step up protocol but the dose is reduced by half when leading follicle is 14 mm. This approach reduces the number of lead follicles.[7]

Mild Stimulation Protocol

Lower number of oocytes retrieved during mild stimulation is associated with favorable pregnancy outcomes as there may be natural selection. The benefits of low cost should be balanced with the decrease in pregnancy rate per cycle. With current recommendation of maximum two embryo transfer there seems to be no need of aggressive stimulation to obtain large number of oocytes at the cost of good quality oocyte selection and adequately primed endometrium. In the recent years mild protocols have been introduced which aim at a low stimulation which gives acceptable results with minimal risks and lower cost. Here the endogenous FSH is also taken advantage of while stimulating. ISMAAR association defines a "mild" IVF cycle either as:

a. A stimulation regimen in which gonadotropins are administered at a lower-than-usual dose and/or for a shorter duration throughout a cycle in which GnRH antagonist is given as cotreatment, or
b. A stimulation in which oral compounds (e.g. antiestrogens) are used either alone or in combination with gonadotropins and GnRH antagonists.[8]

Role of GnRH Antagonist in Mild Stimulation

With use of antagonists down regulation is not needed. The IVF cycle can start with an undisturbed early follicular phase recruitment of follicles by an endogenous FSH rise which occurs in a natural menstrual cycle. The endogenous intercycle FSH rise is taken advantage of rather than suppressed. FSH is added on day 5 to continue FSH elevation and extend the FSH window, for many follicles to develop. This limits the duration and dose of FSH administration. A premature LH surge may occur with rising estradiol levels which act through positive feedback loop. Native GnRH, antagonist has an immediate action blocking the pituitary when estradiol levels start rising and approach threshold levels at which an LH surge can occur. In a analysis of three studies, a flexible GnRH antagonist protocol was compared to the fixed protocol. In stimulated cycles it was seen that intense ovarian response with more number of follicles led to an early rise in estradiol. Thus threshold levels of estradiol which initiates a LH surge are reached earlier before follicles reach an optimum size. In these cases the flexible protocol which is dependent on the size of the follicle on ultrasound to start antagonist to suppress surge, may no longer be accurate to determine time of initiation of GnRH antagonist.[9] This observation might explain the observed lower efficacy of the flexible protocol compared with a fixed protocol in a meta-analysis of four studies.[10] Hence, for patients with a profound ovarian response, early initiation of the GnRH antagonist may be needed.

Clomiphene in Mild Stimulation Protocol

The second mild regime includes using clomiphene 100 mg, delayed low dose gonadotropin and a flexible GnRH antagonist administration for ovarian stimulation protocol. Pregnancy rates comparable to the standard stimulation regimens were obtained, with a significant reduction in the total dose of gonadotropin needed and of the economical costs. The number of recovered oocytes, obtained embryos, transferred embryos, peak of estradiol on the day HCG administration and OHSS were significantly higher in conventional group but there were no significant difference in clinical pregnancy rate and ongoing pregnancy rate between two groups.[11]

MONITORING

Careful monitoring with serum estradiol levels and ultrasonography is needed to achieve the goal of ovulation without hyperstimulation and multiple pregnancy

Serum Estradiol Levels

Follicles with a diameter of less than 10 mm produce relatively little estradiol but its level starts rising exponentially doubling every 2 to 3 days before ovulation. A change in the rate of rise of estradiol suggests a need for increasing or decreasing the dose of gonadotropin. For each mature follicle the level of estradiol is 200 to 300 pg/ml. When the gonadotropin injection is given between 5 and 8 pm the estradiol estimation should be done early morning.

Ultrasonography

A baseline ultrasonography is a must. In case there are residual ovarian cysts (more than 10 mm) treatment should be deferred as stimulation in the presence of a cyst is often unsuccessful. In a gonadotropin stimulated cycle follicle exhibits a linear growth but reaches maturity at a much smaller mean diameter. 40% patients ovulate when follicle is of 15 to 16 mm diameter. The rate of growth is 1 to 3 mm/day. Endometrial thickness measurements are also important. Cycle fecundity increases with endometrial thickness. Results are poor if endometrial thickness is less than 7 mm.

SIDE EFFECTS AND RISKS

1. *Multiple pregnancy:* (10-40%) Twin births have increased by 50% and higher order births have quadrupled. Risk is reduced if ovulation is not triggered when the estradiol level or number of maturing follicles is excessive.
2. *Hyperstimulation syndrome:* It is seen more in young age, low body weight, PCOS and high doses of gonadotropins. Rapidly rising serum estradiol level, concentration over 2,500 pg/ml and observations of a large number of small and intermediate size follicles indicate a high risk for OHSS. Mild forms of OHSS are seen in 8 to 23%, moderate in 6 to 7% and severe in 1 to 2% of cases stimulated with gonadotropins.

3. *Breast and ovarian cancer:* There have been no consistent reports of any causal relationship between gonadotropins and breast or ovarian cancer.
4. *Miscarriage:* (25%) Miscarriage rates are low in hypogonadotropic hypogonadism and much higher in clomiphene resistant anovulatory women.

RECOMBINANT FSH

Recombinant FSH was prepared by transfecting Chinese hamster ovary cell lines with both FSH subunit genes. Starting dose is 50 IU.[12] It was seen that although dose and duration of treatment with FSH was less and significantly more number of oocytes were retrieved with rFSH compared with uFSH, there was no difference in pregnancy rate in the two groups.[13] However, the pregnancy rates improved significantly when using rFSH instead of uFSH in poor responders (33% vs 7%).[14] There was no difference in oocytes recovered, dose and duration of treatment and pregnancy rates between alpha folliculotropin (Gonal F) and beta folliculotropin (Puregon).[15] Clinical choice of gonadotrophin should depend on availability, convenience and costs as no substantive differences in effectiveness or safety was seen on comparing recombinant FSH with other gonadotropins.[16]

The delivery system is a pen shaped device that is either prefilled or can be adjusted to fill variable doses from the vial. They are either lyophilized powder or liquid formulations found in cartridges or pens.

Advantages of Recombinant FSH

1. It has identical amino acids to natural FSH.
2. Consistent.

3. No LH activity.
4. No contamination with urinary proteins.
5. Highly specific and pure.
6. No restriction in supply.
7. Can be administered subcutaneously.

Disadvantages

1. Cost.
2. Increased incidence of OHSS.

RECOMBINANT FSH-CTP IN IVF

The β-subunit of hCG is different from gonadotropic hormones as it has a C-terminal peptide extension which is responsible for reduced clearance resulting in major enhancement of *in vivo* bioavailabilty. Daily injections of FSH have to be given as it has a short half-life. Genes containing the sequence coding the C-terminal peptide (CTP) of hCG is fused with β-subunit of FSH creating an FSH which is long acting with a half-life of 95 hours eliminating need for daily injections. Early follicular phase administration of FSH-CTP avoids the need for daily injections as a single injection enables follicular growth over a period of 7 days. Maximum serum levels are obtained after 36 to 48 hours. A second injection 7 days later may cause hyperstimulation. Hence daily doses of recombinant FSH are given thereafter. It is given as a single subcutaneous injection of 180 mg recombinant FSH-CTP on day 3 followed by daily injections of recombinant FSH 150 IU from day 10 onwards combined with GnRH antagonist 0.25 mg subcutaneously to prevent premature surge of LH.[17] The pharmacokinetics of corifollitropin alfa and rFSH are quite different but their induced pharmacodynamic effects at the dosages used are similar.[18] The safety and efficacy of such regimens is currently being evaluated in large comparative phase III clinical trials.[19] It is recommended that patients should be treated with the appropriate dose of corifollitropin alfa according to their body weight as a lower dose does not result in milder stimulation and a higher dose does not result in an improved ovarian response.

RECOMBINANT LH

It is known that the follicular selection and final stages of follicular maturation are equally if not more dependent on low circulating levels of LH.[20] In addition to stimulating production of thecal androgens as substrate for estrogen synthesis, LH stimulates granulosa cells via LH receptors induced by FSH and estrogen in larger but not smaller follicles. LH then becomes the principal stimulus for final stages of follicular maturation while at the same time declining concentration of FSH starve the smaller more FSH dependent follicles into atresia. Low dose hCG or recombinant LH can promote larger follicles to grow while hastening the regression of smaller follicles.

Recombinant LH can be used for inducing rupture in a single dose of 15,000 or 30,000 IU which is equivalent to reference treatment of 5000 IU hCG. It is superior with regard to incidence of OHSS and has a shorter half-life than hCG. Recombinant LH is also needed in hypogonadotropic hypogonadism in a dose of 75 IU daily for ovulation induction with rFSH for better results.[21]

HUMAN CHORIONIC GONADOTROPIN

Human chorionic gonadotropin (hCG) promotes the final stages of follicular maturation helping the oocyte reach metaphase II. Approximately 36 hours are required for completion of meiotic process and oocyte retrieval should be done within this time. It can be derived from human urine or can be recombinant. Recombinant hCG is available in syringes of 250 µg which is equivalent to 5000-6000 IU of hCG. There is no evidence of difference between rhCG or rhLH and uhCG in achieving final follicular maturation in IVF, with equivalent pregnancy rates and OHSS incidence.[22]

Exogenous gonadotropins have been used since last 4 decades. They are highly effective in ovulation induction but are accompanied with the disadvantage of high cost, extensive monitoring and risks of ovarian hyperstimulation and multiple pregnancy.

REFERENCES

1. ASRM Practice Committee. Gonadotropins Fertil Steril 2008; 90: S13-20
2. Olivennes F, Howies CM, Borini A, Germond M, Trew G, Wikland M, Zegers-Hochschild F, Saunders H, Alam V. Individualizing FSH dose for assisted reproduction using a novel algorithm: the CONSORT study. Reprod Biomed Online. 2011;22 (Suppl 1):S73-82.
3. White DM, Polson DW, Kiddy D. Induction of ovulation with low dose gonadotropins in polycystic ovary syndrome: An analysis of 109 pregnancies in 225 women. J Clin Endocrinol Metab. 1996;81:3821-4.
4. Homberg R, Levy T, Ben-Rafeal Z. A comparative prospective study of conventional regimen with chronic low dose administration of follicle stimulating hormone for anovulation associated with polycystic ovary syndrome. Fertil Steril. 1995;63:729-3.
5. Baird DT. A model for follicular selection and ovulation: Lessons from superovulation. Steroid Biochem. 1987;27:15-23.
6. van Santbrink EJP, Donderwinkel PFJ, van Dassel TJHM. Gonadotropin induction of ovulation using step-down dose

regimen: Single centre clinical experience in 82 patients. Hum Reprod. 1995;10:1048.
7. Hugues JN, Cedrin-Dumerin I, Avril C, Bulwa S, Herve-Fand-Uzan M. Sequential step up and step down regimen: An alternative method for ovulation induction with FSH in polycystic ovarian syndrome. Hum Reprod. 1996;11:2581-4.
8. Nargund J, Fauser BCJM, Macklon NS, Ombelet W, Nygren K, Frydman R. The ISMAAR proposal on terminology for ovarian stimulation for IVF. Hum Reprod. 2007;11(14): 2801-4.
9. Al-Inany HG, Aboulghar M, Mansour R, Serour GI. Optimizing GnRH antagonist administration: meta-analysis of fixed vs flexible protocol. Reprod Biomed Online. 2005;10:567-70.
10. Tarlatzis BC, Fauser BC, Kolibianakis EM, Diedrich K, Rombauts L, Devroey P. GnRH antagonists in ovarian stimulation for IVF. Hum Reprod Update. 2006;12:333-40.
11. Karimzadeh MA, Ahmadi S, Oskouian H, Rahmani E. Comparison of mild stimulation and conventional stimulation in ART outcome. Arch Gynecol Obstet. 2010;281(4):741-6.
12. Calaf Alsina J, Ruiz Balda JA, et al. Ovulation induction with a starting dose of 50 IU of recombinant follicle stimulating hormone in WHO group II anovulatory women: a prospective, observational, multicentric open trial. BJOG 2003;110(12):1072-7.
13. Schats R, Sutter P, Bassil S, et al. Ovarian stimulation during assisted reproduction treatment: A comparison of recombinant and highly purified urinary human FSH. Hum Reprod. 2000;15:1691-7.
14. Deplacido G, Alviggi C, Mollo A, et al. Recombinant follicle stimulating hormone is effective in poor responders to highly purified follicle stimulating hormone. Hum Reprod. 2000;15:17-20.
15. Brinson P, Adagios F, Gibbons L, et al. A comparison of efficacy and tolerability of two recombinant human follicle stimulating preparations in patients undergoing in vitro fertilization-embryo transfer. Fertil Steril. 2001;73:114-6.
16. van Wely M, Kwan I, Burt AL, Thomas J, Vail A, Van der Veen F, Al-Inany HG. Recombinant versus urinary gonadotrophin

for ovarian stimulation in assisted reproductive technology cycles. Cochrane Database Syst Rev. 2011;(2):CD005354.
17. Balen AH, Mulders AG, Fauser BC, Schoot BC, Renier MA, Devroey P, Struijs MJ, Mannaerts BM. Pharmacodynamics of a single low dose of long-acting recombinant follicle-stimulating hormone (FSH-carboxy terminal peptide, corifollitropin alfa) in women with World Health Organization Group II Anovulatory Infertility. J Clin Endocrinol Metab. 2004;89(12):6297-304.
18. Fauser BC, Alper MM, Ledger W, Schoolcraft WB, Zandvliet A, Mannaerts BM. Engage Investigators. Pharmacokinetics and follicular dynamics of corifollitropin alfa versus recombinant FSH during ovarian stimulation for IVF. Reprod Biomed Online. 2010;21(5):593-601.
19. Fauser BC, Alper MM, Ledger W, Schoolcraft WB, Zandvliet A, Mannaerts BM. Engage investigators: pharmacokinetics and follicular dynamics of corifollitropin alfa versus recombinant FSH during ovarian stimulation for IVF. Reprod Biomed Online. 2011;22 (Suppl 1):S23-31.
20. Levy DP, NavarroJM, Schattman GL, Davis OK, Rosenwaks Z. The role of LH in ovarian stimulation; Exogenous LH: lets design the future. Hum Reprod. 2000;15:2258.
21. Schoot DC, Harlin J, Shaham Z, Mannerts BM, Lahlou N, Bouchard P, Bennick HJ, Fauser BC. Recombinant human follicle stimulating hormone and ovarian response in gonadotropin deficient women. Hum Reprod. 1994;9(7): 1237-42.
22. Youssef MA, Al-Inany HG, Aboulghar M, Mansour R, Abou-Setta AM. Recombinant versus urinary human chorionic gonadotrophin for final oocyte maturation triggering in IVF and ICSI cycles. Cochrane Database Syst Rev. 2011;(4):CD003719.

Chapter 5

Role of GnRH Agonists and Antagonists in ART

Surveen Ghumman Sindhu

The GnRH agonists and antagonists have occupied an increasingly important position in the ovulation induction protocols. GnRH analogues are able to suppress gonadotropin release and subsequently, the gonadal function. This is the basis for their clinical applications as it controls the premature endogenous luteinizing hormone (LH) surge and therefore, decreases the cycle cancellation rate.

GnRH AGONIST (GnRH-A)

Substitutions in the GnRH molecule cause enhanced affinity for the GnRH receptors and protects against enzyme degradation increasing half life from 8 minutes to 5 hours.

Decapeptide agonists
- Triptorelin
- Naferelin
- Goserelin

Nonapeptide agonists
- Buserelin
- Lupreolide
- Histerelin

Mechanism of Action

The mechanism of action is a "flare effect", followed by downregulation. Within 12 hours of administration it induces liberation of high amount of FSH and LH and also increases the number of receptors (5-fold increase in FSH, 10-fold increase in LH and 4-fold increase in estradiol receptors). This is the so-called 'upregulation.' A continuous administration of GnRH agonist produces the opposite effect. There is a decrease in level of FSH and LH by internalization of the receptor-agonist complex and a reduction in the number of receptors. This is called 'downregulation' or desensitization of the pituitary. This eliminates any premature LH surge and decreases LH stimulation of ovarian androgen production. The advantage is reduced cycle cancellation, convenient timing of treatment and higher live birth rates. Stimulation is then begun with gonadotropins. Also it can be used as an ovulation trigger to prevent ovarian hyperstimulation syndrome.

Commonly used GnRH agonists are:

Leuprolide	SC 500-1000 mg or IM depot 3.75, 7.5 mg/month.
Buserelin	SC 200-500 mg/day or 300-400 μg intranasaly 3-4 times/day.
Goserelin	SC implant 3.6 mg/month.
Triptorelin	SC 100-500 μg/day or IM depot 3.75 mg/month.

Route of Administration

1. Subcutaneous injections.
2. Sustained release implants.
3. Intramuscular depot injections.
4. Nasal spray.

Subcutaneous: This route is most commonly used because of high bioavailability and low interindividual variation. It results in prolonged and delayed absorption compared to intravenous route.

Intranasal route: Disadvantages of this route include a marked interindividual variation in absorption and considerable losses of peptides by proteolysis and swallowing. Initially preparation like buserelin needed frequent administration (5 times a day) however nasal preparations like naferelin only require twice a day administration.[1] There is an advantage of persistence of drug in the nasal mucosa for up to 24 hours consistent with depot like effects. The drug absorption varies with rhinitis and allergy. It is a more convenient route for the patient as compared to daily injections.

Depot formulation: Since there is more profound suppression of the pituitary gonadal axis with continuous administration of the drug, sustained or continuous release formulations have been developed. Currently available preparations include a suspension of 3.75 mg triptorelin or lueprolide in microcapsules injected intramuscularly once a month or 3.6 mg of goserelin dispersed in a biodegradable polymeric matrix of polyactide-coglycolide as a cylindrical rod implant injected subcutaneously every month. The pharmokinetics of the two differ. In both, the drug is released over 30 to 55 days. The number of follicles developed, E2 levels, oocyte quality, fertilization and pregnancy rates were same as with daily administration.[2] Due to prolonged desensitization the dose of gonadotropins needed is more and stimulation is longer.[2]

Use of GnRH Agonist in COH Protocols

The use of GnRH agonists decreased cancellation rates in IVF cycle from 20 to 2% and improved fertilization and implantation rates.[3] Three protocols have been described:

a. Long protocol.
b. Short protocol.
c. Ultrashort protocol.

Protocols for Administration

Long Protocol

Advantages of long protocol
1. It prevents unwanted LH surge and hence cancellation of cycles.
2. It helps plan the time of ovum pick-up.

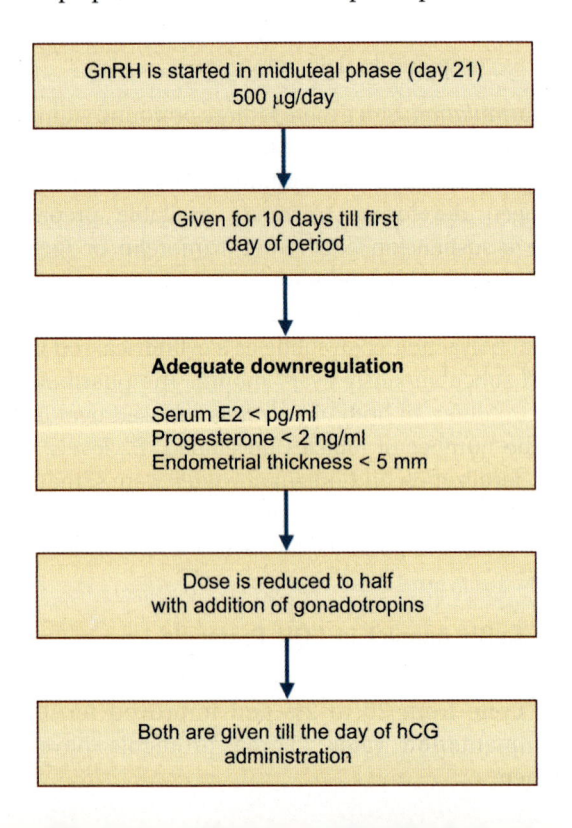

```
┌─────────────────────────────────────────┐
│  GnRH is started in midluteal phase     │
│          (day 21) 500 µg/day            │
└─────────────────────────────────────────┘
                    ↓
┌─────────────────────────────────────────┐
│   Given for 10 days till first          │
│          day of period                  │
└─────────────────────────────────────────┘
                    ↓
┌─────────────────────────────────────────┐
│       Adequate downregulation           │
│                                         │
│   Serum E2 < pg/ml                      │
│   Progesterone < 2 ng/ml                │
│   Endometrial thickness < 5 mm          │
└─────────────────────────────────────────┘
                    ↓
┌─────────────────────────────────────────┐
│   Dose is reduced to half               │
│   with addition of gonadotropins        │
└─────────────────────────────────────────┘
                    ↓
┌─────────────────────────────────────────┐
│   Both are given till the day of hCG    │
│             administration              │
└─────────────────────────────────────────┘
```

3. Improves overall pregnancy rates especially in patients with raised LH levels.
4. Allows synchronization in growth of follicles.
5. Reduces intensive monitoring of cycles to detect premature LH surge.
6. Most studies show a better result with the long protocol than with short or ultrashort protocol.

Disadvantages of long protocol
1. Extends or prolongs treatment cycle.
2. Higher doses of gonadotropins are needed.
3. More expensive.
4. It is associated with symptoms of depression in hypogonadal phase.[4]

Short Protocol

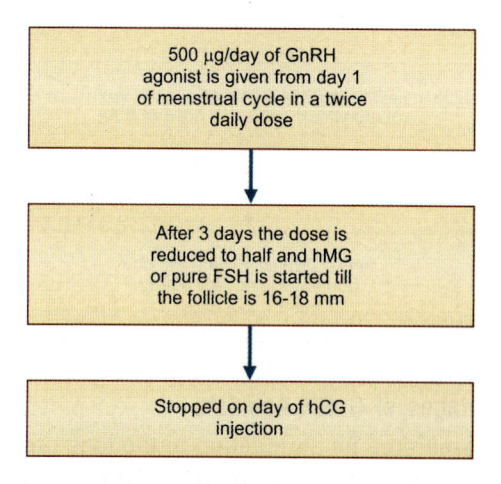

```
500 µg/day of GnRH agonist is given from day 1
of menstrual cycle in a twice daily dose
           ↓
After 3 days the dose is reduced to half and hMG
or pure FSH is started till the follicle is 16-18 mm
           ↓
Stopped on day of hCG injection
```

Advantages of short protocol
1. Better for older patients and poor responders as it causes greater follicular recruitment.

2. The flare effect offers an advantage in hypogonadotropin hypogonadism.
3. Shorter protocol.
4. Less expensive.
5. Less chances of ovarian hyperstimulation because of lower E2 levels.

Disadvantages of short protocol

In PCOS it causes irregular growth of follicle and is not helpful where LH levels are raised.

Ultrashort Protocol

This differs from the short protocol in discontinuing the agonist once it has stimulated the flare. This reduced the doses of both drugs. However this protocol had a poor pregnancy rates as compared to long protocol because of premature LH surge.

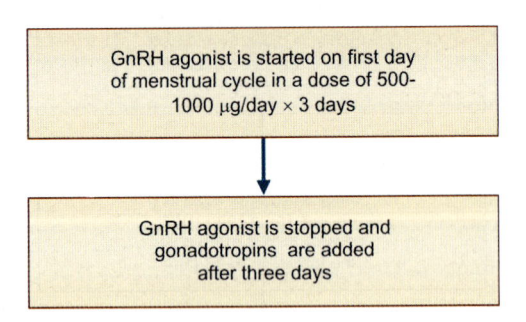

> GnRH agonist is started on first day of menstrual cycle in a dose of 500-1000 μg/day × 3 days

> GnRH agonist is stopped and gonadotropins are added after three days

Disadvantages of GnRH Agonists

1. Increased time for stimulation in the long protocol.
2. Short protocol may increase premature LH surge.
3. Luteal phase support is needed.
4. Increased cost due to increased requirement of gonadotropin.

5. It may cause hyperstimulation due to flare response in luteal phase in the long protocol leading to high estradiol levels and ovarian cyst.[5]

Advantages of GnRH Agonists

1. Decreases the need for close monitoring to detect spontaneous LH surge.
2. Less cycle cancellation.
3. Better response.
4. More flexible schedule.
5. Higher oocyte recovery and pregnancy rate.

Side Effects and Risks of GnRH Agonists

1. *Ovarian cyst:* It is seen in 14 to 29%, more with the short protocol.
2. *Ovarian hyperstimulation syndrome (OHSS):* The increased incidence of OHSS is due to increased pregnancy rate and higher doses of gonadotropins being used.
3. *Luteal phase defect.*
4. Transient neurological disturbances like parasthesia or headaches occur in 5%.

GnRH Agonist for Ovulation Trigger

In patients at risk to develop OHSS, the only option available earlier was to withhold the ovulatory dose of human chorionic gonadotropin leading to cancelled cycles. GnRH agonist, when administered in a single dose, bring about the LH surge and triggers ovulation like hCG, because of its flare effect.

Dose: Leuprolide acetate: 1 mg given either subcutaneously as a single, or two doses 12 hours apart can act as an ovulation trigger.

Probability of pregnancy: After luteal support there is a non-significant difference in delivery rate in favor of hCG triggering.[6]

Advantages

a. Its short duration of action is more physiological unlike extended surge with the use of hCG.
b. Decrease in multiple pregnancy.
c. Prevents OHSS as it has shorter duration of action compared to hCG. Luteotropic action is prolonged in hCG administration leading to development of multiple corpora lutea and supraphysiological levels of E2.
d. Can be used along with antagonist.

Disadvantages

a. Cannot be used in cases of hypogonadotropic hypogonadism.
b. It causes pituitary desensitization making luteal support necessary.
c. Not used for cases downregulated with GnRH agonist as the flare effect of LH release by a single dose of the agonist will not occur because of pituitary downregulation, making ovulation trigger ineffective.

GnRH ANTAGONISTS

Antagonists act by competitive inhibition of GnRH receptors preventing the native GnRH from exerting its stimulatory effect on the pituitary cells, resulting in rapid decline in LH and FSH lasting for 10 to 100 hours. There is no stimulatory phase unlike the GnRH agonists. Due to competitive nature of action this effect is dose dependant and depends on the equilibrium between endogenous

GnRH and the antagonists. Their action is easily reversible. Antagonists neither deplete the LH and FSH stores nor inhibit their synthesis.

Contraindications

1. Hepatic dysfunction.
2. Renal dysfunction.
3. Hypersensitivity to GnRH analogs.

Protocols

Antagonist can be given in two ways:

a. *Lubeck protocol* (*Multidose protocol*): Gonadotropins are started as usual. When follicle reaches 14 mm or on a fixed day of protocol, antagonist is added at a dose of 0.25 mg/day until the day before ovulation (Fig. 5.1). This protocol can be either fixed or flexible.
   i. *Fixed protocol:* Daily injections of small doses initiated on a fixed day of stimulation till hCG administration.
   ii. *Flexible protocol:* Daily injections of small doses initiated depending on the size of the dominant follicle (14 mm) or on estradiol levels till hCG administration.
b. *French protocol* (*Single dose protocol*): Gonadotropins are started as usual. Antagonist is given in a single dose of 3 mg when E2 is about 150 to 200 pg/ml and follicular size is 14 mm (Fig. 5.2).

Single versus multiple dose GnRH antagonist protocol

Advantage of single dose protocol was lesser injections but if hCG needs to be delayed additional daily doses are given. About 10% women require additional doses.

Cochrane review 2002 has concluded that both protocols were equally effective in preventing premature

Fig. 5.1: Lubeck protocol

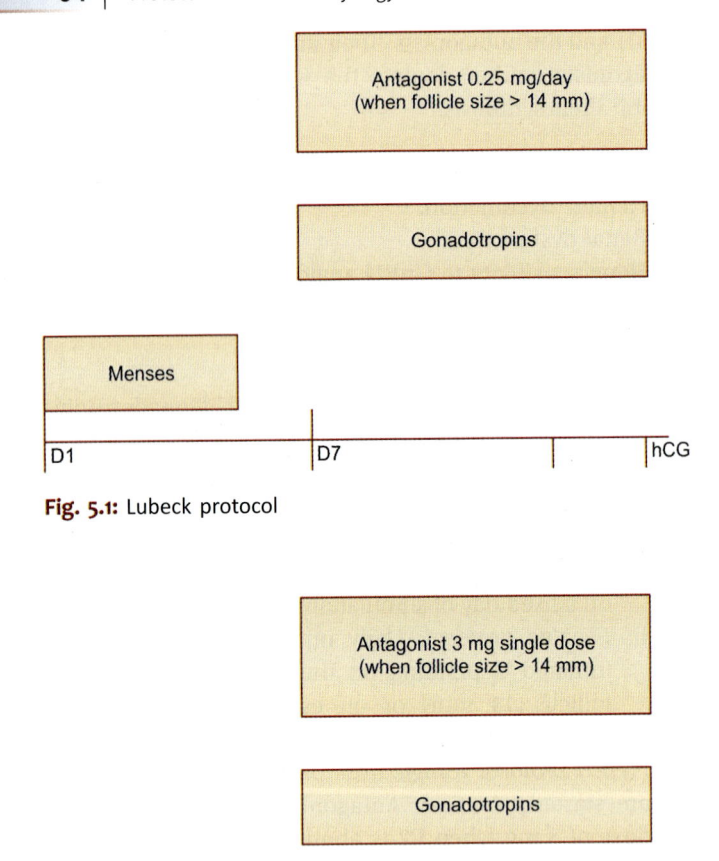

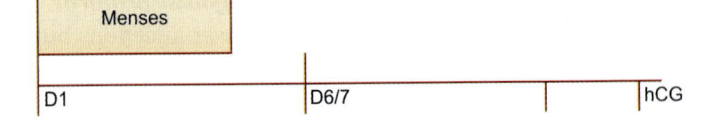

Fig. 5.2: French protocol

LH surge.[7] It was seen that the single dose protocol may lead to extreme suppression of LH but pregnancy rates were similar with both protocols.[8]

Fixed versus flexible antagonist administration
In an analysis of three studies, a flexible GnRH antagonist protocol was compared to the fixed protocol. In stimulated cycles it was seen that intense ovarian response with more number of follicles led to an early rise in estradiol. Thus threshold levels of estradiol which initiates a LH surge are reached earlier before follicles reach an optimum size. In these cases the flexible protocol which is dependent on the size of the follicle on ultrasound to start antagonist in order to suppress surge, may no longer be accurate to determine time of initiation of GnRH antagonist.[9] This observation might explain the observed lower efficacy of the flexible protocol compared with a fixed protocol in a meta-analysis of four studies.[10]

Hence, for patients with a profound ovarian response, early initiation of the GnRH antagonist may be needed.

Which GnRH antagonist is to be used?
Cetrorelix and ganirelix effectively prevented LH surges however, cetrorelix required significantly fewer injections, increasing patient convenience.[8]

Should FSH dose be increased in antagonist cycle?
Although with antagonist cycles gonadotropin dose needed is lower as there is no pituitary suppression, however a reduced oocyte recovery was notice. An initial higher dose of FSH gave a higher oocyte recovery but there was no difference in pregnancy rates.[11] It was seen that increasing dose of FSH or HMG after starting antagonist did not increase pregnancy rates.[12,13]

Role of oral contraceptive pill pretreatment in ovarian stimulation with GnRH antagonists

Pretreatment with an oral contraceptive (OC) in antagonist cycle has been suggested to allow greater control over patient response rate and to avoid follicular asynchrony. Scheduling of cycle is no longer based on menstruation but on discontinuation of OCP. A meta-analysis proved that no increase in pregnancy rate was seen with OC.[14] However, it has been associated with increased duration of treatment and higher doses of gonadotropin.[15]

LH supplementation with GnRH antagonist

An abrupt suppression of endogenous LH by GnRH antagonist occurs in the mid-follicular phase, at a critical stage for follicular development. However studies have shown no increase in pregnancy rate with LH supplementation or increase of hMG dose on initiation of antagonist.[16,17] The decision to add LH must be individualized. It has been seen that the direction and rate of change in LH concentrations are the important factors governing the follicular unit development, not the LH concentration itself.[18] It was found in a study that in 12 to 14% of downregulated patients the initial response to FSH is suboptimal (in terms of follicular growth and estradiol rise) and their day 8 LH concentration decreased from 1.2 to 0.7. It was suggested that these patients are the candidates for hLH supplementation. Normal responders increased their mean LH concentrations from 1.5 to 4.3 after 8 days of stimulation. It was suggested that the follicular unit is sensitive not necessarily to the current concentration of LH, but rather to the dynamics of the change in these concentrations and hence LH supplementation must be individualized.[19] In women on antagonist-based cycles for the first time, it is preferable to add recombinant LH or partly switch to HMG on the day of antagonist administration.[20]

Luteal support

It is seen that pituitary suppression may continue into luteal phase with poor development of endometrium. Hence luteal support is a must and has shown to improve pregnancy rates.

Advantages of GnRH Antagonists over GnRH Agonist in ART

1. Short, simple and convenient method of stimulation, which is well tolerated by the patient.
2. There is immediate suppression with no stimulatory phase. So no ovarian cyst formation takes place as in agonist cycle.
3. There are no symptoms of estrogen deprivation.
4. Minimal local reactions.
5. Decreased risk of OHSS: A recent Cochrane (2011) showed a decreased risk of OHSS but similar live birth rates compared to GnRH agonists.[21]
6. Clinical results of IVF cycles are comparable in both (Cochrane 2011).[21]
7. Decrease in the overall cost of treatment.
8. Immediate reversibility.
9. Reduced dose of gonadotropins.
10. Effect on endometrium: Simón et al (2005) observed that the endometrial development after GnRH antagonist mimics the natural endometrium more closely than after GnRH agonist.[22]

GnRH antagonists administration during the late follicular phase resulted in lower serum LH levels and better embryo quality in comparison to GnRH agonists. Studies have concluded that antagonists should be the first choice in IVF treatment, with less of the complications and risks of controlled ovarian hyperstimulation and an acceptable success rate.[23]

Disadvantages of Antagonists

1. Easy patient scheduling is lacking, due to the reliance on spontaneous menstrual cycles.
2. Lack of stimulatory effects on folliculogenesis typical of GnRH agonist regimens.
3. Need to replace LH if recombinant FSH is used.

Thus to conclude the GnRH antagonist reduces the dose and duration of gonadotropin treatment as it does not nullify FSH or LH secretion but interrupts the premature LH surge. It has the disadvantage of loss of easy patient rescheduling due to reliance on natural recruitment of follicles, lack of stimulatory effect on folliculogenesis unlike GnRH agonists and need for replacement of LH if recombinant FSH is used.

Recommendations for GnRH antagonist use in IVF cycle[24]
1. Increase in the starting dose of gonadotropins or to increase gonadotropin dose at antagonist initiation is not necessary
2. OCP pretreatment can be used for scheduling IVF cycles
3. Addition of LH with initiating antagonist not necessary
4. Fixed protocol appears to be superior to flexible initiation by a follicle of 14–16 mm
5. Results with single dose and multiple dose protocols were similar but single dose led to more profound LH suppression although convenience of a single injection administration was there.

GONADOTROPIN RELEASING HORMONE

It is mainly used in WHO group I anovulatory women but can be used in PCOS patients. The advantages are that significant follicular monitoring is not needed and it has less risk for OHSS and multiple pregnancy. It can be given either subcutaneously in a dose of 20 μg or intravenously 5 μg at 90 min interval through a portable programmable mini pump worn by the patient throughout. If there is no response in weekly estradiol level the dose is increased by increments of 5 μg. Luteal phase support can be given by continuation of the pump. Problems encountered are malfunction of the pump and local effects like thrombophlebitis, cellulitis, urticaria or anaphylaxis. Ovulation rates of 90%, conception rates of 20 to 30% per cycle and cummulative pregnancy rate of 80 to 90% after 12 months are seen in WHO group 1 women.[25] In PCOS cumulative pregnancy rate is 30 to 40%. Abortion occurs in 20% cases and multiple pregnancies in 5%.

REFERENCES

1. Anik ST, McRae G, Narenberg C, et al. Nasal absorption of naferelin acetate, the decapeptide (p-Nal{2}6) LHRH, in rhesus monkeys. J Pharm Sci. 1984;73:684-5.
2. Albuquerque LE, Saconato H, Maciel MC. Depot versus daily administration of gonadotrophin releasing hormone agonist protocols for pituitary desensitization in assisted reproduction cycles. Cochrane Database Syst Rev. 2005 Jan 25;(1): CD002808.
3. Akagbosu FT. The use of GnRH agonists in infertility. In Brinsden R (Ed). A textbook of In Vitro Fertilization and Assisted Reproduction (2nd edn): London: Parthenon Publishing; 1999. pp. 83-9.

4. Bloch M, Azem F, Aharonov I, Ben Avi I, Yagil Y, Schreiber S, Amit A, Weizman A. GnRH-agonist induced depressive and anxiety symptoms during in vitro fertilization-embryo transfer cycles. Fertil Steril. 2011;95(1):307-9.
5. Depenbusch M, Diedrich K, Griesinger G. Ovarian hyperresponse to luteal phase GnRH agonist administration. Arch Gynecol Obstet. 2010;281(6):1071-2.
6. Humaidan P, Kol S, Papanikolaou EG. Copenhagen GnRH Agonist Triggering Workshop Group GnRH agonist for triggering of final oocyte maturation: time for a change of practice? Hum Reprod Update. 2011;17(4):510-24.
7. Al-Inay H, Aboulghar M. GnRH antagonist in assisted reproduction: a Cochrane review. Hum Reprod Update. 2002;17(4):874-85.
8. Wilcox J, Potter D, Moore M, Ferrande L, Kelly E. CAP IV Investigator Group Prospective, randomized trial comparing cetrorelix acetate and ganirelix acetate in a programmed, flexible protocol for premature luteinizing hormone surge prevention in assisted reproductive technologies. Fertil Steril. 2005;84(1):108-17.
9. Al-Inany HG, Aboulghar M, Mansour R, Serour GI. Optimizing GnRH antagonist administration: meta-analysis of fixed vs flexible protocol. Reprod Biomed Online. 2005;10:567-70.
10. Tarlatzis BC, Fauser BC, Kolibianakis EM, Diedrich K, Rombauts L, Devroey P. GnRH antagonists in ovarian stimulation for IVF. Hum Reprod Update. 2006;12:333-40.
11. Out HJ, Rutherford A, Fleming R, Tay CC, Trew G, Ledger W, Cahill D. A randomized, double-blind, multicentre clinical trial comparing starting doses of 150 and 200 IU of recombinant FSH in women treated with the GnRH antagonist ganirelix for assisted reproduction. Hum Reprod. 2004;19:90-5.
12. Propst AM, Bates GW, Robinson RD, Arthur NJ, Martin JE, Neal GS. A randomized controlled trial of increasing recombinant follicle-stimulating hormone after initiating agonadotropin-releasing hormone antagonist for in vitro fertilization-embryo transfer. Fertil Steril. 2006;86(1):58-63.
13. Aboulghar MA, Mansour RT, Serour GI, Al-Inany HG, Amin YM, Aboulghar MM. Increasing the dose of human

menopausal gonadotropins on day of GnRH antagonist administration: randomized controlled trial. Reprod Biomed Online. 2004;8:524-7.
14. Griesinger G, Venetis CA, Marx T, Diedrich K, Tarlatzis BC, Kolibianakis EM. Oral contraceptive pill pretreatment in ovarian stimulation with GnRH antagonists for IVF: a systematic review and meta-analysis. Fertil Steril. 2008;90(4): 1055-63.
15. Bendikson K, Milki A, Speck-Zulak A, Westphal L. Comparison of GnRH antagonist cycles with and without oral contraceptive pill pretreatment in poor responders. Fertil Steril. 2003;80 (Suppl. 3):s188.
16. Griesinger G, Schultze-Mosgau A, Dafopoulos K, Schroeder A, Schroer A, von Otte S, Hornung D, Diedrich K, Felberbaum R. Recombinant luteinizing hormone supplementation to recombinant follicle stimulating hormone induced ovarian hyperstimulation in the GnRH antagonist multiple-dose protocol. Hum Reprod. 2005a;20:1200-6.
17. Aboulghar MA, Mansour RT, Serour GI, Al-Inany HG, Amin YM, Aboulghar MM. Increasing the dose of human menopausal gonadotropins on day of GnRH antagonist administration: randomized controlled trial. Reprod Biomed Online. 2004;8:524-7.
18. Huirne JA, van Loenen AC, Schats R, et al. Dose-finding study of daily GnRH antagonist for the prevention of premature LH surges in IVF/ICSI patients: optimal changes in LH and progesterone for clinical pregnancy. Hum Reprod. 2005;20: 359-67.
19. De Placido G, Alviggi C, Perino A, et al. Recombinant human LH supplementation versus recombinant human FSH (rFSH) step-up protocol during controlled ovarian stimulation in normogonadotrophic women with initial inadequate ovarian response to rFSH. A multicentre, prospective, randomized controlled trial. Hum Reprod. 2005;20:390-6.
20. Kol S. To add or not to add LH: consideration of LH concentration changes in individual patients Reprod BioMed Online. 2005;11:664-6.

21. Al-Inany HG, Youssef MAFM, Aboulghar M, Broekmans FJ, Sterrenburg MD, Smit JG, Abou-Setta AM. Gonadotrophin-releasing hormone antagonists for assisted reproductive technology. Cochrane Database of Systematic Reviews 2011, Issue 5. Art. No.: CD001750. DOI: 10.1002/14651858.CD001750.pub3
22. Simon C, Oberye J, Bellver J, Vidal C, Bosch E, Horcajadas JA, Murphy C, Adams S, Riesewijk A, Mannaerts B, Pellicer A. Similar endometrial development in oocyte donors treated with either high- or standard-dose GnRH antagonist compared to treatment with a GnRH agonist or in natural cycles. Hum Reprod. 2005;20(12):3318-27.
23. Xavier P, Gamboa C, Calejo L, Silva J, Stevenson D, Nunes A, et al. A randomised study of GnRH antagonist (cetrorelix) versus agonist (buserelin) for controlled ovarian stimulation: effect on safety and efficacy. Eur J Obstet Gynecol Reprod Biol. 2005;120:185-9.
24. Tarlatzis BC, et al. GnRH antagonists in ovarian stimulation for IVF. Hum Reprod Update. 2006;12:333-40.
25. Ghosh C, Buck G, Priore R, Wende JW, Severino M. Follicular response and pregnancy among infertile women undergoing ovulation induction and intrauterine insemination. Fertil Steril. 2003;80:328-35.

Chapter 6

Embryo Transfer and Troubleshooting

Pankaj Talwar

INTRODUCTION

All the diverse steps in an IVF cycle can proceed successfully till this stage in about 80% of the IVF center's.[1] Embryo transfer, the final step in ART, is the most crucial procedure which decides the pregnancy outcome.[2]

FACTORS AFFECTING EMBRYO TRANSFER

Varied factors affect results of Embryo Transfer (Table 6.1). These issues could be pertaining to those addressed before, during or after the embryo transfer. Each step in embryo transfer is important and all IVF lab protocols should be followed closely.

RELEVANT ISSUES TO BE ADDRESSED BEFORE EMBRYO TRANSFER

Embryo transfer is usually performed 48-72 hours after oocyte insemination/ICSI (4-8 cell stage). There are many issues like embryo selection after grading, choice of the transfer catheter, relevance of mock transfer and ultrasound before ET, relaxation of patient, injury to endometrium, and experience of the clinician.

Table 6.1

Factors affecting embryo transfer outcome

Relevant issues to be addressed before embryo transfer
1. Relevance of embryo selection and grading
2. Choices of the catheter and outcome of embryo transfer
3. Relaxing the patient before the procedure
4. Role of ultrasound and mock before embryo transfer before the procedure
5. Damage to the endometrium
6. Experience of the clinician

Relevant issues to be addressed during embryo transfer
1. Position of the patient during embryo transfer
2. Gentle and atraumatic technique
   i. The use of a Volsellum in cervix manipulation during ET
   ii. Role of uterine contractility in success of embryo transfer
3. Cervical mucus removal
4. Use of ultrasound-guidance during embryo transfer
5. Type of embryo transfer medium used during embryo transfer
6. Air bubble technique during embryo transfer
7. Time interval between embryo loading and transfer
8. Place of embryo deposition in the uterine cavity
9. Retained embryos and repeat embryo transfer

Relevant issues to be addressed post embryo transfer
1. Bed rest after embryo transfer
2. Sexual intercourse post transfer
3. Medication after embryo transfer

Relevance of Embryo Selection and Grading

Many studies have shown that morphological features in the embryo may be used as biomarkers of quality and for superior embryo selection which may enhance pregnancy rates and potentially reduce further the number of embryos needed for transfer. A recent Cochrane review stated that delaying transfer from day 2/3 to the blastocyst stage (days 5–6) may offer a window of opportunity to select better quality embryos and gives better pregnancy rate.[3] The embryo quality can be assessed by various methods.

i. *Morphological parameters:* Most of the existing scoring systems are based on several morphological parameters such as.
   - Cleavage stage
   - Embryonic fragmentation
   - Blastomere uniformity and number.

   The newer techniques, which work without compromising embryo quality that would occur as a result of increased handling time outside the incubator, include multilevel digital recording of embryo images and software programs that allow detailed interpretation of the embryo pictures.

ii. *Embryo metabolics:* Micromethods for assessing the metabolism of embryos were developed in order to improve the selection of embryos with the best developmental potential. These include the:
   - Embryos' respiratory rate
   - Glucose consumption
   - Nitric oxide levels
   - Amino acid turnover pace.

   These techniques are cumbersome and are in experimental stage.

Choices of the Catheter and Outcome of Embryo Transfer

The ideal ET catheter should be soft enough to avoid any trauma to the endocervical canal or endometrial cavity. It should be pliable enough to negotiate through the cervical canal into the endometrial cavity. Additionally, its tip should be smooth and nontraumatic. Ideal catheters are of co-axial variety. The outer sheath should also be malleable and inserted till internal os very gently. A recent meta-analysis of 10 studies comparing soft ET catheters with more rigid ones revealed that the clinical pregnancy rate was significantly better when using the soft catheters.[4]

Relaxing the Patient During the Procedure

It has been proposed that various methods of analgesia or even anesthesia during ET may be associated with higher pregnancy rates. Acupuncture and hypnosis during ET, have shown a better implantation and pregnancy rate in some studies.[5,6] We routinely administer diazepam 10 mg IM one hour before the procedure.

Role of Ultrasound and Mock Embryo Transfer Before the Procedure

Ultrasonography is very essential in measuring and evaluating the cervico-uterine angle, length, and direction before ET.[7] Nearly 30% of patients had a difference of 1 cm in the cavity length from trial ET compared of US-guided ET, suggesting a benefit of US-guided ET. Assessment of endometrial thickness and pattern by ultrasonography should be done before ET. An endometrium of more than 8 mm with a triple line pattern is associated with higher chances of pregnancy. Likewise, the endometrial volume, measured with 3D ultrasound, of less than 2.5 ml on the day of transfer showed poor probability of implantation.[8] A markedly thick endometrium also deters implantation.

Damage to the Endometrium

Injury caused by tricky embryo transfers due to cervico-uterine angulations or the lack of experience by the clinicians may disrupt the endometrium with a consequent negative impact on the endometrial receptivity and implantation rates.[9] This may be due to:

- Bleeding in the uterine cavity
- Inflammatory changes in the endometrial lining
- Plugging of the embryo transfer catheter, which in turn may retain the embryos and lead to grade two transfer
- Initiation of uterine contractions, which eventually may expel the embryos from the uterine cavity.

The damage may be avoided by thorough clinical assessment of the case before actual embryo transfer.

Experience of the Clinician

Nontraumatic embryo transfer which influences the final outcome and avoids of uterine contractions depends upon technical skills of the clinician. It is likely that the clinician's experience has an influence upon the outcome.[10]

RELEVANT ISSUES TO BE ADDRESSED DURING EMBRYO TRANSFER

The important issues to be addressed during transfer would include position of patient, atraumatic technique, cervical mucus removal, ultrasound guidance, media used for transfer, time interval between loading and transfer, place of embryo deposition and policy for retained embryos.

Position of the Patient During Embryo Transfer

The preferable position for embryo transfer is lithotomy. Bladder should be partially full.

Gentle and Atraumatic Technique

The embryo transfer should be atraumatic, painless and gentle, characterized by the lack of blood, mucus, endometrial cells on the catheter tip, suggestive of injury to the endometrium. Even the insertion of the vaginal speculum should be done gently as it can initiate uterine contractions. Nearly 30% of embryo transfers may be difficult thus reducing the chance of conception.[11]

i. *The use of a volsellum in cervix manipulation during ET:* Cusco's speculum is recommended to be used in embryo transfers as this makes the procedure atraumatic and gentle. Holding the cervix with a volsellum during ET was found to increase oxytocin release and junctional zone contractions which remain high till the end of the procedure and can lead to the expulsion of the embryos.[12]

> *Note:* Volsellum should be used only in order to negotiate the cervical canal angulation with the catheter tip when necessary as it induces uterine contractions and prostaglandin release.

ii. *Role of uterine contractility in success of embryo transfer:* Due to the embryo transfer procedure antegrade waves may be generated in the uterine cavity, which may lead to expulsion of the embryos.[13] To avert these unwelcome uterine contractions the clinician should:
- Avoid the use of tenaculum
- Use a soft coaxial embryo transfer catheter
- Avoid touching the uterine fundus
- Manipulate gently while performing the transfer procedure.

> *Note:* If during the procedure the tip of the catheter touches the uterine fundus, and contractions are initiated the patient will present with suprapubic pain/heaviness.

Cervical Mucus Removal

Mucus plug may:
1. Form dense network along the catheter tip akin to a spider's web preventing embryos to get expelled.

2. Entangle the embryos and may pull them out like Chinese yo-yo leading to high rate of expelled embryos.
3. It was also found that cervical mucus culture tested positive in 71% of patients and 49% of patients had positive culture of the catheter tip. They showed reduced pregnancy rates.[14,15]

Cleaning the cervical os of the mucus before ET is advisable to avoid these common complications.

Use of Ultrasound-guidance During Embryo Transfer

Transabdominal ultrasound-guided embryo transfer offers the clinician an opportunity to visualize the echogenic tip of the catheter and decide the exact site of embryo deposition. It also ensures that the Embryo Column and air bubble interface is not displaced after ET. Ultrasound may be useful in difficult cases to visualize the uterocervical angle negotiate the catheter accordingly in order to minimize trauma to the cervical canal and/or the endometrium.[16] Benefit of this technique as compared with clinical touch transfer has been shown in a meta-analysis of Buckett.[17] In contrast, a recent randomized study could not confirm this finding.[18]

Type of Embryo Transfer Medium Used During Embryo Transfer

Embryos should be transferred in any media with high protein content in physiological concentration, which has similar milieu to the uterus on the day of implantation. Wide variety of macromolecules like fibrin sealants and hyaluronan (Embryo Glue) are suggested now days to improve the implantation rate. RCT found that treating the embryo with fibrin glue (Embryo Glue) prior to ET resulted in a significant improvement in clinical, implantation, and ongoing pregnancy rates.[19] We do day 2 embryo transfer in G2 (Vitrolife)/ISM 1 (Medicult)/cleavage media (cook) pre-equilibrated media.

Air Bubble Technique During Embryo Transfer

Embryos are transferred in culture media bracketed between 2 small air columns. It was suggested that the air bubbles mark the position of the embryos inside the catheter. Air is seen as hyperechoic shadows during ultrasound guided embryo transfer as compared hypoechoic embryo column. This makes the visualization of the embryo column easy as it is seen sandwiched between two hyperechoic areas during embryo transfer. Thus, embryo column is protected against inappropriate placement, and prevents entanglement of the embryos to the mucus plug during embryo transfer.

Time Interval Between Embryo Loading and Transfer

Embryos are adversely affected by the fall in temperature, humidity, pH changes and air currents, which the embryo culture plates and loaded catheters encounter outside the incubator. It was found that the longer is this time interval, the lower is the pregnancy and implantation rate and that an interval of more than 2 minutes carries an adverse prognosis. It is proposed to carry out the procedure as quickly as is possible and to load the catheter only when patient is positioned, cleaned and draped with ultrasound focused on uterine cavity.[20]

Place of Embryo Deposition in the Uterine Cavity

The ideal site for embryo deposition has been an issue of debate, but the majority of the studies appear to concur that depositing the embryos in the mid cavity is correlated with better implantation rate. A study using 3D ultrasound revealed that embryos deposited at the maximum implantation potential point (MIP) were associated with good implantation and pregnancy rates.[21] MIP is a point of intersection of the two imaginary lines formed by extending the fallopian tube course inside the uterine cavity.

Retained Embryos and Repeat Embryo Transfer

A study revealed that 3.9% of all transfers were complicated by retained embryos.[22] Embryos are considerably more likely to be retained when the transfer catheter has been difficult and the catheter tip was detected to be contaminated with mucus or blood. Retained embryos may be transferred again immediately or after some time, without any adverse effect on the pregnancy outcome.[23]

RELEVANT ISSUES TO BE ADDRESSED POST EMBRYO TRANSFER

Bed Rest after Embryo Transfer

Recent studies have shown that this is not necessary and immediate ambulation following the ET has no adverse effect on the pregnancy rate as compared to bed rest for one to two hours.[24]

Sexual Intercourse Post-transfer

Large number of studies have revealed that the pregnancy outcome does not differ between the couples who avoided and those who did not avoid intercourse during the peritransfer period.[25]

Medication After Embryo Transfer

Routine use of low dose aspirin, sildenafil and antibiotics have not been recommended by any RCT. Progesterone is beneficial but starting its administration on the day of pickup did not have additional improved PR as compared to starting it on the day of ET.[26] Nonsteroidal anti-inflammatory drugs (NSAIDs) inhibit the production of prostaglandin. Administration of 10 mg of piroxicam one to two hours before the procedure demonstrated significant improvement of implantation and pregnancy rates.[27] Administration of 10 mg diazepam to ally anxiety, 30 minutes to 1 hour before the procedure, did not reveal any statistical difference in the outcome.

EMBRYO TRANSFER STEP BY STEP (FIGS 6.1 TO 6.10)

A. *Counseling:* The patient is informed of the fertilization rate, the number of available embryos, and the number of embryos selected for the transfer. We transfer two embryos (4–6 cell stage) or single blastocyst during the procedure. Spare embryos are graded and patients are informed about the embryo's being frozen. All the communications are done as per Indian Council of Medical Research (ICMR) guidelines and patients are appropriately counseled.

B. *Embryology pertaining to the embryo transfer:* Always work on the heated platform, with aseptic measures. All disposables should be labeled and efforts should be made to work quickly as embryos are now outside the CO_2 environment.

1. *Preparation of transfer plates:* Transfer plates (4 well, Falcon/Nunc) are prepared 2 hours before the embryo transfer. A point to be remembered is that Medicult media work best at pH of 5-5.5 and Vitrolife/Cook media at pH of 6.

Embryo Transfer and Troubleshooting

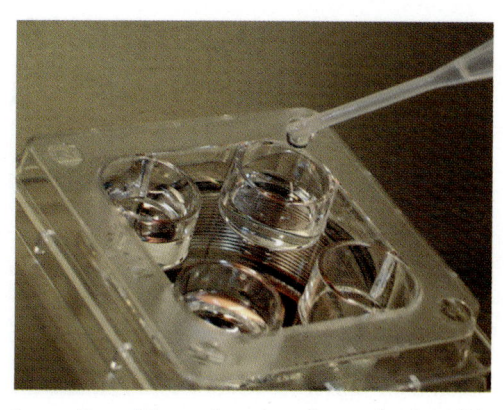

Fig. 6.1: Preparation of the embryo transfer media plate. We use four well NUNC IVF plate for the procedure. Embryo transfer is done at 4–6 cell or at blastocyst stage. Dispense 500 microliter of G1 PlUS/universal/ fertilization media in well 1. Dispense same volume of cleavage media/ blastocyst/embryo glue media in well 2 and well 3 of the 4 well plate. The media is equilibrated for minimum 18–20 hours before dispensing and the plate prepared minimum 30 minutes before the embryo transfer

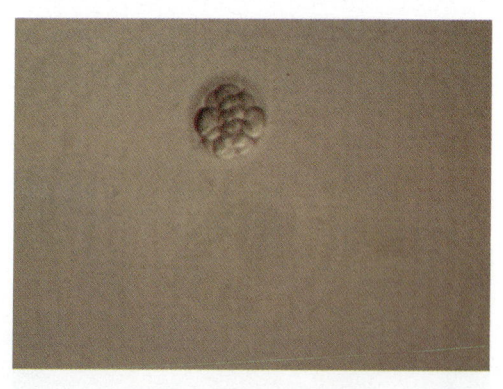

Fig. 6.2: Day three, grade 1, 8-cell embryo. We prefer to carry out single embryo transfer in young patients and freeze the supernumerary embryos; this embryo is presently in cleavage media and is planned for embryo transfer

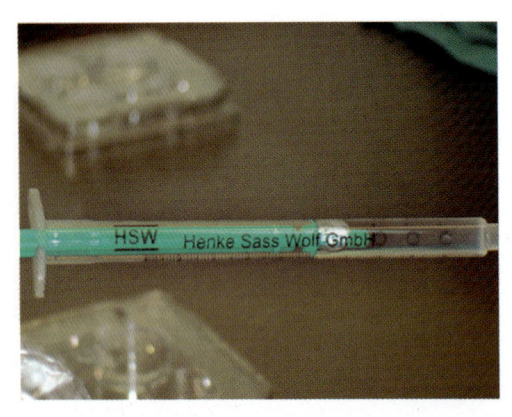

Fig. 6.3: One ml syringe, without rubber plunger is used for embryo transfer. The nozzle of the syringe is attached to the embryo transfer catheter. We fill the syringe with 500 microliters of embryo transfer media—either blastocyst or embryo glue for flushing the catheter. Ensure that the syringe does not contain any air bubbles. Syringes are loaded with transfer media 30 minutes before the embryo transfer and kept in incubator for equilibration

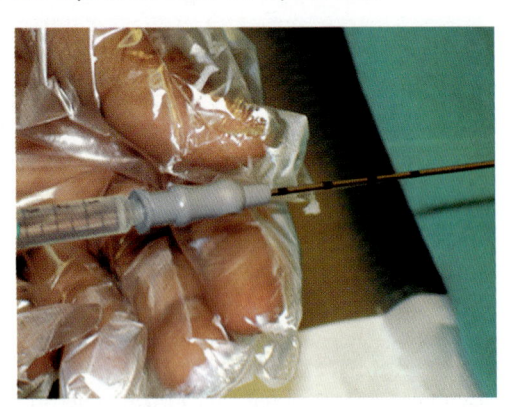

Fig. 6.4: Now we attach the 1 ml syringe with the inner soft embryo transfer catheter. Ensure that the fitting is tight otherwise the assembly may detach at the critical period of flushing the embryo transfer catheter

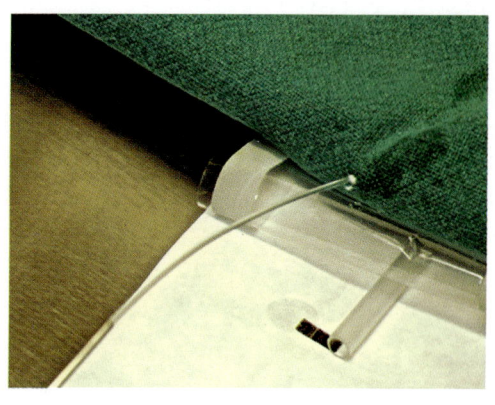

Fig. 6.5: Inner soft embryo transfer catheter being flushed with the media. This will equilibrate the inner lining of the ET catheter with the media column loaded with the embryos. This avoids sudden shock to the embryo. The syringe should be flushed with same media in which we transfer the embryos

> *Precaution:* Care should be taken to not mix media from different companies as they all have different constituents and pH requirement.

    i. Well 1: Dispense Well 1 of the transfer plate with 0.5 ml pre-equilibrated G1 media (Vitrolife)/Universal media (Medicult)/Cleavage media (cook).
    ii. Well 2 and 3 of the 4: In these, we dispense 400–500 microliter of pre-equilibrated G2 (Vitrolife)/ISM 1 (Medicult)/cleavage media (cook).
2. *Preparation of flushing syringes:* It is recommended that 1 ml syringe without a rubber plunger be used. These are filled with 500 microliters of pre-equilibrated G2 media (Vitrolife)/ISM media (Medicult)/Cleavage media (cook). These syringes are prepared

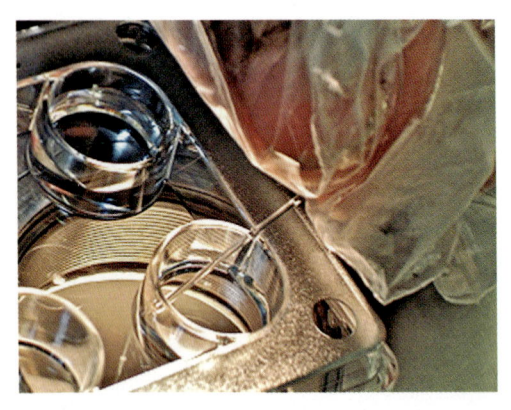

Fig. 6.6: Embryos are selected from the cleavage plate and the ones planned for the transfer are moved from cleavage plate to the well 1 of 4 well plate for rinsing and removing the traces of oil. These are quickly moved to well 2 and then to well 3. The selected embryo/embryos are placed in the middle of the well 3 and brought into focus using a stereo zoom microscope at low magnification. These are now quickly loaded in the inner soft catheter in minimal volumes of the media

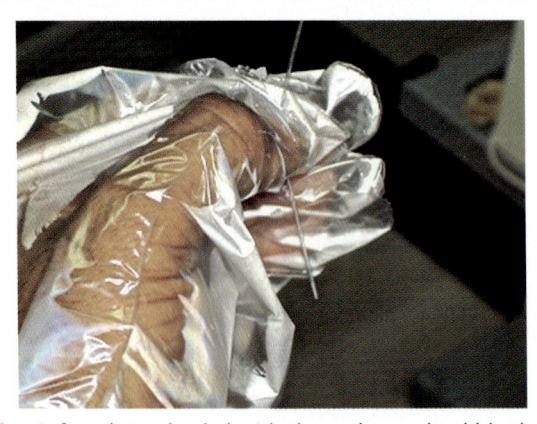

Fig. 6.7: Soft catheter loaded with the embryos should be handled carefully. Gloves should be worn and the catheter tip should be kept horizontal. The catheter tip should be kept cupped to avoid exposure to the cold air currents

Embryo Transfer and Troubleshooting

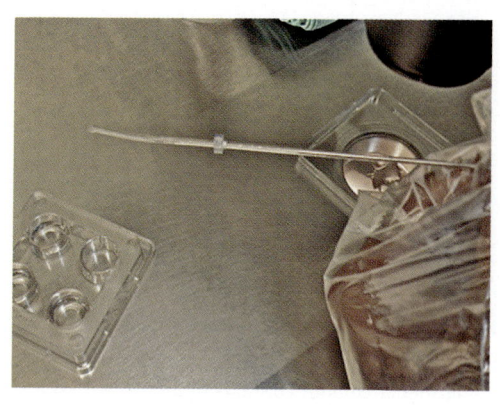

Fig. 6.8: After the embryos have been transferred, the catheter is handed back to the embryologist. The catheter should be kept horizontal and catheter tip cupped with hand. Now the syringe is gently removed and media allowed to flow on a clean warm plate

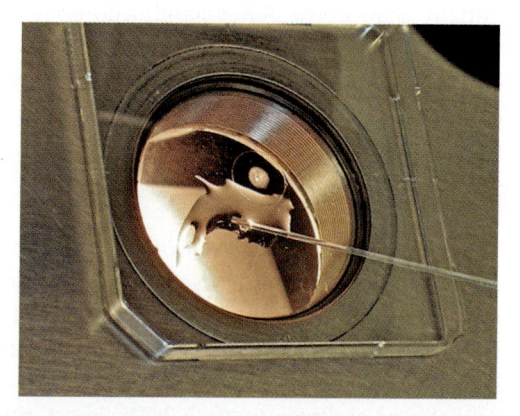

Fig. 6.9: Returning media is observed for the retained embryos. The catheter tip is rolled on the plate to release any entrapped embryos on the catheter tip. Check the mucus plug for entrapped embryo's. If retained embryos are seen, these are transferred back to the cleavage media, equilibrated for 15 minutes and transferred again

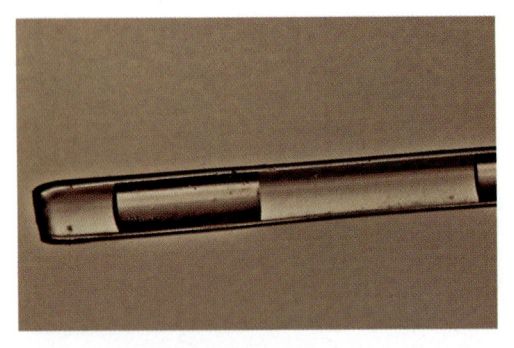

Fig. 6.10: A close up view of the tip of the soft embryo transfer catheter. The media column contains embryos

      minimum 2 hours prior to the embryo transfer and kept in the incubator at the required pH.
3. *Visualization of embryos and grading:* Embryos are initially seen at 20–30X magnifications in a single well culture plate. After these have been visualized and focused, the magnification should be increased to 40–50X to carry out embryo grading.

> Tip: Working at low light gives better results although it is a strain on the eyes.

4. *Transfer of embryos to well 1 of the 4 well dish:* 170 microns Cook flexipet is used to transfer embryos from the single well culture plate to the well 1 of 4 well plate, which contains G1 (Vitrolife)/universal/cleavage media (Cook).
5. *Transfer of embryos to well 2:* We must rinse the embryos gently in well 1 to remove all traces of oil and old culture media. Here, we must work at low magnification and light as grading as been carried out already before shifting the embryos. Well 2 contains

more physiological media and will now act as our reservoir for embryo transfer and spare embryos.

> Note: Minimum 3-4 rinses are carried out before transferring the embryos to the well 2 with minimal media.

    6. *Selection of embryos for transfer to well 3:* The top 2 embryos are selected and further transferred to well 3. Embryos are loaded in the Embryo transfer catheter from well 3 in G2 (Vitrolife)/ISM 1 (Medicult)/ cleavage media (cook) as they are physiological more akin to the uterine milieu.

    7. *Cryofreezing:* The balance of the embryos in well 2 are used for cryofreezing.

C. *Pre-procedure requirement:* There are certain requirements which should be adhered to before taking her for ET.

    1. *Preprocedure medication:* We administer 10 mg diazepam injection intramuscular with 0.6 mg atropine intramuscular 1 hour before the procedure. If she is very stressed, it is better to perform ET under general anesthesia.

    2. *Fluid intake:* She is advised to drink fluids and inform the nurse when her bladder is full.

    3. *Ultrasound for bladder status:* Check the status of the bladder before taking the patient to the transfer room. We prefer bladder to be filled till the fundus of the uterus, so as to get satisfactory acoustic window during embryo deposition.

        i. *Record:* The previously taken ultrasound picture of the uterus and the dummy ET is revised to get an idea about the length and direction of the uterus and the degree of cervicouterine angulation.

        ii. *Position:* Put the patient in the lithotomy position and drape with sterile towels as in other operative cases. Cusco's speculum is gently inserted and cervical os visualized. Rarely we may have to hold the cervix with the volsellum.

iii. *Cleaning cervical mucus:* The cervix and the vaginal vaults are cleaned of cervical mucus and vaginal secretions using tissue culture media and sterile gauze. Sterile gauze is left at the os for two minutes. It will stick to the mucus plug and pull it out very effectively. We have used warm normal saline to clean the cervix in over 5000 embryo transfers with no compromise in the internationally accepted pregnancy rate.

iv. *Ultrasound to visualize cervical canal and uterine cavity:* Inspection of the cervical canal by ultrasound with special emphasis on the cervical uterine angulations and abnormal curvatures is of prime importance.

v. *Insertion of outer sheath:* Insert the outer sheath of the cook catheter in the cervical canal and stop just above the internal os. If we go further we can damage the endometrium, as the outer sheath is firm and can avulse the endometrial lining.

In case of difficulty in traversing the canal:
- If the outer sheath is introduced beyond internal os in the endometrial cavity it may disrupt the endometrium as it is firm in nature. The stimulus of the outer sheath of ET catheter passing through the internal cervical canal and cavity may also initiate uterine contractions.
- Gentle uterine sounding may be carried out and catheter outer sheath may be inserted till internal os.
- If because of adhesions one cannot negotiate the os, cryofreezing of all the embryos is recommended followed by transfer after dilatation and office hysteroscopy.

vi. *Loading the embryos in the inner catheter:* Meanwhile the embryologist will firmly fix the preloaded syringe with the inner soft cook catheter and flush it with its contents—G2 (Vitrolife)/ISM 1 (Medicult)/cleavage media (cook) pre-equilibrated media. Now the 4 well plate is taken out of the incubator and all the embryos' in well 3 are collected together using 170 flexipet. The catheter tip is brought near the embryos' are these are loaded with a continuous column (20 μl) of culture media followed by very small column of air followed by 10 microliters of culture media.

Tip: It is important to place the embryos close as this will help in loading them in minimal volume of culture media which is very important for good outcome after the embryo transfer.

vii. *Deposition of embryo transfer into uterine cavity:* The inner catheter containing the embryos at the tip are carried to the transfer room and the inner sheath is inserted in the outer cannula, which is already in the cervical canal. Inner catheter is always carried cupped in the left palm for (right handed) clinicians so that the unnecessary exposure to the air currents and light is avoided. The inner catheter is gently pushed inside and as it transverses the outer sheath and comes to lie around 1 cm from the fundus the plunger is pressed to release the embryo's gently. Now gently withdraw the outer and inner sheath. The inner sheath tip is always kept in the outer sheath to avoid sudden temperature changes.

> *Tip:* Once the plunger is pushed it is kept pressed so that there is no negative suction and rotated 360 degrees to release any sticking embryos and mucus plug before withdrawing.

viii. *Inspection for retained embryos:* The catheter is immediately handed over to the embryologist who releases the contact between the syringe and the catheter and the contents of the catheter are emptied on the sterile dish cover. The catheter tip is gently rolled on the lid and inspected for retained embryos, blood, and mucus.

ix. *Protocol for retained embryos:* If we have retained embryos they are immediately rinsed in G1 (Vitrolife)/universal (Medicult)/cleavage media (Cook) and transferred to fresh well with G2 (Vitrolife)/ISM 1 (Medicult)/cleavage media (cook) pre-equilibrated media. The embryos are allowed to equilibrate for approximately 1 hour before these are transferred again.

Growing tendency towards transferring less embryos, preferably a single embryo has motivated the ART teams to alter their methodologies as ET has lately been acknowledged as a decisive step in an IVF cycle.

REFERENCES

1. Human Fertilisation and Embryology Authority, Fifth Annual Report. London: Human Fertilisation and Embryology Authority, 1996.
2. Sallam HN. Embryo transfer: factors involved in optimizing the success. Curr Opin Obstet Gynecol. 2005;17:289-98.
3. Blake DA, Farquhar CM, Johnson N, Proctor M. Cleavage stage versus blastocyst stage embryo transfer in assisted conception. Cochrane Database Syst Rev. 2007;4:CD002118.

4. Abou-Setta AM, Al-Inany HG, Mansour RT, Serour GI, Aboulghar MA. Soft vs. firm embryo transfer catheters for assisted reproduction: a systematic review and meta-analysis. Hum Reprod. 2005;11:3114.
5. Paulus WE, Zhang M, Strehler E, El-Danasouri I, Sterzik K. Influence of acupuncture on the pregnancy rate in patients who undergo assisted reproduction therapy. Fertil Steril. 2002;77:721-4.
6. Levitas E, Parmet A, Lunenfeld E, Bentov Y, Burstein E, Friger M, Potashnik G. Impact of hypnosis during embryo transfer on the outcome of *in vitro* fertilization-embryo transfer: a case-control study. Fertil Steril. 2006;85:1404-8.
7. Shamonki MI, Spandorfer SD, Rosenwaks Z. Ultrasound-guided embryo transfer and the accuracy of trial embryo transfer. Hum Reprod. 2005;3:709.
8. Zollner U, Zollner KP, Specketer MT, et al. Endometrial volume as assessed by three-dimensional ultrasound is a predictor of pregnancy outcome after *in vitro* fertilization and embryo transfer. Fertil Steril 2003;80:1515–7.
9. Poindexter AN 3rd, Thompson DJ, Gibbons WE, et al. Residual embryos in failed embryo transfer. Fertil Steril. 1986;46:262–7.
10. Angelini A, Brusco GF, Barnocchi N, El-Danasouri I, Pacchiarotti A, Selman HA. Impact of physician performing embryo transfer on pregnancy rates in an assisted reproductive program. J Assist Reprod Genet. 2006;23:329-32.
11. Mansour R, Aboulghar M, Serour G. Dummy embryo transfer: a technique that minimizes the problems of embryo transfer and improves the pregnancy rate in human *in vitro* fertilization. Fertil Steril. 1990;54:678-81.
12. Kovacs GT. What factors are important for successful embryo transfer after *in vitro* fertilization? Hum Reprod. 1999;14:590.
13. Fanchin R, Righini C, Olivennes F, et al. Uterine contractions at the time of embryo transfer alter pregnancy rates after *in-vitro* fertilization. Hum Reprod. 1998;13:1968-74.
14. Egbase PE, Al-Sharhan M, Al-Othman S, Al-Mutawa M, Udo EE, Grudzinskas JG. Incidence of microbial growth from the tip of the embryo transfer catheter after embryo transfer

in relation to clinical pregnancy rate following *in vitro* fertilization and embryo transfer. Hum Reprod. 1996;11:1687.
15. Fanchin R, Harmas A, Benaoudia F, Lundkvist U, Olivennes F, Frydman R. Microbial flora of the cervix assessed at the time of embryo transfer adversely affects *in vitro* fertilization outcome. Fertil Steril 1998;70:866.
16. Sallam HN, Agameya AF, Rahman AF, et al. Ultrasound measurement of the uterocervical angle before embryo transfer: a prospective controlled study. Hum Reprod. 2002;17:1767-72.
17. Buckett WM. A meta-analysis of ultrasound-guided versus clinical touch embryo transfer. Fertil Steril. 2003;80:1037-41.
18. Drakeley AJ, Jorgensen A, Sklavounos J, et al. A ran-domized controlled clinical trial of 2295 ultrasound-guided embryo transfers. Hum Reprod 2008;23:1101-6.
19. Valojerdi MR, Karimian L, Yazdi PE, Gilani MA, Madani T, Baghestani AR. Efficacy of a human embryo transfer medium: a prospective, randomized clinical trial study. J Assist Reprod Genet. 2006; 23:207-12.
20. Matorras R, Mendoza R, Exposito A, Rodriguez-Escudero FJ. Influence of the time interval between embryo catheter loading and discharging on the success of IVF. Hum Reprod. 2004;19:2027-30.
21. Gergely RZ, DeUgarte CM, Danzer H, Surrey M, Hill D, DeCherney AH. Three dimensional/four dimensional ultrasound-guided embryo transfer using the maximal implantation potential point. Fertil Steril. 2005;84:500-3.
22. Leeton HC, Seifer DB, Shelden RM. Impact of retained embryos on the outcome of assisted reproductive technologies. Fertil Steril. 2004;2:334.
23. Lee HC, Seifer DB, Shelden RM. Impact of retained embryos on the outcome of assisted reproductive technologies. Fertil Steril. 2004;82:334-7.
24. Bar-Hava I, Kerner R, Yoeli R, Ashknazi J, Shalev Y, Orvieto R. Immediate ambulation after embryo transfer: a prospective study. Fertil Steril. 2005;83:594.
25. Tremellen KP, Valbuena D, Landeras J, et al. The effect of intercourse on pregnancy rates during assisted human reproduction. Hum Reprod. 2000;15:2653-8.

26. Baruffi R, Mauri AL, Petersen CG, Felipe V, Franco JG Jr. Effects of vaginal progesterone administration staring on the day of oocytes retrieval on pregnancy rates. J Assist Reprod Genent. 2003;20:517.
27. Moon HS, Park SH, Lee JO, Kim KS, Joo BS. Treatment with piroxicam before embryo transfer increases the pregnancy rate after *in vitro* fertilization and embryo transfer. Fertil Steril. 2004;8:816.

Chapter 7

Ovum Pickup and Troubleshooting

Pankaj Talwar

INTRODUCTION

The elementary part of any IVF-ET procedure is the harvesting of mature oocyte cumulus complexes in the minimal traumatic way and the ensuing development and transfer of an embryo. Laparotomy, laparoscopy and transabdominal scans were used initially, but discarded swiftly because of the morbidity associated with it.[1] Now, transvaginal ultrasound guided aspiration of oocyte cumulus complexes is well accepted and presently it has become the most extensively used practice in ART units all over the world.

RELEVANT ISSUES

Pertaining to oocyte retrieval pertain to timing, anesthesia, type of transducer and pickup needle.

Timing

Ovum pickup (OPU) is performed approximately 36 hours after 10,000 IU of hCG injection, i.e. just before the time of ovulation. Study carried out with OPU done at 34 and 38 hours revealed no significant difference in the frequency of spontaneous ovulation, number of oocytes retrieved, oocyte cumulus complex quality, embryo quality, implantation and pregnancy rates.[2]

Preparation of Vagina

Initially Betadine was used but it was found that the pregnancy rate was significantly higher in the normal saline group (17.2% versus 30.3% clinical pregnancies per embryo transfer).[3] There was no increase in infection risk in the saline group. Today, most IVF units use only normal saline at 37°C for vaginal preparation before oocyte retrieval.

Anesthesia/Analgesia

Anesthesia is necessary for the comfort of the patient and for the gynecologist to maximize the harvesting of oocytes, and plays an important role in a successful outcome. General anesthesia, monitored sedation with or without local anesthesia, and regional technique have all been used and studied. The anesthetic agents must be short acting, with minimal side effects and little penetration into the follicle, so that oocyte is not harmed by their presence. The key is short exposure to the least toxic agent. The majority of anesthetic agents have been deemed safe for use.

> *Caution:* Neuroleptanesthesia is not recommended, and there remains some controversy over the use of nitrous oxide and the inhalatory agents.[4]

Equipment

Any high-resolution ultrasound equipment with a vaginal transducer can be used for safe and accurate puncture of follicles during ovum pickup procedure.

Ultrasound and Probe

a. *Frequency:* The probe should have frequency of 5–7 MHz giving the equipment a sufficient penetration depth and enough resolution for accurate visualization of the uterus and the adenxa.

b. *Biopsy guide:* The vaginal transducer should have a snuggly fitting biopsy guide, which should allow easy gliding movement of the ovum pickup needle through the needle channel.
c. *Length:* The probe should be long (total length of approximately 40–50 cm) with a gentle curve, which allows for easy handling for the clinician and also does not cause discomfort to the patient during the scan (Fig. 7.1).
d. *Shape:* The transducer probe should have a shape that is easy to place into a sterile probe cover, which are commercially available and should also permit firm

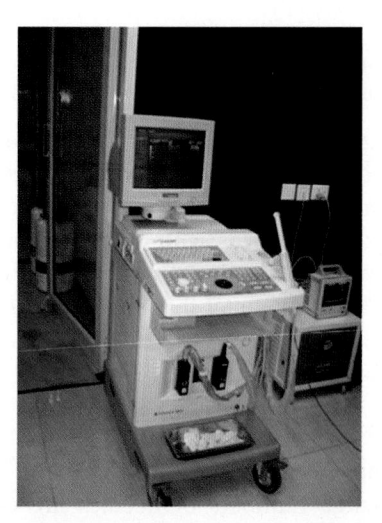

Fig. 7.1: Ultrasound machine with TVS probe. Probe and the exterior of the machine should be cleaned in the morning of the ovum pickup using 70% alcohol followed by normal saline

fixation of biopsy guide after the sterile cover has been placed over the vaginal probe.

Suction Apparatus

In the initial days, manual aspiration of follicular fluid was often performed by means of a syringe connected to the pickup needle. This technique created, uneven pressures which was harmful to oocyte.[5] Creating a negative pressure by means of a suction pump where the pressure can be controlled in a standardized manner is probably the safest and the best way. Today there are several such suction pumps available with foot-pumps specifically designed for oocyte complex aspiration (Figs 7.2 and 7.3). Sophisticated suction pumps with adjustable aspiration pressure are widely available commercially.

> *Caution:* High negative or uneven pressure in the aspirating system might cause damage to the oocyte cumulus complexes.

Suction pressure: It was shown earlier that a negative pressure of 90–120 mm Hg seems to be optimal for a good recovery and exerts no harm on the oocyte cumulus complex when aspirating mature follicles with intrafollicular volume of 3-4 ml. However, aspirating an immature oocytes from follicles of 5-8 mm diameter that have a very small volume of follicular fluid needs less negative pressure, in range of 40–60 mm Hg.[6,7]

Ovum Pickup Needle (Figs 7.4 to 7.7)

Ovum pickup needle play an important role in the procedure. Large numbers of needles are commercially available to us. A number of factors have to be considered while choosing a needle.

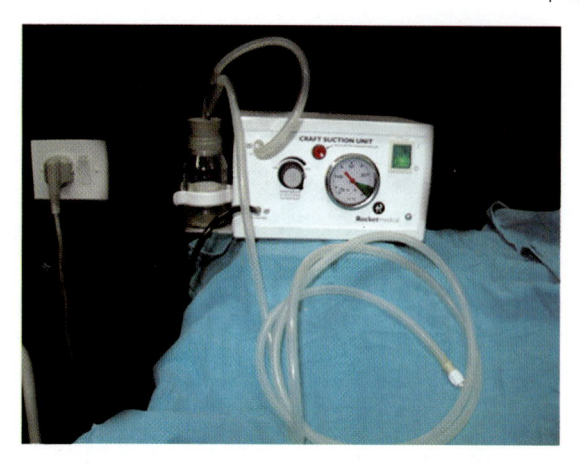

Fig. 7.2: Rocket suction pump. Vacuum source for oocyte aspiration. It provides smooth, low volume vacuum at pre-determined negative pressures thus allowing safe, simple, low turbulent flow oocyte recovery. Mas simple, safe operation with air-operated foot controls. High vacuum foot control is available on Duo-Vac suction pumps. Their super quiet diaphragm pumps make it easy to live with in the OR and means low maintenance service. The pump can build up fully variable vacuum from 0-400 mm Hg and single use water trap set provides cost-effective solution to regular processing of reusable water traps and tubing. We use negative suction between 90-100 mm Hg for aspiration of the mature oocyte cumulus complex

a. *Needle sharpness:* The sharpness of the needle is the most important factor. A sharp needle means less trauma to the ovarian cortex and follicles, thus reducing postoperative pain and bleeding from the ovarian surface (Fig. 7.6).
b. *Echogenic tip:* It is important that the surface of needle tip has etchings, making the tip echogenic sonologically. Echogenic tip is easy to identify while doing ovum pickup procedure allowing us to know the position of

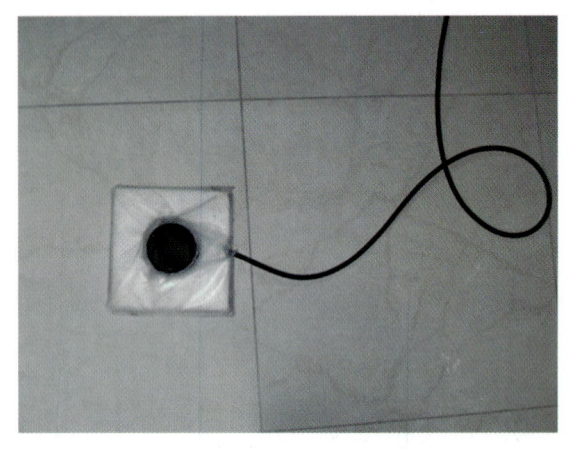

Fig. 7.3: Foot control of the rocket suction pump

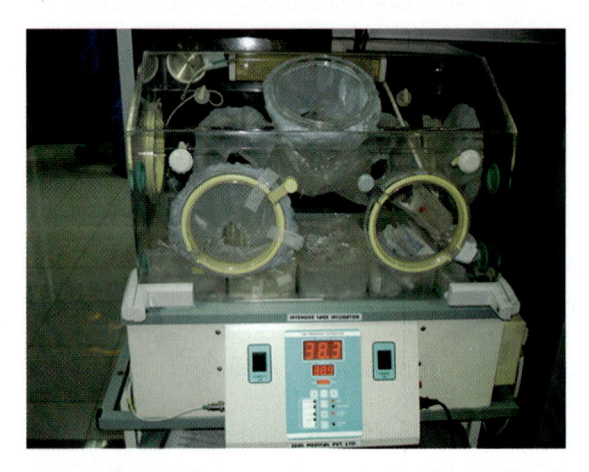

Fig. 7.4: A baby incubator to warm up the disposables for the embryology laboratory. This ensures that the tubes and plates are at 37°C before the ovum pickup procedure

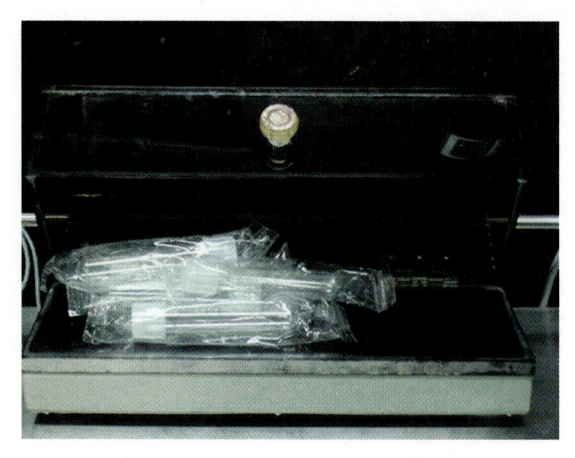

Fig. 7.5: Test tube warmer. For preheating of slides, petri dishes, pipettes, etc. at desired temperatures. The dimensions of anodized aluminum heating plate are 300 mm (L) x 100 mm (W) x 40 mm (H). Bigger size plate also can be supplied with separate digital temperature controller. The temperature range is from ambient to 110°C. The tubes are kept here just before the OPU procedure. Roughly we require 1 tube for 2-3 follicles. Only the calculated no of tubes should be opened

the needle with respect to the follicle, ovarian tissue and pelvic viscera (Fig. 7.7).

c. *Diameter:* The diameter of the needle is significant for two reasons. A thin needle 18-20 gauge means less pain when analgesia only is used. However, a needle with too small inner diameter may be harmful to the oocyte cumulus complex.[8] As long as the inner diameter of the needle is 0.8-1 mm, it seems as if the oocyte cumulus complex is unaffected, provided that the aspiration pressure is less than 120 mm Hg. In our opinion, a needle with an outer diameter of 18 gauge and an inner diameter of 20 gauge is ideal for OPU.

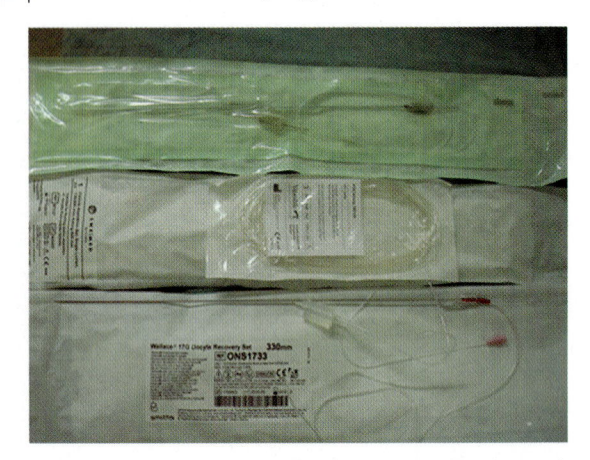

Fig. 7.6: The ovum pickup needles. These needles have sharp, noncoring bevel, have highly echogenic markings at the needle tip for easy identification on ultrasound, smooth internal lumens and external surfaces to prevent damage to the oocyte cumulus complex and for easy insertion through the vaginal wall and ovarian stroma. Tight fitting PTFE tubing ensures no changes in lumen diameter between the needle cannula and aspiration tubing which could cause turbulence in the fluid flow. Ergonomically designed handle allows rotation of the needle tip to "curette" the follicle wall to improve oocyte recovery rates. Extensive washing processes followed by proven sterilization methodology is fully validated by endotoxin (LAL) testing and mouse embryo testing, to ensure a sterile, nontoxic finished product

> *Caution:* Too thin a needle often causes problems by deviating away from the puncturing line, particularly if the ovary is situated high up in the pelvis and the ovaries have a thick stroma. They may also damage oocyte cumulus complex if negative pressure is too high.

d. *Needle handle:* An adequately shaped fingertip handle on the distal end of the needle is preferable because it allows follicle puncture with good clinical touch.

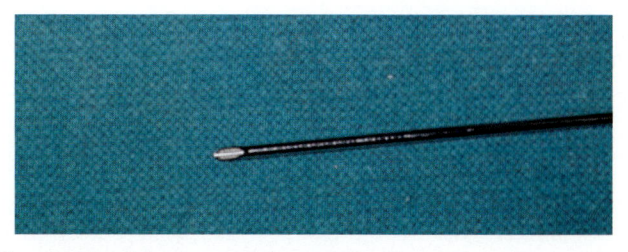

Fig. 7.7: Tip of the ovum pickup needle. The tip has got serrations to make it echogenic

e. *Connecting tubing:* To increase the recovery, it was shown earlier that Teflon tubing between the needle and the polysterene tube was important. Commercially available follicle aspiration needles do have such sampling tube which is sterile and mouse embryo tested. The set is ready to use and only needs to be connected to the suction pump. The set is made for single use and thereby guarantees sterility and nontoxicity to the oocyte. Over the last 15 years, our group has used such follicle aspiration sets and found them to be very convenient.

Temperature Control

Another important point is to transport oocytes to the laboratory in the best condition. The clinician should be aware of sudden pH and temperature changes that the oocytes undergo during and immediately after they have been harvested. It has been documented that the temperature of the follicular fluid dropped by 7.7 ± 1.3°C upon aspiration as the fluid is transported to the collection tubes via the needle and the tubing. Dissolved oxygen levels rose by 5 ± 2 vol% and the pH increased by 0.04 ± 0.01. They concluded that these changes could be detrimental to the oocyte's survival, and attempt should be made to minimize these detrimental changes.[9]

> *Recommendation:*
> 1. The collection tubes must be kept in a test tube warmer while they are waiting to be connected to the collection system.
> 2. The tubes should not be filled above the level of alloy blocks (Fig. 7.11).
> 3. These should be transported immediately to the embryologist.

Follicle Flushing

Initial randomized trials demonstrated that when performing transvaginal ultrasonically guided oocyte recovery, there were no significant differences in number of oocytes retrieved, fertilization rate, or pregnancy rate between those where flushing had been used as compared to no flushing.[10] Also, the time taken for the procedure and the amount of anesthesia required was significantly more. It was soon recognized that most oocyte can be recovered by just aspirating, and that the follicular fluid from the next follicle will often flush the oocyte into collection tube. This was called the ROC technique (Rapid oocyte recovery). In our IVF program, we do not flush follicles and have had a recovery rate of 80-90% per punctured follicle and routine flushing would seem redundant in modern day IVF practice. It is important to carry out flushing of the needle and the tubing before the procedure to remove dead space in the aspiration set. This avoids frothing in the collected follicular fluid. Reflushing of the needle and the tubing with the suitable media should follow egg collection. Standard needle and tubing has nearly 1 ml of dead space and till the follicular fluid being aspirated does not exceed this quantity dead space will remain. This is important when we do ovum pickup in IVM as the fluid contained in a follicle 6-8 mm is 0.1-0.2 ml and multiple follicles have to be emptied before we can obliterate this dead space and collect fluid in the collecting tube.

> *Recommendation:* Instead of flushing the follicles, the oocyte could the recovered by rotating the ultrasound probe and maintaining suction until the last drop of follicular fluid is aspirated, and the follicular wall hugs, the needle tip.

OPU STEP BY STEP

1. *Initial check:* Before commencing oocyte collection, the system is tested by aspirating some culture medium. This also provides a column of fluid to collect the follicular fluid, thus encouraging laminar flow (Figs 7.8 to 7.16).

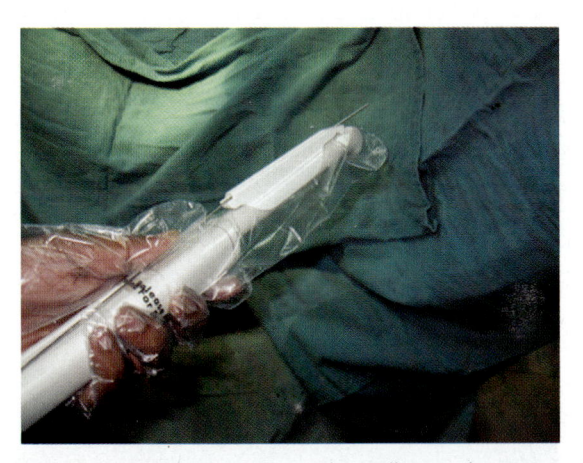

Fig. 7.8: Mounted biopsy guide and needle on the TVS probe. Biopsy guide should be attached firmly so that the needle always follows the desired path in the ovary. Probe is always covered with polyethylene and designed with a welded seam along its length to inhibit accidental breakage. Each cover is individually wrapped and packaged in a sterile barrier with two cable clips. The covers are e-beam sterilized

138 *Protocols in Clinical Embryology and ART*

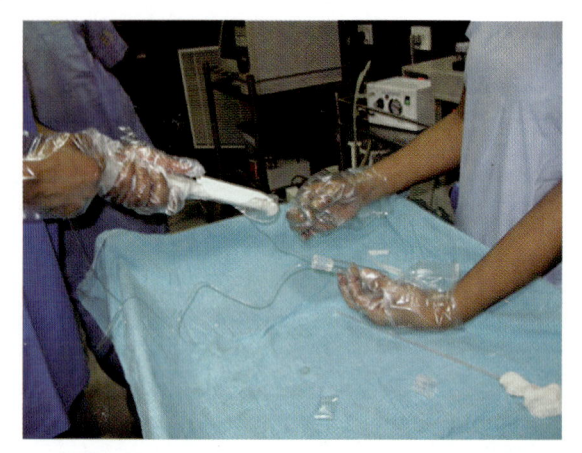

Fig. 7.9: HEPES/MOPS based media being aspirated in the needle to rinse the interior of the needle. This will protect the oocyte complex from the temperature and osmotic shock

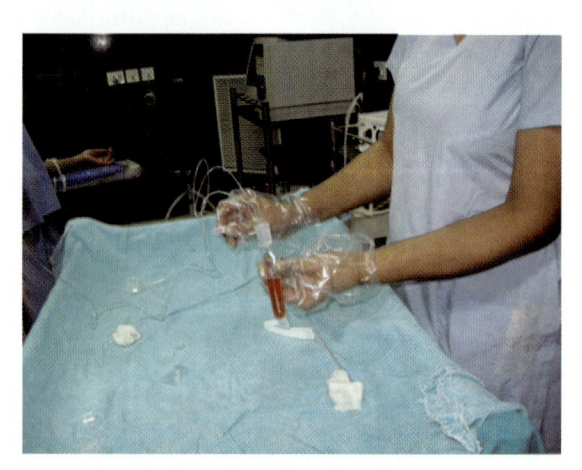

Fig. 7.10: Aspirate being collected in the tube

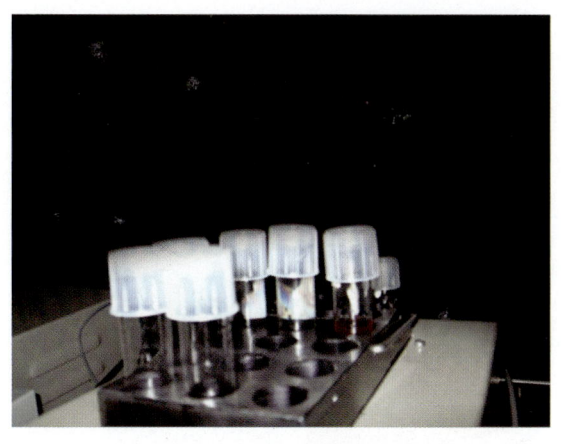

Fig. 7.11: Tubes with aspirate are placed in the tube warmer till the embryologist sees them. This should be done quickly to avoid the shock to the eggs. A replacement of messy water bath for heating all sizes of test tubes in removable, autoclavable anodized aluminum blocks, ideal for transporting samples from one place to another with minimum of temperature loss. Digital display and control of temperature with +/–0.2°C accuracy from ambient to 110°C comes with anodized aluminum blocks of 75 × 50 × 50 mm to accommodate specified test tubes

2. *Identifying follicles:* The ovaries are visualized on transvaginal sonography and ovarian follicles should be differentiated from other pelvic anatomical structures that may give the impression of being similar. Both, the preovulatory ovarian follicles and iliac vessels look hypoechoeic (dark), and thus iliac vessels on cross-section may be confused with a follicle. The aim should be to view the vessels in the longitudinal view with ovaries lying in the plane adjacent to them. The bowel lumen is echogenic and will show peristaltic movements if observed for few seconds. Encysted

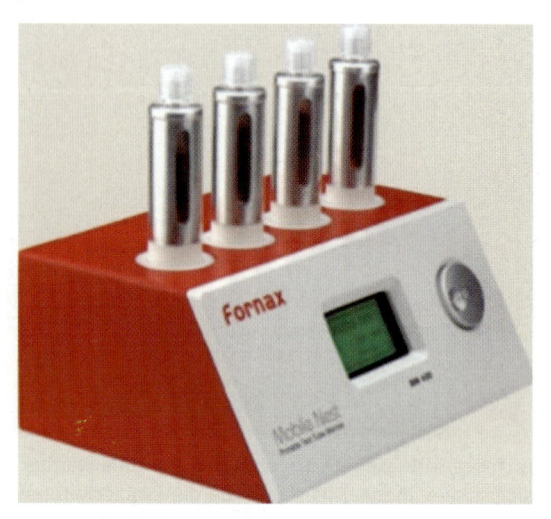

Fig. 7.12: Fornax test tube warmer. Base station for four portable warmers. The warmer is a handheld device with Li-ion rechargable battery. It is equipped with heating element, digital sensor, microcontroller, nonvolatile memory and LED indicators. When placed on base station, it gets connected electrically by its contacts. These contacts help base station and the mobile device communicates with each other and also charge the battery. The mobile nest when in mobile mode continuously monitors the temperature with a 14 bit accuracy, corrects it several times a second. This yields a rock steady temperature profile even in varying surroundings. The mobile nest continues to log for the power consumption index and temperature abnormalities. These are downloaded to the base station when the nest is docked. With monitoring and reporting features, the user can be assured about the mobile nest working accurately at every step. A transparent window facilitates easy viewing of the follicular fluid

peritoneal collections, hydrosalphinx and persistent ovarian cysts would have been documented on previous scans and do not cause any confusion.

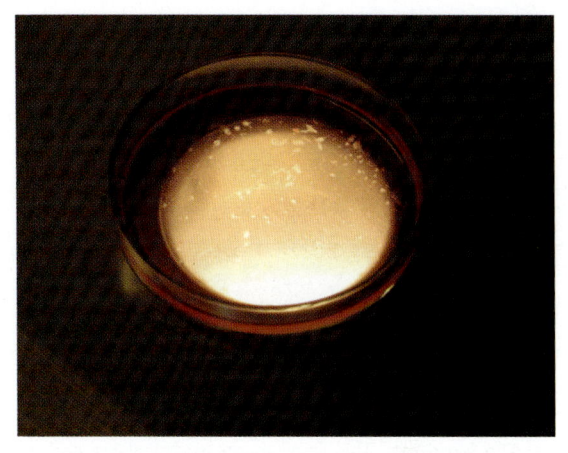

Fig. 7.13: Aspirated follicular fluid. OCC's are being identified

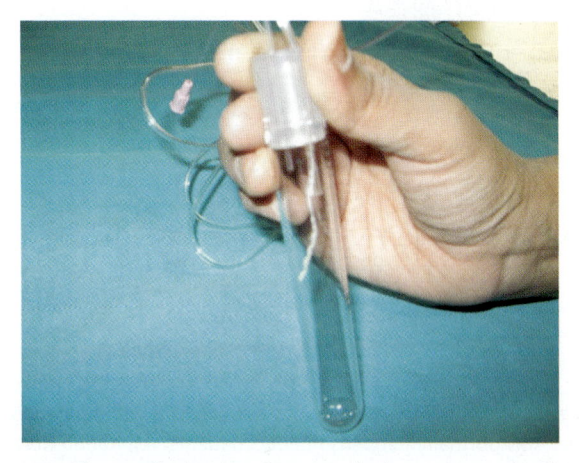

Fig. 7.14: The cracked tube. Pressure leakage occurs leading to nonaspiration of the fluid

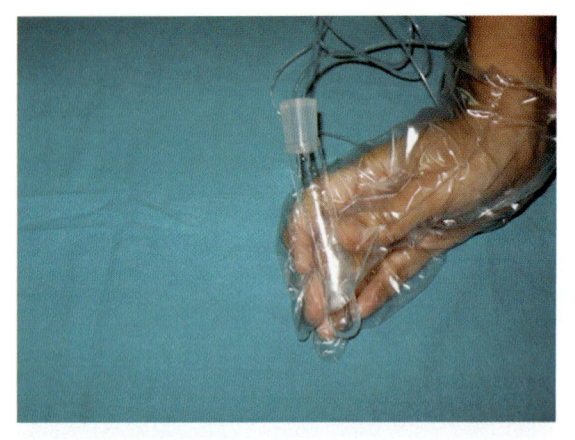

Fig. 7.15: The loose cap. This leads to pressure leakage and follicular fluid is not aspirated. Whenever we realize that the pressure is not building up we must check the cap connection and tighten it if required

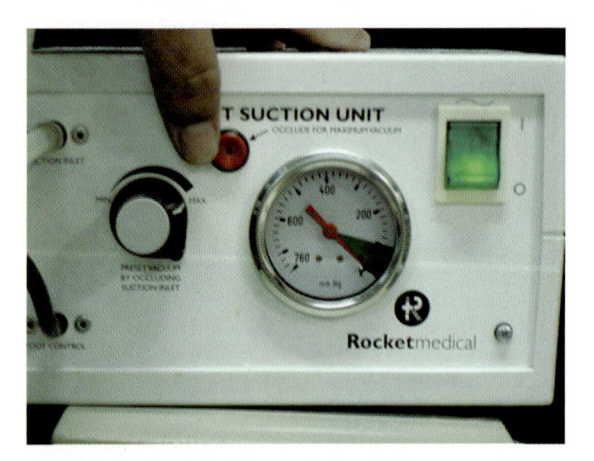

Fig. 7.16: Sometime the needle may get chocked with blood clots or tissue. This normally happens in PCOS patients. Aspiration may stop at this moment. The red button is pressed on the pump to increase the negative pressure thus dislodging the clot

> *Caution:*
> - Puncture of iliac vessels is avoided by differentiating them from a follicle by their minimal echogenic contents and by changing the plane of the transducer by 90°.
> - Puncture of dermoid cyst and endometrioma should be avoided as they may spill the contents leading to localized chemical reaction and also serve as a nidus for pelvic infection.

3. *Preparation of needle and tubing:* Needle is inserted in the biopsy guide fixed over the vaginal transducer, which has been covered with the sterile vaginal probe cover. We flush the needle with MOPS/HEPES based media to eradicate the dead space.
4. *Aspiration of follicle:* Transducer is inserted in the vagina and ovary is brought in the focus. We ensure that very minimal tissue lies between the follicles and the transducer. In situation where the ovaries are adherent and follicles cannot be approached, perforation of endometrial cavity should be avoided. It is our practice to always commence with the right ovary, and then to aspirate follicles sequentially. It is best to keep the needle within the ovary if possible minimizing the amount of trauma to the ovarian capsule. When all follicles within the right ovary are aspirated, the needle is withdrawn, probe rotated and moved in the vagina and we aspirate the ovary in similar manner. Follicle is focused in direction of biopsy guide probe line. Needle is briskly inserted in the nearest follicle. The pressure within the follicle, before penetration, varies, depending on the size, shape, and position of the follicle. The internal pressure of the increases, correlating with size. However, due to the pressure caused by the needle deforming the surface of the follicle at the time of puncture, the pressure within the follicle may be much higher. The more blunt the needle,

the higher will be the resultant pressure. Suction pressure should be on during thus movement. Allow the suction to occur uniformly. Keep the needle tip under vision in the middle of the follicle. Always keep the pressure on and allow the follicle to collapse around the needle tip till the time follicle is completely emptied.

> *Note:*
> Negative suction during the time of entry ensures that even if fluid spills out during the time of entry, which is common with the blunt tip needle, fluid is aspirated and the oocyte cumulus complex is not lost in the peritoneal cavity.
>
> If the pressure was deactivated while the needle was still in the follicle (and there were no leaks), the pressure within the needle and collecting tube drops, and there is, often backflow towards the follicle. This can result in the oocyte being sucked back and possibly lost. The amount of backflow depends on how much air enters the system and how much higher the collection tube is above the patient's pelvis.

5. *Suction pressure:* It is recommended that pressures be kept less than 120 mm Hg. The higher the speed of travel, the more are the chance of damage to the oocyte. Apart from the speed of travel, turbulent nonlaminar flow can also damage the oocyte, either by stripping its cumulus mass or fracturing the zona. It is believed that an intact cumulus may be important in preventing damage to oocytes.

COMMON PROBLEMS ENCOUNTERED DURING OVUM PICKUP

Failure to Aspirate the Follicular Fluid

Before the ovum pickup is commenced we must flush the needle and the tubing with suitable (HEPES/MOPS) based media. This ensures that there is no air in the aspiration system and we have laminar flow of the follicular fluid throughout the procedure.

If rarely fluid aspiration suddenly stops, without wasting any time the steps in Flow chart 7.1 should be carried out.

Flow chart 7.1: Management of failure to aspirate the follicular fluid

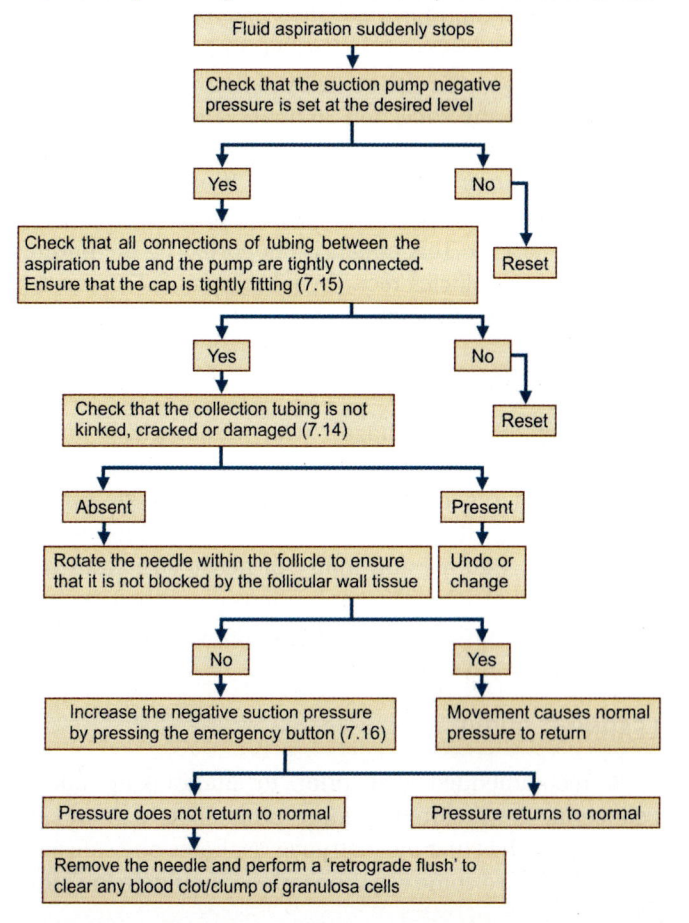

```
Fluid aspiration suddenly stops
        ↓
Check that the suction pump negative
pressure is set at the desired level
    ↓               ↓
   Yes              No → Reset
    ↓
Check that all connections of tubing between the
aspiration tube and the pump are tightly connected.
Ensure that the cap is tightly fitting (7.15)
    ↓               ↓
   Yes              No → Reset
    ↓
Check that the collection tubing is not
kinked, cracked or damaged (7.14)
    ↓               ↓
  Absent          Present
    ↓               ↓
Rotate the needle within the follicle to ensure     Undo or
that it is not blocked by the follicular wall tissue  change
    ↓               ↓
   No              Yes
    ↓               ↓
Increase the negative suction pressure    Movement causes normal
by pressing the emergency button (7.16)    pressure to return
    ↓               ↓
Pressure does not return to normal    Pressure returns to normal
    ↓
Remove the needle and perform a 'retrograde flush' to
clear any blood clot/clump of granulosa cells
```

No Oocytes Retrieved

Sometimes, post aspiration no oocytes are harvested. In such cases, the fluid collected is clear and devoid of cells (granulosa and cumulus). This can be due to two reasons:

i. *Empty follicle syndrome:* Such clinical condition occurs if the patient has not taken her ovulation trigger and normally should have negative pregnancy card test. If the test is negative, it is feasible to forsake the ovum pickup from the other ovary, administer hCG, and reschedule the collection 36 hours later.

ii. *Follicles that have an adequate exposure to hCG and do not contain retrievable oocytes:* It may be due to an intrinsic defect in folliculogenesis that leads to early oocyte atresia. This notion is supported by the finding that empty follicles recur in subsequent IVF cycles for some affected women.

COMPLICATIONS

Despite all the advantages with transvaginal oocyte retrieval during IVF treatment, the aspiration needle may injure pelvic organs and structures leading to serious complications. The most common complications are hemorrhage, trauma, and injury of pelvic structures and pelvic infection. Other complications described include adnexal torsion, rupture of endometriotic cysts, and even vertebral osteomyelitis[11] (Table 7.1).

LEARNING CURVE

It is recommended that prior to undertaking oocyte collection, a structured training program is carried out. One approach is that the instructor aspirates one side and, having collected some eggs, the trainee should do the other

Table 7.1

Diagnosis and management of complications occurring during OPU

	Diagnosis	Management
Vaginal hemorrhage	Bleeding from the vaginal vault is the most common consequence and has been reported to occur between 1.4 and 18.4%.[12]	However, such a bleeding generally ceases spontaneously at the end of the procedure. Sometimes, the bleeding site needs to be identified and application of a pressure with a sponge is necessary.
Pelvic hemorrhage	Injury to intraperitoneal or retroperitoneal pelvic blood vessels and subsequent bleeding have been reported to occur from 0 to 1.3%. Retroperitoneal bleeding can be difficult to diagnose due to the absence of free fluid in the pouch of Douglas and can be present several hours after oocyte pickup.[13]	Acute severe intra-abdominal bleeding is often detected by symptoms like weakness, dizziness, dyspnea, abdominal pain, tachycardia, and low blood pressure typical for any severe bleeding, immediately after the OPU. In such cases, early hemodynamic monitoring with serial measurement of hemoglobin concentrations is needed.
Trauma to pelvic structures	Rare. Can occur if the gut is adherent due to chronic pelvic infections or endometriosis.	Antibiotics. Laparoscopic evaluation and surgical intervention may be required.

Contd...

Contd...

	Diagnosis	Management
Pelvic infection, tubo-ovarian or pelvic abscess.	Pelvic infections after TVOR have been reported to occur between 0.2% and 0.5%	Antibiotics and treatment for tubo-ovarian abscess.
Acute abdomen	Commonly occurs due to injury to ovarian tissue.	Painkillers and observation for features of hemodynamic instability is necessary.
Postoperative nausea and vomiting	Commonly occur due to effect of anesthesia	IV fluids and ondensetron.

side. The number of supervised collections probably varies between 20 and 40 before trainees should be allowed to perform collections on their own. The collection rates, time taken for the oocyte collection and the complication rate, are available for analysis.

TVS guided oocyte recovery is safe method for oocyte retrieval. It is simple and is done with minimal risk. Complications are few.

REFERENCES

1. Lapata A. Johnston IMH, Leeton JF, et al. Collection of human oocytes at laparoscopy and laparotomy. Fertil Steril. 1974;25:1030-4.
2. Bjercke S, Tanbo T, Dale PO, et al. Comparison between two hCG to-oocyte aspiration intervals on the outcome of *in vitro* fertilization, J Assist Reprod Genet. 2000;17(6):319-22.

3. Van Os HC, Roozenderg BJ, Janseen Caspers HAB, et al. Vaginal disinfection with povidone iodine and the outcome of *in vitro* fertilization. Hum Reprod. 1992;7(3):349-50.
4. Coetsier T, Dhont M, De Sutter P, et al. Propofol anaesthesia for ultrasound-guided oocyte retrieval: accumulation of the anaesthetic agent in follicular fluid. Hum Reprod. 1992;7:1422-4.
5. Choen J, Avery S, Campbell S. Follicular aspiration using a syringe suction system may damage zona pellucida. J *In Vitro* Fertil Embryo Transf. 1986;4:224.
6. Mikkelsen AL, Smith S, Lindenberg S. Possible factors affecting the development of oocytes in *in vitro* maturation. Hum Reprod. 2000;15(suppl 5):11.
7. Papanikolaou EG, Platteau P, Albano C, et al. Immature oocyte *in vitro* maturation: clinical aspects. Reprod Biomed Online. 2005;10:587.
8. Awonuga A, Waterstone J, Ovesanya O, et al. A prospective randomized study comparing needles of different diameters for transvaginal ultrasound-directed follicle aspiration. Fertil Steril 1996;65:109.
9. Redding GP, Bronlund JE, Hart AL. The effects of IVF aspiration on the temperature, dissolved oxygen levels, and pH of follicular fluid. J Assist Reprod Genet. 2006;23:37-40.
10. Kingsland CR, Taylor CT, Aziz N, Bickerton N. Is follicular flushing necessary for oocyte retrieval? A randomized trial. Hum Reprod. 1991;6:382.
11. El-Shawarby S, Margara R, Trew G. A review of complications following trans-vaginal oocyte retrieval for *in vitro* fertilization. Hum Fertil (Camb). 2004;7:127.
12. Tureck RW, Garcia CR, Blasco L, Perioperative complications arising after transvaginal oocyte retrieval. Obstet Gynecol. 1993;81:590.
13. Azem F, Wolfey Y, Botchan A. Massive retroperitoneal bleeding: a complication of transvaginal ultrasonography-guided oocyte retrieval for *in vitro* fertilization-embryo transfer. Fertil Steril. 2000;74:405.

Chapter 8

Embryo Selection

Ved Prakash, Pankaj Talwar

INTRODUCTION

In vitro fertilization (IVF) is a technique in Assisted Reproduction (AR) that has been continuously improving over the part few decades. Despite progress in the IVF technique itself, only a minority of the *in vitro*-generated embryos have the ability to implant and to give a viable pregnancy, probably because of intrinsic characteristics of the gametes. The success rate of human *in vitro* fertilization (IVF) remains relatively low when the number of pregnancies is considered in proportion to the number of embryos transferred. The low pregnancy rates per embryo transferred leads to a need to transfer more than one embryo, which in turn increases the chance of multiple pregnancy. To increase the probability of implantation, several embryos are usually transferred at the same time in each patient.[1]

As ARTs procedures have been simplified and are being used worldwide, there has been an increase in the reported number of multiple pregnancies. Such births result in greater problems for both mother and infants, including an increased rate of cesarean section, premature births, low birth weight, neonatal death and disability.[2] To increase pregnancy rates and limit the occurrence of multiple births, a more efficient and rigorous procedure for embryo selection prior to transfer is therefore needed.[3] In order to transfer two, or even one, embryos(s) without markedly lowering the pregnancy rate, it is important to increase our knowledge of how to select the optimal cleavage-stage embryos or blastocysts.[4]

Although the advent of '-omics'-based technologies may ultimately enhance the non-invasive assessment of human embryos *in vitro*, there are still no routinely applicable techniques or analytical devices available to grade concepts, thus the IVF clinics worldwide continue to select embryos for transfer based on their development rate and morphological features as assessed by light microscopy. However, the many variations in embryo grading schemes applied by different clinics make inter-clinic comparisons extremely difficult, if not impossible.[5]

In the past two decades, a great deal of effort has been made to correlate the morphological appearance of embryos with the implantation rate and successful pregnancy outcome. Amongst the alternative prognostic parameters that have been introduced by reproductive specialists, screening embryo's morphology aids the embryologist in selecting the best embryos for embryo transfer (ET).[6]

Embryo scoring is performed in different ways, with each center having its own scoring system. However, since all current systems are based on morphological evaluation, most parameters evaluated are the same between centers, albeit with different emphases being placed on each parameter.

The current practice in most IVF laboratories is to score cleavage-stage embryos on day 2 or 3 after oocyte retrieval, evaluating the grade of fragmentation, cytoplasmic appearance and number of blastomerers per embryo. These variables can be collectively counted as a cumulative embryo score (CES = grade × number of blastomeres). In addition, variation in the zona pellucida thickness, presence of multinucleated blastmeres, location of fragment and size of blastomeres in relation to each other may be analyzed. Embryo quality has also been reported to correlate with oocyte and zygote morphology, e.g. appearance of the cytoplasm, pronuclei and polar bodies.[7]

EMBRYO ASSESSMENT

As a result of improved embryo culture techniques, ART centers may produce better quality embryos, with equivalent cell numbers and morphological scores. Elective single-embryo transfer is increasingly undertaken inorder to prevent adverse outcomes related to multiple pregnancies. Thus, selecting embryos with high implantation potential is one of the most important challenges in the field of Assisted Reproduction. Moreover, it is important to identify healthy viable and non-viable embryos and cryopreserve only the former. Such identification needs to be accurate in order to avoid massive and useless cryopreservation and to improve the chances of achieving a pregnancy for IVF couples.

Various methods have been proposed to evaluate embryo viability in IVF programs. A limiting factor in such evaluations is that they should be neither invasive nor time consuming. Selection of the most viable cleavage stage embryo is usually based on embryo morphology on day 2 or day 3, with the rate of development in culture as a guide. New parameters such as zygote morphology have recently been proposed to identify embryos with a good prognosis for implantation.

Extended embryo culture until the blastocyst stage (day 5/6) was successfully proposed as a means to select the most developmentally competent embryos. Delaying transfer until the blastocyst stage should increase the potential for self-selection of viable embryos since only a small proportion of embryos reach this stage, as the embryonic genome is activated between the four- and eight-cell stage. When embryos are cultured *in vitro*, about 50% will cease development during the first week. The reasons for this high rate of embryo loss during early development are not fully understood. They might include chromosomal abnormalities, suboptimal culture conditions or inadequate oocyte maturation.

Although the best way to evaluate embryo viability is its ability to implant, assessment of embryo development *in vitro* might make it possible to remain independent of the uterine receptivity that clearly influences implantation success.[8]

FERTILIZATION ASSESSMENT

The oocytes are observed in between 18 to 20 hours after the insemination to look for the signs of fertilization. Fertilization is the fusion between an oocyte and a sperm cell, with the resulting fusion of haploid nuclear material of both. The result of fertilization is a diploid zygote. Signs of fertilizations includes the expulsion of second polar body and formation of two pronuclei (2PN), one containing the male and another the female chromosomes. Both the pronuclei migrate towards the center and unite to form a new set of chromosomes.

PRONUCLEI SCORING

Fertilization scoring involves careful analysis of the pronuclei and NPBs within the nuclei in a single observation at 18 hours after fertilization. Hoffman's contrast module is recommended for accurate scoring of fertilization. Normally, fertilized eggs should have two pronuclei, two polar bodies, regular shape with intact zona pellucida, and a clear healthy cytoplasm. The cytoplasm can be slightly granular and healthy, brown or dark and degenerated.

Pronuclei should be of approximately the same size. Fertilized oocytes that have pronnuclei of different size have an incidence of chromosomal abnormalities.[9] Two pronuclei stage scoring include the size, number and alignment of the nuclei in vertical row of each pronuclei, in a single observation (Figs 8.1A and B).[10]

EVALUATION OF EMBRYO QUALITY

The embryos are examined carefully at intervals to ensure that the division is continuing at the right pace.

The ideal features of embryos at different timing of postinsemination are:

Cleavage	Stages	Timing of postinsemination
1st Cleavage	2-cell stage without fragmentation	25–26 hours
2nd Cleavage	4 or more cell with <20% fragmentation	42–44 hours
3rd Cleavage	8 or more cell with <20% fragmentation	66–68 hours

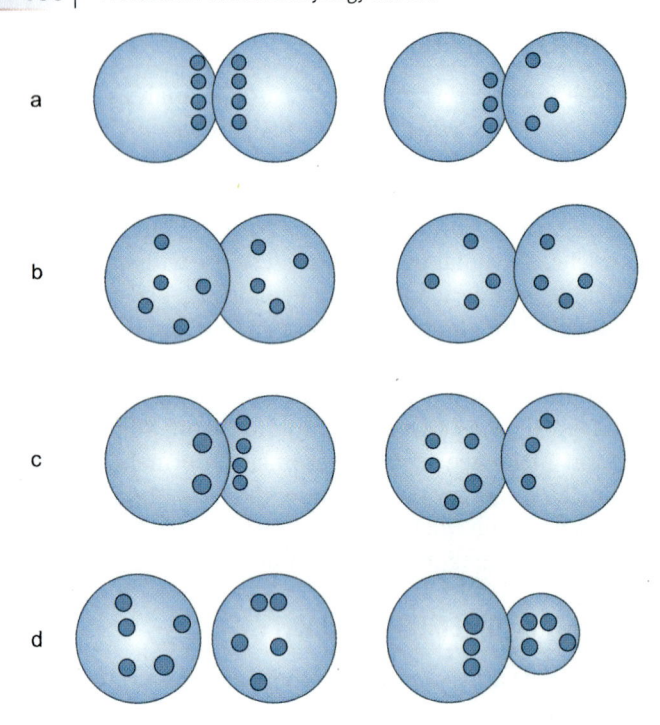

Fig. 8.1A: Pronuclei stage scoring: (a) It has equal number of nucleoli and aligned at pronuclei junction, (b) Equal number of scattered, (c) Unequal sized and unequal number of nucleoli, (d) Unequal sized nucleoli with unequal number of nucleoli

After 3rd day it becomes difficult to count the cells. The embryo is now referred to as morula. In a normally growing embryo, blastocyst stage is achieved at 5 to 6 days postinsemination (Fig. 8.2).

Laboratories have developed grading methods to judge oocyte and embryo quality. In order to optimize pregnancy rates, there is a significant evidence that a morphological

| Grade I | Grade II |
| Grade III | Grade IV |

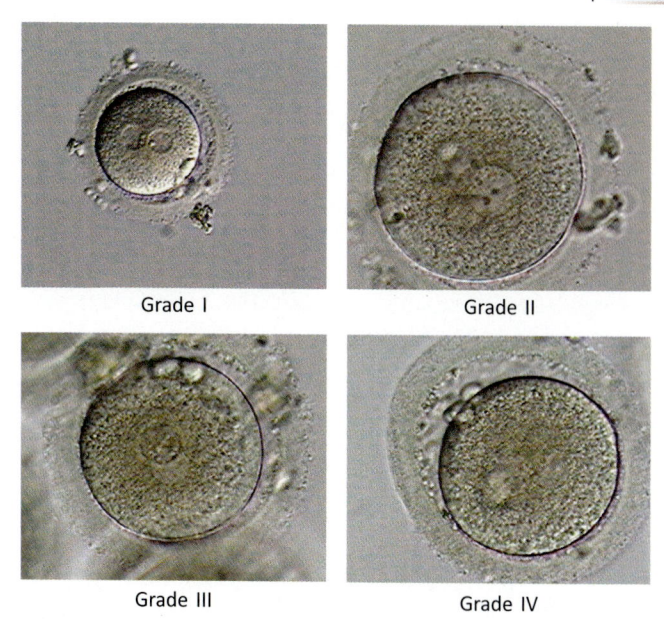

Fig. 8.1B: Types of grades

scoring system and cell number is the best strategy for the selection of embryos.[11] The limitations of evaluating embryos based on morphological criteria alone are well recognized as the correlations between gross morphology and implantation are weak and inaccurate, unless the embryos are clearly fragmenting.[12]

Embryo morphology is determined by the number and size of the blastmeres, the proportion of the fragments and the presence of multi nucleated blastomeres. It has been demonstrated that after 2 days of culture, the 4-cell stage is the optional cleavage stage.[13,14] Embryos at this cleavage stage with little or no fragmentation and multinucleated

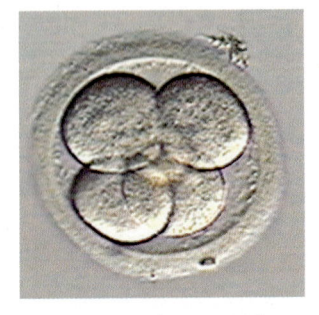

2-Cell stage after 25–26 hours

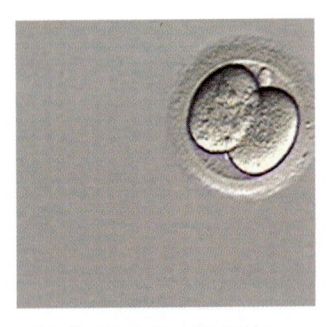

4-Cell stage after 42–44 hours

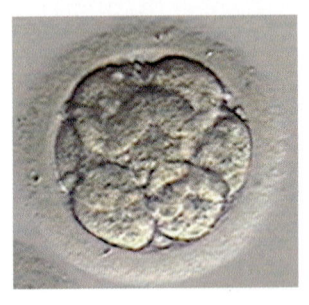

8-Cell stage after 66–68 hours

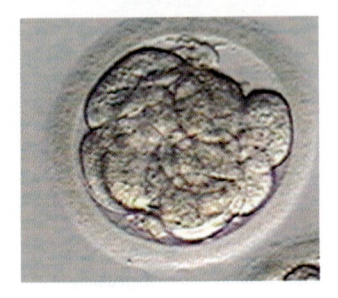

Morula stage on day 4

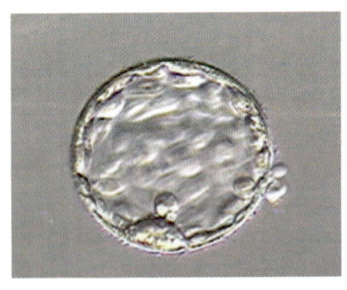

Blastocyst on day 5

Fig. 8.2: Ideal features of embryo at different timing of post-insemination

blastomeres are associated with a higher implantation rate compared to embryos at other cleavage stages with fragmentation or multinucleated blastomeres. However, there is an evidence that embryos selection on day 2 to 3, based on morphological criteria may be unreliable, resulting in the transfer of embryos that are abnormal or that arrest at later developmental stages.[15-18]

Based upon these criteria, embryos may be classified (Figs 8.2 and 8.3):

Grade I (Good): Grade I embryos have stage-specific cell size. These embryos have an even number of equal sized blastomeres with intact zona. If the number of blastomeres is uneven because one still has to divide, then grade I one still applies. Grade one embryo have no, or very few, fragments (less than 10%), with no multinucleation.

Grade II (Fair): These embryos have stage-specific cell size for majority of cells and no evidence of multinucleation, uneven or irregularly-shaped blastomeres, accompanied by fragmentation, but not more than 25 percent of volume.

Grade III (Poor): The amount of fragmentation increases to 10 to 50 percent with unequal size blastomeres with evidence of multinucleation.

Sometimes different criteria are used in different laboratories for the scoring, which make it difficult to compare the results regarding the relationship of embryo quality to pregnancy chances. About 20 percent of transferred embryos of grade 1 to 2 become implanted in the uterus. The chances of ongoing pregnancy per good quality embryo transferred is about 10 to 15 percent.[18]

Protocols in Clinical Embryology and ART

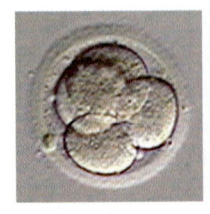

Grade I
(Equal number of blastomeres No fragmentation)

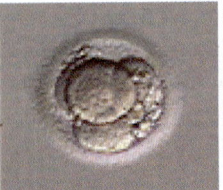

Grade II
(Uneven number of blastomeres with >10% fragmentation)

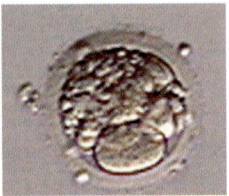

Grade IV
(Scarcely recognizable blastomeres with >50% fragmentation)

Fig. 8.3A: Embryo grading

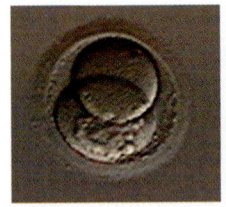

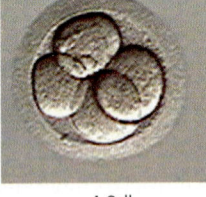

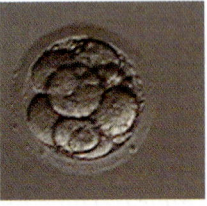

2-Cell
4-Cell
8-Cell

Fig. 8.3B: Grade I (Good) embryos at various cell stages

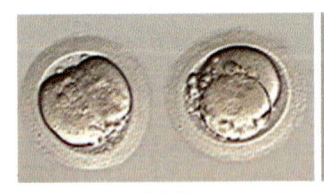

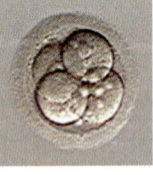

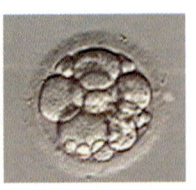

2-Cell
4-Cell
8-Cell

Fig. 8.3C: Grade II (Fair), at various cell stages

2-Cell   4-Cell   8-Cell

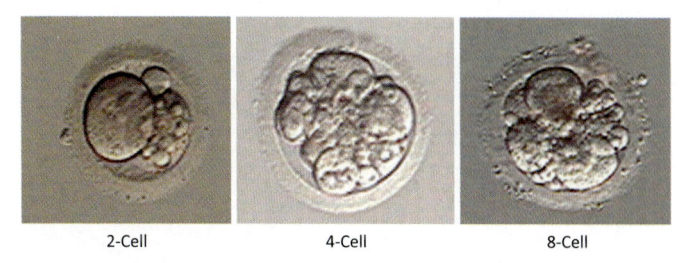

Fig. 8.3D: Grade III (Poor), at various cell stages

BLASTOCYST SCORING

The blastocyst scoring assessment is based on the expansion state of the blastocyst and on the consistency of the inner cell mass and trophectoderm cells.[19] Using such a grading system, it was determined that when a high scoring blastocyst with expanded blastocoel, compacted inner cell mass and cohesive trophectoderm epithelium is transferred, the clinical pregnanacy and implantation rate of >80 percent and 69 percent, respectively, may be attained (Figs 8.4 and 8.5).

162 | *Protocols in Clinical Embryology and ART*

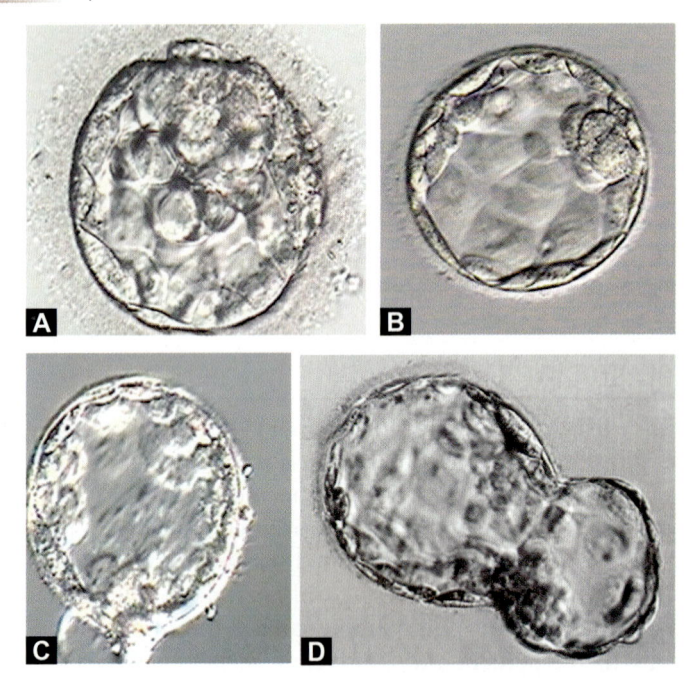

Figs 8.4A to D: Blastocyst embryos: (A) Early blastocyst, (B) Blastocyst (fully expanded), (C) Beginning of hatching and (D) Intermediate phase of hatching

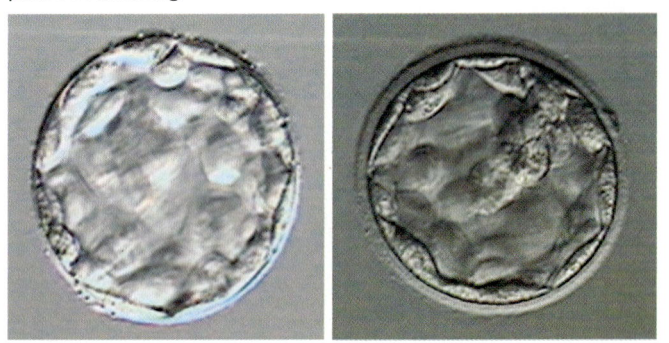

Fig. 8.5A: Grade I blastocyst

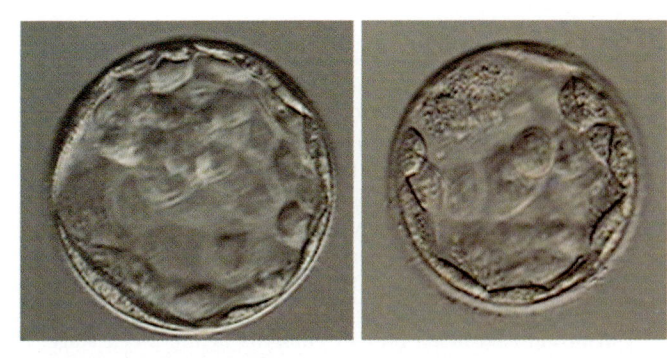

Fig. 8.5B: Grade II blastocyst

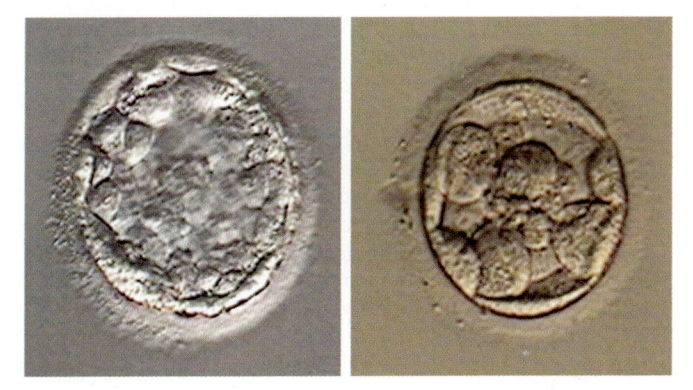

Fig. 8.5C: Grade III blastocyst

Blastocyst[20]

Grade I: Fully expanded blastocyst healthy inner cell mass and tropectoderm.

Grade II: Unhealthy inner cell mass, cavity partially expanded.

Grade III: Collapsed blastocode cavity unhealthy inner cell mass.

REFERENCES

1. Beuchat P, The´venaz, Unser M, Ebner T, Senn A, Urner F, Germond M, Sorzano COS. Quantitative morphometrical characterization of human pronuclear zygotes. Human Reproduction. 2008;23(9):1983-92.
2. Neuber E, Rinaudo P, Trimarchi JR, Sakkas D. Sequential assessment of individually cultured human embryos as an indicator of subsequent good quality blastocyst development. Human Reproduction. 2003;18(6):1307-12.
3. Shoukir Y, Campana A, Farley T, Sakkas D. Early cleavage of *in vitro* fertilized human embryos to the 2-cell stage: a novel indicator of embryo quality and viability. Human Reproduction. 1997;12(7):1531-6.
4. Lundin K, Bergh C, Hardarson T. Early embryo cleavage is a strong indicator of embryo quality in Human IVF; Human Reproduction. 2001;16(12):2652-7.
5. Alpha Scientists in Reproductive Medicine and ESHRE Special Interest Group of Embryology. The Istanbul consequences workshop on embryo assessment: proceeding of an expert meeting. Human Reproduction. 2011;26;(6);1270-83.
6. Khalili MA, Razavi V, Mardanian F, Esfandiari N. The predictive value of pronuclear morphology screening on embryo development and pregnancy outcome in ART cycles. Middle East Fertility Society Journal. 2008;13:1.
7. Lundin K, Bergh C, Hardarson T. Early embryo cleavage is a strong indicator of embryo quality in Human IVF; Human Reproduction. 2001;16(12):2652-7.
8. Guerif F, Le Gouge A, Giraudeau B, Poindron J, Bidault R, Gasnier O, Royere D. Limited value of morphological assessment at days 1 and 2 to predict blastocyst development potential: A prospective study based on 4042 embryos. Human Reproduction 2007;22(7):1973-81.
9. Munne S, Cohen J. Chromosome abnormalities in human embryos. Hum Reprod Update. 1998;4:842-55.
10. Scott L. Pronuclear scoring as a predictor of embryo development. Reprod Biomed Online. 2003;6:57-70.
11. Cummins J, Breen T, Harrison K, et al. A formula for scoring human embryo growth rates in *in vitro* fertilization: its value

in predicting pregnancy and in comparison with visual estimates of embryo quality. J *In Vitro* Fert Embryo Transf. 1986;3:284-95.

12. Brian Dale; Kay Elder (Eds). Oocyte retrieval and embryo culture (Eds): *In vitro* fertilization, Reprinted Cambridge University Press 1999.pp.102-127

13. Giorgetti C, Terriou P, Auquier P, Hans E, Spach JL, Salzmann J, Roulier R. Embryo score to predict implantation after *in vitro* fertilization: based on 957 single embryo transfers. Hum Reprod. 1995;10:101-5.

14. Ziebe S, Petersen K, Lindernberg S, Andersen AG, Gabreilsen A, Andersen AN. Embryo morphology or cleavage stage: how to select the best embryos for transfer after *in vitro* fertilization. Hum Reprod. 1997;12:1545-9.

15. Rijnders PM, Jansen CAM. The predictive value of day 3 embryo morphology regarding blastocyst formation, pregnancy and implantation rate after day 5 transfer following *in vitro* fertilization or intracytoplasmic sperm injection. Hum Reprod. 1998;13:2869-73.

16. Graham J, Han T, Porter R, Levy M, Stillman R, Tucker M. Day 3 morphology is a poor predictor of blastocyst quality in extended culture. Fertil Steril. 2000;74:495-7.

17. Milki AA, Hinckley MD, Gebhart J, Dasig D, Westphal LM, Behr B. Accuracy of day 3 criteria for selecting the best embryos. Fertil Steril. 2002;77:1191-5.

18. Lens JW, Rijnders PM. The embryos. In Laboratory aspects of *in vitro* fertilization. Bras M, Lens JW, Piederiet MH, Rijnders PM, Verveld M, Zeilmaker GH (Eds). Publication NV Organon. 1996.pp. 177-203.

19. Gardner D, Schoolcraft W. *In vitro* culture of human blastocyst. In Jansen R, Mortimer D (Eds). Towards reproductive certainty: infertility and genetics beyond Carnforth. Parthenon Press; 1997.pp.378-88.

20. Gardner DK, Lane M, Stevens J, Schlenker T, Schoolcraft WB. Blastocyst score affects implantation and pregnancy outcome: towards a single blastocyst transfer. Fertil Steril. 2000;73:1155-8.

Chapter 9

Culture Media in IVF and Embryo Culture

Pankaj Talwar

INTRODUCTION

In Assisted Reproductive Technology embryo culture is one of the cornerstones of the success of reproductive procedures (Fig. 9.1) Overtly, it is a simple procedure of using appropriate culture media formulations, but in reality it requires a combination of quality control and quality assurance programs, sufficient number of incubation chambers, and optimal environment for the development *in vitro* and maintaining the viability of concepts. Oocytes and embryos

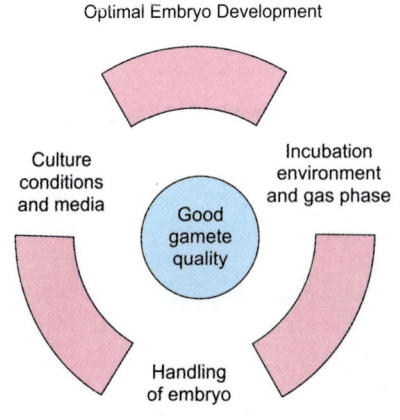

Fig. 9.1: Essential prerequisites for embryo growth

are very sensitive, and should not be exposed to big differences in temperature or pH. Human conceptus prefer a temperature of 37°C and neutral pH for multiplication and growth various media products are formulated with the same core salt concentration, to minimize osmotic or pH stress when moving from one medium to another[1] (Fig. 9.1 and Table 9.1). It has been shown that the detrimental effects of stress applied at the early stage of development during handling and culture of the oocyte and 2PN may not be evident until the blastocyst stage. We can deduce that lack of morphological abnormalities does not mean that no damage has occurred to the cells at cellular level. The damage may reveal itself at the blastocyst stage or at the time of implantation.

ESSENTIAL CONCEPTS

pHo and pHi

We must understand the concept of pHi and pHo before starting with the embryo culture. The actual pH of the surrounding medium (pHo-7.4) is different from that

Table 9.1

Constituents of culture media

1. Water—99%
2. Pyruvate, lactate, glucose
3. Amino acids
4. Ions—Potassium, sodium, calcium
5. Extrinsic buffer system
6. Macromolecules
7. Vitamins
8. Antioxidants

inside the embryo (pHi, 7.2) and these both follow a gentle gradient. Various media components' like bicarbonate, L lactate and amino-acids play an important role in driving this gradient. Of the two isomers of lactate, D and L, only the L-form is biologically active and is recommended for use in culture media. Amino acids increase the intracellular buffering capacity and further help in maintaining the pHi at around 7.2.

Presently, we have the technology to record direct external pH (pHo) using ph meters or using various devices to check CO_2 concentrations in the incubator with fyrite kit and infrared sensors, which will give us indirect record of the pHo. Adding phenol red to the culture medium allows visual estimation of a medium's pH within a tube in the incubator. It is recommended that once a pH measurement demonstrates a pH near the level desired, and assuming no changes in medium composition, or CO_2 concentration levels it is practical to monitor and control the pH by recording the CO_2 levels in the incubator by using methods that yield more precise levels of CO_2 (Fyrite/hand held digital devices) thereby maintaining the pH to range of 0.025–0.05 pH units.

Buffer systems form an important control of pH.

Buffer System

An important part of the media is the buffer system it uses. *In vivo* oocyte and early embryo are protected by surrounding cumulus cells and are not required to regulate pH themselves till 8–10 hours after fertilization when transport systems are initiated. Early embryos and denuded oocytes for ICSI are susceptible to pH changes when manipulated. Amino acids must be present in media to facilitate the buffering of pH. Media may be buffered with:

- HEPES
- MOPS
- Phosphate
- Bicarbonate

Buffers are added depending on the intended use of the media. Those with bicarbonate buffer should be equilibrated in CO_2 incubator while media with HEPES and MOPS can be used after warming to 37°C.

Sodium Bicarbonate

Bicarbonate is an important intracellular buffer and has been shown, to be essential for embryo development. CO_2 is part of the bicarbonate buffer system as appreciated with the equilibrium reaction:

$$CO_2 + H_2O \rightleftharpoons H_2CO_3 \rightleftharpoons H^+ + HCO_3^-$$

It is required in small amounts in the oocytes and early embryos. For those procedures requiring a bicarbonate buffered medium, the formulations have been designed to maintain a pH of 7.2–7.4 in an atmosphere of 5–6% CO_2 to yield a medium pH (pHo) of around 7.3–7.4, at 37°C for laboratories located at or near sea level. For laboratories located at higher altitudes, the CO_2 percentage should be increased by approximately 0.6% CO_2 per 1000 meters. When handling bicarbonate-buffered medium it is essential to minimize the amount of time the culture dish is out of a CO_2 environment to prevent increases in pH.

HEPES [4-(2-Hydroxyethyl)-1-piperazineethanesulfonic Acid]

HEPES is a zwitterionic, organic chemical buffering agent widely used in culture. This can maintain physiological pH despite changes in carbon dioxide concentration due cellular metabolism. HEPES buffered media have been formulated to give a pH of 7.3–7.5 in air, at 37°C. This makes it possible to handle gametes outside the incubator for a period of 15–20 minutes.

Phosphate Buffer

Cryopreservation of cleavage stage embryos is performed in phosphate buffered solutions, which will keep a pH of 7.2–7.4 in air.

MOPS [3-(N-morpholino)propanesulfonic Acid]

A zwitterionic buffer active in the pH range of 6.5 to 8.0. It is an excellent buffer for many biological systems at near-neutral pH. G-MOPS™/G-MOPS™ PLUS are MOPS buffered media and must be used at 37°C in ambient atmosphere. Such buffering systems do not require a CO_2 environment and may give us 10–15 minutes to handle the gametes outside the incubator.

> *Caution:* MOPS should not be exposed to a CO_2 environment and covered by paraffin oil equilibrated in a CO_2 environment, as the pH of the media will go down below the specification range.[2]

Quality of Water

High quality water is used for the preparation of the media. Ultrapure water is produced from a state of art water purification system producing more than 18.2 mega Ohm pyrogen free water with a very low total organic carbon content. All products are membrane filtered through a 0.2 µm retentive filter in a fully validated process.

THE PHYSIOLOGY OF SEQUENTIAL CULTURE MEDIA

The requirement of the gametes and embryo at different stages of development differ in terms of nutritional and metabolic microenvironment. The conditions which support the blastocyst differentiation are different from those that enhance zygote development. Human oocytes and embryos are unique for culturing, as they are quiescent at the beginning but in 2–3 days of culturing have sudden surge in physiological requirements, molecular regulation, and metabolism as they multiply to 250–300 cells in 4 days. It has been seen that the Metaphase stage II oocyte and pronucleus stage conceptus has a relatively low levels of oxygen consumption and has a preference for carboxylic acids, such as pyruvate, as its primary energy source with very minimal requirements of glucose. As the embryo proceeds to the blastocyst stage with ICM and trophectoderm, the embryo exhibits high biosynthetic activity and high oxygen consumption and has an ability to metabolize glucose preferentially, along with other energy sources with increased requirement of protein synthesis and requiring both nonessential and essential amino acids. Sequential media caters to the changing day-to-day biosynthetic quotient of the gametes and conceptus (Figs 9.2 and 9.3).

Physiology of IVF Fertilization Medium

The fertilization medium provides the environment for the retrieved egg in the presence of cumulus cells during conventional *in vitro* fertilization.

A. Carbohydrates and Energy
- The medium is driven by glucose, which is converted by cumulus cells to pyruvate via glycolysis to generate ATP. ATP flows directly into the egg cytoplasm through microvilli as it completes meiosis 1 and is prepared for fertilization.
- The freshly ovulated or retrieved egg cannot itself metabolize glucose. *In vivo*, cumulus cells

Culture Media in IVF and Embryo Culture

Difference in embryo physiology before and after compaction

Before compaction:
- Low biosynthetic activity
- Low QO2
- Pyruvate and lactate preferred
- Nonessential amino acids beneficial
- Maternal genome
- Individual cells–single cell physiology
- One cell type
- More susceptible to environment

After compaction:
- High biosynthetic activity
- High QO2
- Glucose preferred
- Both nonessential and essential amino acids needed
- Embryonic genome
- Transporting epithelium–somatic cell physiology
- 2 cell types–ICM and trophectoderm

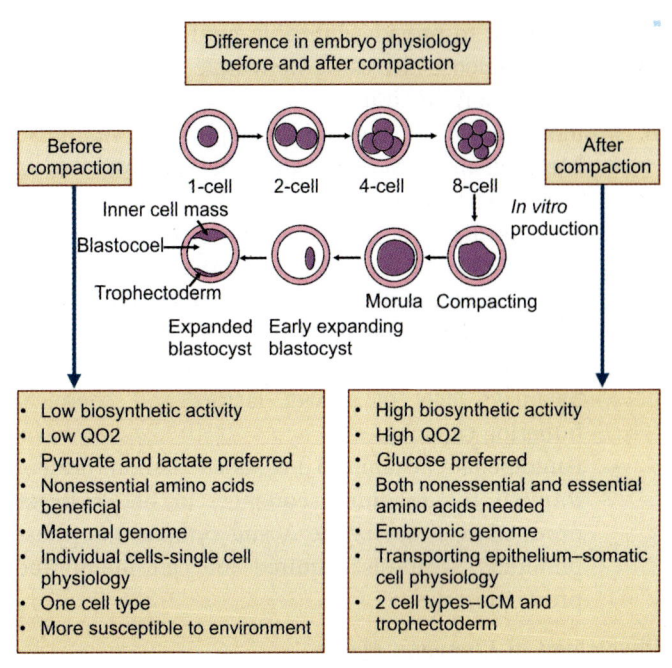

Fig. 9.2: Changing requirements of developing conceptus

IVF/Fertilization media → Cleavage media → Blastocyst media

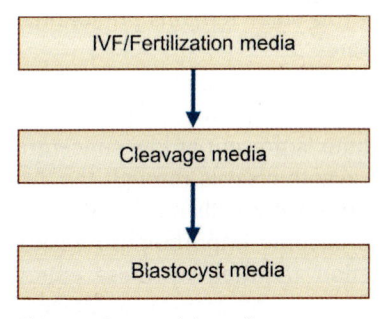

Fig. 9.3: Sequential media

continue to provide diffusible pyruvate to the egg. Thus, glucose drives carbohydrate metabolism in fertilization medium.

B. Protein, nucleic acids, membrane lipids and vitamins
- Metabolism is catabolic and the egg lives on its accumulated reserves.
- The fertilization medium provides nonessential amino acids for metabolic purposes.
- Albumin concentration has been reduced to limit the potential for breakdown into ammonium while retaining its benefits in delivering a physiologically balanced level of growth factors and chemical buffering capacity.
- Pantothenate (Vitamin B_5) is added vitamin, present through the medium sequence, to better foster production of coenzyme A and cytoplasmic phospholipids synthesis required for cell membrane production.

Physiology of Cleavage Media

Cleavage medium should be introduced when cumulus cells are removed, i.e. for the injection step in ICSI cases or at the fertilization check in non-ICSI cases. Metabolism in the embryo at this stage remains predominantly catabolic

A. Carbohydrates
- Pyruvate predominates and glucose has been included at a low concentration.
- Phosphate is present at low concentrations.
- As the zygote cleaves through the 2-cell and 4-cell stages to reach 8-cells on day 3, anabolic pathways start to become important. To ensure the NADPH production required by these emerging anabolic pathways, a small amount of glucose is present to drive the pentose phosphate shunt.

- Pantothenate is added to aid in the crucial third cell cycle.

B. Protein, nucleic acids, membrane lipids and vitamins
- As anabolic pathways become active for cell membrane components and nuclear structures a low concentration of essential amino acids has been introduced to better anticipate new protein production.

Physiology of the Blastocyst Media

As the embryo blastulates, the massive increase in cell number requires a new order of activity for anabolic synthetic pathways and the energy required to drive rapid differentiation. As the new embryonic genome replicates and becomes active, controlling REDOX stresses becomes even more important. For REDOX balance, stable mitochondria and abundant NADPH constitute the important electron sinks. A low level of oxygen favors glycolysis, with rapid production of ATP.

A. Carbohydrate
- Glucose returns at a higher concentration to support glycolysis.
- Lactate concentration has been reduced to encourage pyruvate's reduction to lactate when ATP is plentiful.

B. Protein, nucleic acids and membrane lipids
- The new embryonic genome is alternately replicating and being transcribed, producing new DNA, RNA, proteins and enzymes.
- Essential and nonessential amino acids are fully provided for by the medium. Nucleic and salvage pathways are no longer enough for the massive requirements the embryo has for DNA and RNA, which now demand *de novo* purine and pyrimidine synthesis.

USE OF OIL OVERLAY IN ART

Oil overlay has several advantages and is necessary:
- Prevents evaporation of media
- Reduces change in pH caused by loss of CO_2 from media. An oil overlay also reduces the speed of CO_2 loss and the associated increase in pH.
- Serves as trap for embryotoxins
- Protective barrier
- Should be bought in smaller bottles
- Incubation with IVF media before use.

QUALITY CONTROL TESTING FOR THE CULTURE MEDIA

All media products are produced in a specially designed production facility certified to Good Manufacturing Practice (GMP) by ISO standards. Independent QC checks are made both during the production process and prior to release. Twice monthly production runs ensure that fresh media are always available.

The following quality control methods are used in media manufacturing units.

pH, Osmolality, Viscosity Measurement

The pH, osmolality and viscosity measurement is performed and the range of acceptance for each product is kept as small as possible, considering the nature of the product and its intended use (Table 9.2).

Mouse Embryo Assay (MEA)

Mouse embryo assay (MEA) is a functional test method. All media, medium components, oil for overlaying, consumables and critical devices used for media manufacturing are tested

> **Table 9.2**
>
> **Common prerelease specifications recommended for the IVF culture media**
>
> - pH: 7.3–7.5
> - Osmolarity: 285–295 mOsm/kg
> - Mouse embryo assay (MEA) > 80%
> - Endotoxins: < 0.4 EU/ml
> - Shelf life: 8 weeks from date of manufacture
> - Sterile: Filtered sterility assurance level (SAL 10^{-3}).

by culturing one-cell stage mouse embryos to the expanded blastocyst stage. The safety and efficacy of the media is determined by observing the number of embryos that develop to defined developmental stages with appropriate cell numbers in a predetermined time period, as cell numbers of the blastocysts are linked to their subsequent viability upon transfer to the uterus.[2-4]

Fresh one cell or two cell mouse embryos are cultured in test medium and control medium for 72 hours (for two cell) or 96 hours (for one cell) respectively. FDA guidelines require 70% formation rate to expanded blastocysts. Sensitivity of the MEA increases with use of 1-cell mouse embryos as opposed to 2-cell stage.[5]

Endotoxin Level

The absence of toxic levels of endotoxins is verified for all raw materials and each lot manufactured. The validated bacterial endotoxin test (LAL assay) is the most sensitive of the currently used methods for endotoxin testing with a minimum sensitivity of 0.005 EU or IU/ml. Endotoxin level should be as low as possible, (less than 125 IU/ml).

Sterility Test

The sterility of all media is confirmed by a membrane filtration as they can neither be autoclaved or heat sterilized due to sensitivity to high temperatures. The test period for media is 2 weeks and for oil 3 weeks. After 7 and 14 days the medium is examined for the content of microorganisms. The sterility is checked in each batch by microbiological methods and should give a sterility assurance level (SAL) of 10^{-3}.

Hybritest™

The patented Hybritest™ is employed under protein free conditions. This increases the test's sensitivity to toxic substances without any "masking" effects from proteins, particularly albumin. Hybridoma cells are cultured in test media with a minimum of 10-fold increase in cell count after 4 days. Critical raw materials are subjected to the Hybritest™ at incoming inspection.

Sperm Survival Test

This test is intended to demonstrate the absence of substances that will reduce the viability of spermatozoa. The sperm survival test is based on CASA (computer automated semen analysis) in determination of VAP (path velocity), VSL (mean progressive velocity), VCL (track speed) and beat frequency. Incubation in media takes up to 18 hours.

Sperm Immobilization Test

Sperm with normal motility characteristics are mixed with the media. To pass the test, the VAP, VSL and VCL of the sperm suspended in the media must be below 30 μm/sec.

Functionality Test

This test is done for Sperm Slow™. Sperm with normal motility characteristics are mixed with the Sperm Slow™ medium. Sperm Slow™ is tested for the ability to reduce the velocity of the sperm cells. This reduced velocity is necessary to catch the sperm cells used for ICSI.

ESSENTIALS OF HANDLING MEDIA AND LAB EQUIPMENT

There are many do's and don't's in handling media:

1. *Lab equipment:* Organize and prepare in advance. Ensure that all equipment is correctly maintained and regularly checked.
2. *Incubator handling:* Minimize the number of door openings by having separate incubators for media equilibration and culture. Try to use multicompartment incubators as they maintain the CO_2 levels and temperature better as compared to single door ones. If possible use bench top incubators for embryo culture as these equilibrate quickly and maintain better environment. The time that gametes (especially oocytes) and embryos are handled outside the incubator should be kept to a minimum.

   Carbon dioxide and oxygen concentration in incubator: Majority of culture media contains HCO_3^- in a concentration corresponding to pH 7.2-7.4 when equilibrated in 5-6% CO_2. When making a decision about the CO_2 concentration it must be remembered that the more the incubator is opened and closed the lower is the actual CO_2 concentration in the incubator and the longer is the equilibration time. It is therefore recommended to have separate incubators for media equilibration and culture, and increasing the CO_2

concentration to 6% as the workload increases. We strongly recommend the use of 6% CO_2 at sea level to improve equilibration times and ensure the optimal pH for embryo culture. The O_2 concentration in the oviduct is 40% or less than that found in the atmosphere. The uterus has an even lower O_2 concentration. We recommend using 5% O_2 as constituents of triple gas mixture as better embryo growth is seen.

Measurement of CO_2: The amount of CO_2 in the incubation chamber can be calibrated with a Fyrite kit, although such an approach is only accurate to ±1%. The Fyrite device uses Bacharach solution (potassium hydroxide) that absorbs CO_2 from the incubator air. The partial volume of gas removed by absorption and dissolution of CO_2 is recorded, indicating the percentage of the gaseous volume occupied by CO_2. Care must be taken to avoid saturation of the Bacharach solution with CO_2 and the solution should be replaced after 300 determinations. A more suitable method is to use a hand-held digital infrared metering system that can be calibrated and is accurate to around 0.2%.

3. *Air handling:* Carbon filters to purify incoming gas supplies are recommended. Laminar flow with HEPA filters are essential.

4. *Aseptic conditions:* Wipe all surfaces with milli-Q water and clean periodically with 70% alcohol. All handling is done under laminar air flow. When using gloves, make sure they are nontoxic.

5. *Disposables:* Use only quality-controlled products for all ART procedures and keep a log of all products and procedures performed. Preferably use MEA tested products.

6. *Temperature maintenance:* Temperature loss occurs rapidly and is related to the amount of time a culture dish stays out of the incubator. Using heated stages and pads, e.g. heated microscope stages, can to some extent compensate for this. Switch on the stage at least 30 minutes before to ensure the temperature is appropriate. AC vents and door should not face laminar flow or incubator. Ambient temperature of 24°C should be maintained.
7. *Humidity:* Changes in osmolality occur slowly and it is therefore important to keep the media in a correctly humidified environment and/or covered with liquid paraffin.

> Do not incubate HEPES buffered media in a CO_2 enriched atmosphere as carbon dioxide can hamper the buffering capacity of the HEPES based media.

Precautions to be taken while dispensing media and opening the media bottles (Figs 9.4 to 9.15).

1. Wash and disinfect your hands before handling any product.
2. Take necessary precautions when handling any biological fluid such as blood, follicular fluid and semen.
3. All procedures should be performed in a clean, dedicated work environment. Open all products in a clean laminar air flow (LAF) cabinet.
4. Before bringing bottles into the LAF cabinet, ensure that the bottles are clean on the outside. It is recommended that the bottles be wiped with a lint free cloth and ethanol.
5. Identify the product and check the expiry date. Break the tamper-evident seal and discard.

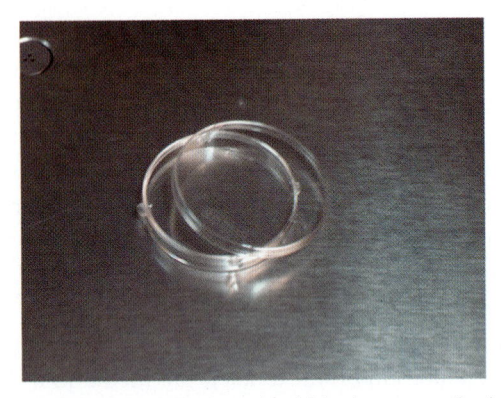

Fig. 9.4: The lid of the IVF plate should be kept over the base dish to avoid contamination of the edges of the lid

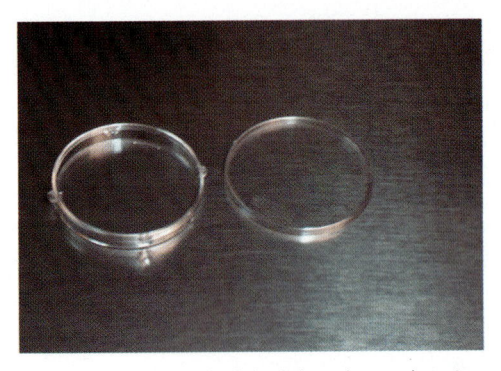

Fig. 9.5: Keeping the open end of the lid on the workstation may lead to contamination of the lid edges and may effect the IVF outcome

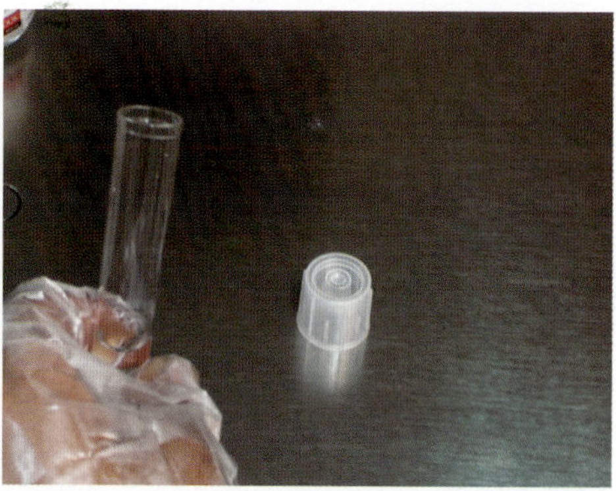

Culture Media in IVF and Embryo Culture | **183**

Fig. 9.6: Wrong way of keeping the test tube cap on the table. The cap edges may get contaminated and cause cross contamination

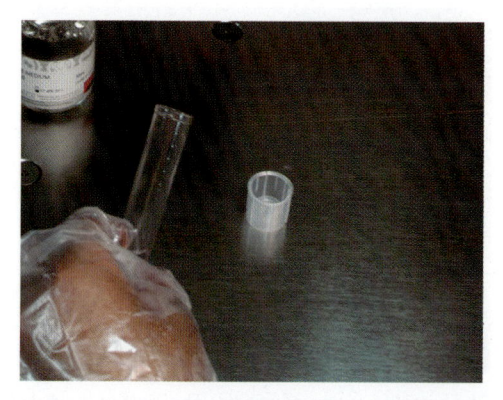

Fig. 9.7: The correct way of keeping the cap on the workstation

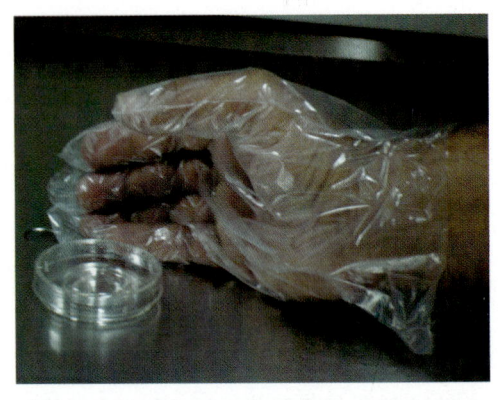

Fig. 9.8: Always work using powder, odour and Latex free gloves

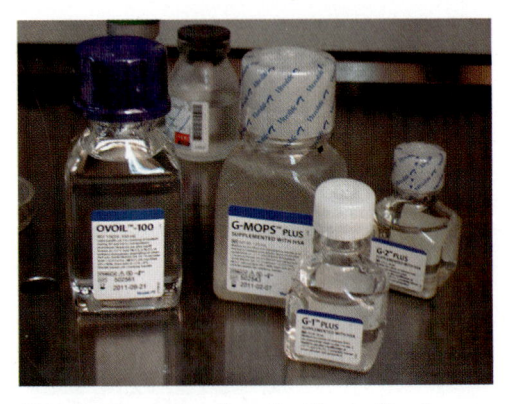

Fig. 9.9: The vitrolife range of media. The bottles have screw caps and are thus easy to handle

Culture Media in IVF and Embryo Culture | **185**

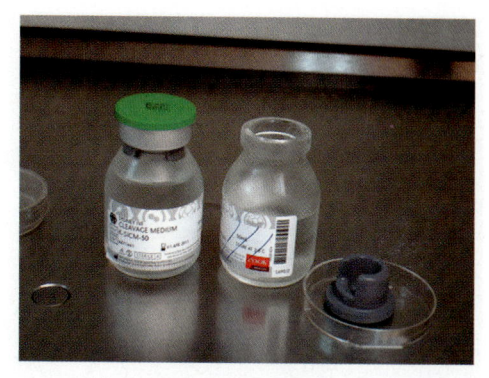

Fig. 9.10: The cook's cleavage media bottle have rubber stopper. The cap should be kept on the sterile IVF plate lid to avoid contamination

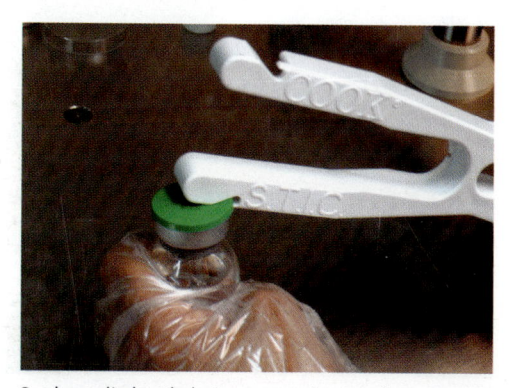

Fig. 9.11: Cook media bottle being opened using the specially designed opener. This avoids fingers touching the corners of the rubber cap and thus contamination is avoided

186 | *Protocols in Clinical Embryology and ART*

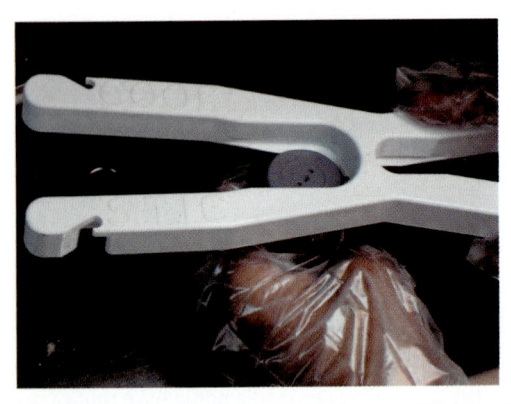

Fig. 9.12: The opener being used to remove the cap of the media bottle

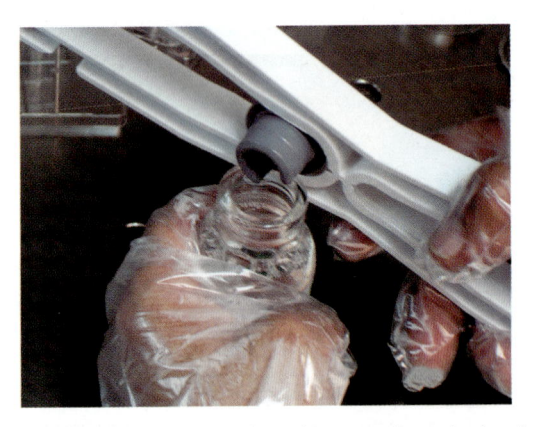

Fig. 9.13: Safe way of removing the rubber cap from the bottle. This avoids contamination

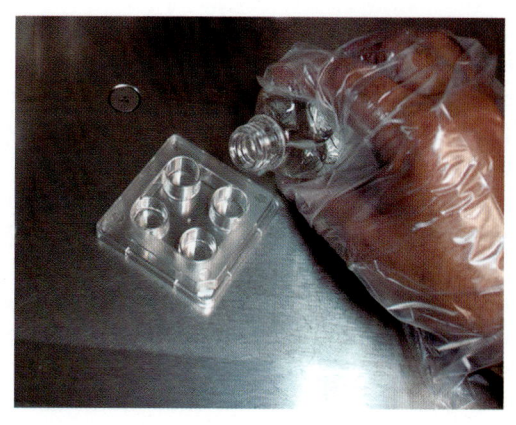

Fig. 9.14: Media should not be poured from the bottle directly. This can cause contamination of the mouth of the bottle

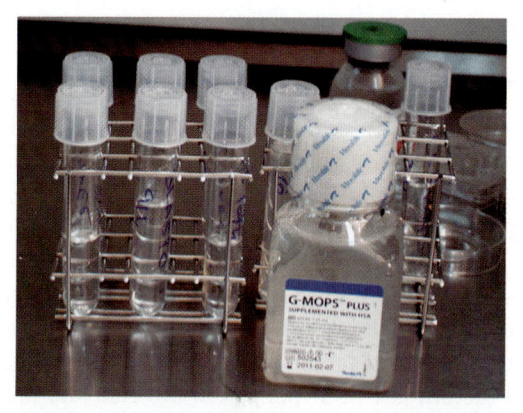

Fig. 9.15: Media dispensed in the tubes. Bicarbonate media should be stored with cap half opened. MOPS or HEPES based media should be stored with cap tightly closed in CO_2 free incubator

6. Remove the cap and place the cap face down in a sterile petri dish.
7. Remove the desired volume with a sterile nontoxic pipette. Replace bottle cap and screw on firmly.
8. Do not touch the inner sides of the cap.
9. Keep the media as cool as possible.
10. Prepare dishes immediately after the bottles have been removed from the refrigerator.
11. Media bottles should not be left at ambient temperature for a longer period of time than it takes to prepare dishes or tubes.
12. Never pour the contents out of the bottle directly, the may lead to media contamination.

Note: Bicarbonate media should be stored in incubator with cap half opened. MOPS or HEPES based media should be stored with cap tightly closed in CO_2 free incubator.

MEDIA PREPARATION AND PREEQUILIBRATION

1. All media should be prepared and preequilibrated in the incubator an evening before. Incubation time should optimally be kept as short as possible, while still allowing time for the CO_2 to equilibrate properly. In practice, minimum 2 hours, equilibration of open well dishes and dishes with microdroplets covered with pre-equilibrated liquid paraffin is required. For equilibration of larger volumes (e.g. a 60 ml/120 ml) the dictum is 1 hour per cm in the vial/ the bottle.

Note: The time of equilibration should not exceed 16 hours ("over night") as degradation of the amino acids, the Human Serum Albumin and the antibiotics will occur.

2. First label the dishes with patient ID and then add the media and liquid paraffin using sterile pipettes.
3. Media for embryo culture is dispensed in either wells of a four well plate, single well plate or 30/60 mm plates with 10–100 µl microdroplets covered with liquid paraffin.
4. When preparing microdroplets, make sure they are covered immediately with liquid paraffin in order to avoid evaporation.
5. Culture media should be replaced every 48 hours to maintain optimum culture conditions.

STORAGE OF THE MEDIA

Commercially available culture media have many unstable components making the media vulnerable to changes in its composition due to prolonged storage at room temperature and exposure to light. It is therefore essential for us to know, how to handle and store such solutions (Table 9.3). Two of

Table 9.3

Precautions to prevent breakdown of amino acids into ammonia which hamper embryo growth

- Open media bottle should be in the refrigerator at 2–8°C, and used within 7 days.
- The date of opening of the media bottle should be written on the label.
- We recommend setting up media dishes for equilibration the afternoon before the day they will be used to minimize heat-induced degradation of media components.
- Renewal of media after 48 hours of culture
- Replace glutamine - the most labile – by a more stable alanyl-glutamine

the most labile components in the culture media are amino acids and vitamins. Glutamine is the most labile amino acid and produces the highest levels of ammonium for any amino acid. These high levels of ammonium impair embryo development during culture and post implantation due to altered genomic impression. It is thus essential that when using culture media containing amino acids the medium plates are placed in the incubator for the minimum time required for equilibration and culture. Fortunately, glutamine can be replaced with alanyl-glutamine, a dipeptide that is stable at 37°C. Vitamins are light sensitive and therefore care should be taken to minimize exposure to light while handling the media droplets.

SHELF LIFE AND PACKAGING

1. Different media have different shelf life. Most products have a shelf life of 8 weeks from shipment. Media without HSA or other biological material have the longest shelf life – 52 weeks.
2. Ideally the media are packaged in small units for primarily single day use.

> *Caution:* Ensure that the opened vials and bottles should be used within 7 days after opening and discard excess media.

Media is one of the most important aspects which lead to the success of IVF. Understanding the science behind it helps in proper handling of the media to ensure good results.

CONCLUSION

1. Crucial considerations for gamete handling and fertilization are temperature, pH and osmolality.

2. Temperature loss occurs rapidly and is related to the amount of time a culture vessel stays out of the incubator and whether the table surface is heated, or not.
3. Changes in osmolality depend, on volume, temperature and presence or absence of oil overlay. Changes in osmolality will occur slowly and is often an undetected parameter. The culture system should be correctly humidified and culture should be done, under oil.
4. Changes in pH occur rapidly and, like temperature, is related to the time the culture vessel stays out of the incubator and the time of exposure to air.
5. Ensure that all surfaces are warmed and that all materials that may come in contact with the oocytes are sterile, non-toxic and of tissue culture quality, preferably mouse embryo tested.

DISPOSABLES IN ART

This is the age of plastic laboratory ware. Charts showing the annual plastic production since the beginning of the 20th century are impressive. Almost flat until 1950 the production-curve has taken off in the seventies to reach nearly 250 million tons today. Though only a small portion of the annual production is used for lab plastic ware, plastic is to be found everywhere in the lab.

Most disposable cell culture dishes and plates are made of polystyrene, since some of its features perfectly meet the needs of cell culturing. Polystyrene is biologically inert, has excellent optical clarity and is hard and tough enough to withstand the daily use in incubators and other cell culture apparatus. Untreated polystyrene surfaces are, however, very hydrophobic, rendering them difficult for cells to attach. To overcome this drawback they are often modified with hydroxyl, keton, aldehyde, carboxyl or amine groups to increase the surface hydrophily and to introduce a negative or positive charge. Due to the low heat distortion point of polystyrene between 64°C and 80°C, polystyrene plastic wares would melt if autoclaved; hence they are the classic lab disposables. Polystyrene is a good choice for a lot of applications from cell culturing to ELISA.

The common plastics used in the ANT laboratory are:

1. Polypropylene (PP)
2. Polystyrene (PS)
3. Polyethylene (PE)
4. Polybutadiethylene (PBE)

QUALITY CONTROL TESTS

1. *Sterility assurance level (SAL):* Sterility assurance level (SAL) is a term used in microbiology to describe the *probability* of a single unit being non-sterile after it has been subjected to the *sterilization* process. For example, medical device manufacturers design their sterilization processes for an extremely low SAL (10^{-6}), "one in a million" devices should be non-sterile. SAL is also used to describe the killing efficacy of a sterilization process, where a very effective sterilization process has a very high SAL.

In microbiology it's impossible to prove that all organisms have been destroyed because: 1) they could be present but undetectable simply because they're not being incubated in their preferred environment and 2) they could be present but undetectable because their existence has never been discovered. Therefore, SALs are used to describe the probability that a given sterilization process has destroyed all of the microorganism.

Mathematically, SALs referring to probability are usually very small numbers and so are properly expressed as negative exponents. SALs referring to the sterilization efficacy are usually much larger numbers and so are properly expressed as positive exponents ("The SAL of this process is ten to the six"). In this usage, the negative effect of the process is sometimes inferred by using the word "reduction". ("This process gives a six-log reduction"). SALs can be used to describe the microbial population that was destroyed by the sterilization process. Each log reduction (10^{-1}) represents a 90% reduction in microbial population. So a process shown to achieve a "6-log reduction" (10^{-6}) will reduce a population from a million organisms (10^{6}) to very close to zero, theoretically. It is common to employ overkill cycles to provide greatest assurance of sterility for critical products such as implantable devices.

2. *Nonpyrogenicity* is another aspect which is important for the plastic lab ware in the IVF laboratories. It should not be reactive against heat and fire.

3. *USP Class VI and Elution test:* Protocols are certificate tests which confirms quality. The US pharmacopeia tests suitability of plastic ware before use in the laboratory. Class 6 testing is important for testing and validation of medical lab ware. It includes toxicity, intra cutaneous, systemic injection testing using one or more of four extracting media. The class 4 and class 6 test also include the USP Implantation test.

4. *Mouse embryo assay (MEA) test:* Blastocyst formation ratio larger than 80% for fully expanded blastocysts both in test and control is the desired outcome. The

embryo toxicity test is a release test and the product will only be sold if it has passed the test.

5. *Human sperm motility bioassay testing (HSSA-test) only for IVF tubes:* To pass the HSSA-test, the test samples motility of human sperm should be ≥70% after 24 hours of sample preparation. The control sample motility must be at least 50% of the initial swim-up motility for the test to be acceptable. The HSSA-test is a release test and the product will only be sold if it has passed satisfactorily.

6. *Limulus amebocyte lysate (LAL)* is an aqueous extract of blood cells *(amoebocytes)* from the *horseshoe crab*, Limulus polyphemus. LAL reacts with bacterial *endotoxin* or *lipopolysaccharide* (LPS), which is a membrane component of *Gram negative bacteria.* This reaction is the basis of the LAL test, which is used for the detection and quantification of bacterial endotoxins. *Fred Bang* reported in 1956 that gram-negative bacteria, even if killed, will cause the blood of the horseshoe crab to turn into a semi-solid mass. It was later recognized that the animal's blood cells, mobile cells called *amoebocytes,* contain granules with a *clotting factor* known as coagulogen. This is released outside the cell when bacterial endotoxin is encountered. The resulting *coagulation* is thought to contain bacterial infections in the animal's semi-closed *circulatory system.*

In 1970, the *US Food and Drug Administration (FDA)* approved LAL for testing drugs, products and devices that come in contact with the blood. Prior to that date, much slower and more expensive tests on *rabbits* had been used for this purpose.

Blood is removed from the horseshoe crab's pericardium and the crabs are returned to the water.

The blood cells are separated from the serum using *centrifugation* and are then placed in distilled water, which causes them to swell up and burst ("lyse"). This releases the chemicals from the inside of the cell (the "lysate"), which is then purified and *freeze-dried*. To test a sample for endotoxins, it is mixed with lysate and water; endotoxins are present if coagulation occurs.[2]

There are three basic LAL test methodologies: gel-clot, turbidimetric, and chromogenic. The primary application for LAL is the testing of parenteral pharmaceuticals and medical devices that contact blood or cerebrospinal fluid. In the United States, the FDA has published a guideline for validation of the LAL test as an endotoxin test for such products.

The LAL cascade is also triggered by $(1,3)$-β-D-glucan. Both bacterial endotoxins and $(1,3)$-β-D-glucan are considered "Pathogen-Associated Molecular Patterns", or PAMPS, substances which elicit inflammatory responses in mammals.

7. *Odor examination:* An example using the MEA and HSSA control tests.

    Odor from irradiated polystyrene and other plastics should not have any effect on embryo and sperm survival and this has been validated using the MEA and HSSA tests as mentioned below.

8. *MEA acceptance criterion:* ≥80% embryos have developed to blastocysts within 96 hours after fertilization.

TYPES OF DISPOSABLES

The various types of disposbley used in the ART Laboratory are petri dishes, pipettes, movettes, centrifuge tubes, culture dishes, 4 well dishes, etc. (Figs 9.16 to 9.31).

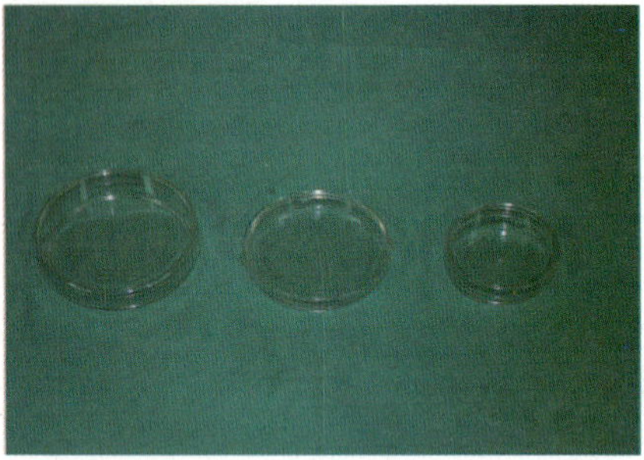

196 | *Protocols in Clinical Embryology and ART*

Fig. 9.16: *IVF petri dishes of various sizes for intended use is in vitro fertilization, procedures* used for insemination, culture and ICSI. CE marked according to Medical Devices Directive 93/42/EEC and produced in compliance with the FDA demands for IVF products

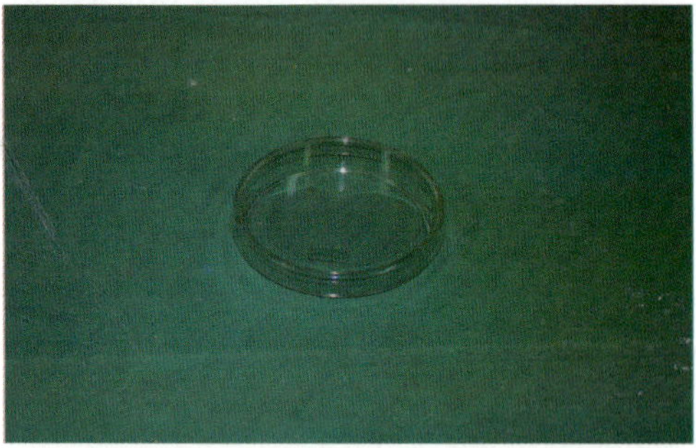

Fig. 9.17: 35×10 mm IVF grade plate-used commonly for insemination of oocyte cumulus complexes and droplet culture. May also be used for OCC harvesting from follicular fluid, TESE sample collection, for rinsing of OCC with culture media to wash oocytes free of of RBCs while harvesting from follicular fluid. Oil overlay is recommended as these plates have large surface area, which may lead to evaporation of the culture media thus bringing changes in the osmolarity and pH. Large surface area may lead to increased chances of contamination and sudden loss of temperature of the droplets if they are not covered with oil

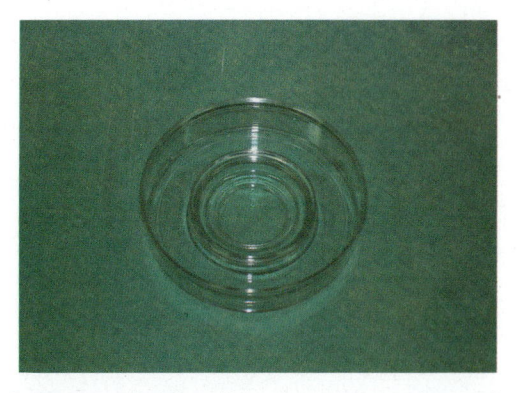

Fig. 9.18: Single well dishes (falcon)-used for embryo culture and for group insemination. Also used for rinsing of OCC in bicarbonate-based media and short incubation of oocytes. The well has volume of 1 ml and oil overlay is recommended

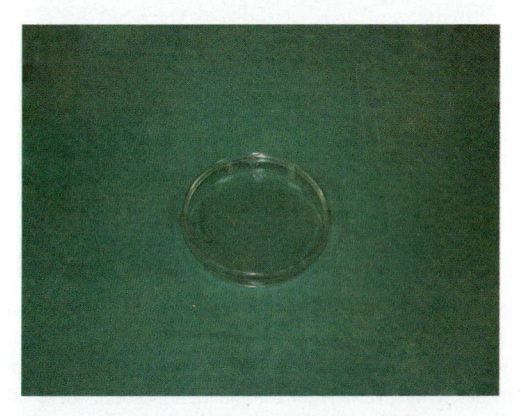

Fig. 9.19: ICSI dish (Falcon)-the dish has edges, which can snugly fit into the micromanipulator. This allows for easy handling of the droplets and the ICSI procedure. Always cover the ICSI drops with oil so as to avoid contamination pH and temperature changes of the media droplets

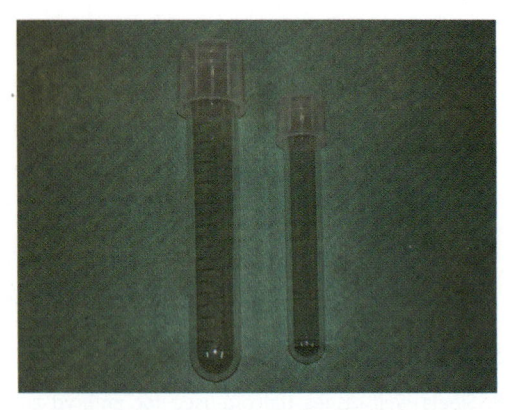

Fig. 9.20: *Falcon polystyrene IVF test tubes.* 17x100 mm, 14 ml and 5 ml polystyrene round bottom test tube with a 1400 RCF rating. They are used during egg harvesting, cyst aspiration, storing and dispensing media, and preparation of semen sample

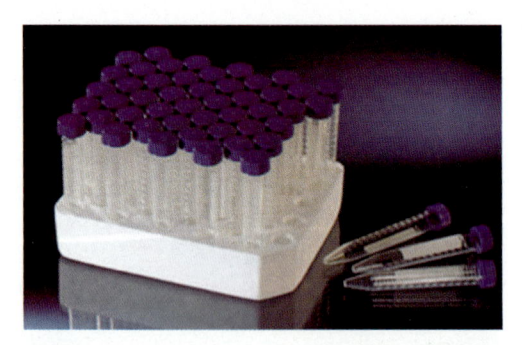

Fig. 9.21: IVF conical test tubes - used for centrifugation. These have printed volume graduations along length of tube with moulded graduations at conical section. Tubes meets USP Class VI. Flat cap and frosted area on tube provides writing surface for sample identification. These tubes have leak-proof closure. Polybutadiene styrene (PBS) tube has excellent optical clarity and rated at 3,000 x g relative centrifugal force (RCF), withstands temperatures to 90°C and are non-pyrogenic. Polypropylene (PP) tubes has excellent chemical resistance, rated at 7,800 x g RCF, withstands temperatures up to 125°C and are RNAse/DNAse free

Culture Media in IVF and Embryo Culture | **199**

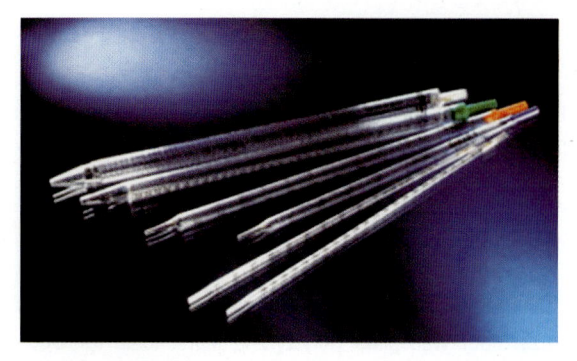

Fig. 9.22: Disposable polysterene pipettes. Accurate, disposable plastic pipettes, cotton plugged and sterilized have color-coded packaging for ease in sorting and selecting the correct size. These individually wrapped in paper-peelable bags, have convenient extra graduations to full pipette volume, printed with a black scale

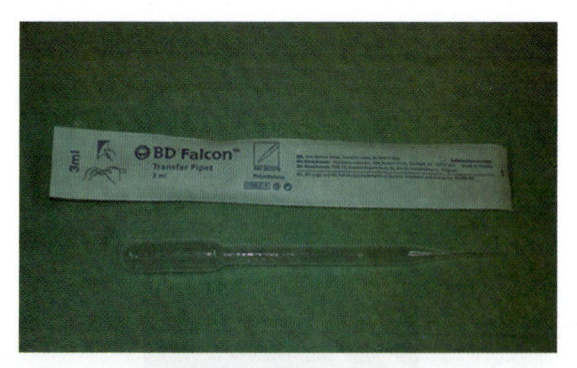

Fig. 9.23: 3 ml polypropylene falcon pipettes. Highly durable one-piece polyethylene individually packed pipette. One squeeze draws 3 ml into this 6-inch transfer pipette. Small tip ensures consistent reproduction of drop size. These are graduated at 1 ml and 2 ml. Commonly used for oocyte cumulus complex handling, media dispensing and for semen preparation

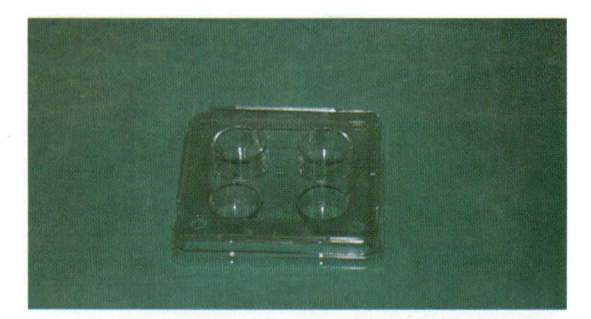

Fig. 9.24: Four well plate polystyrene plate. Ideal for OCC-sperm co-incubation for embryo culture either in 0.5 ml volume or microdroplet culture under oil and embryo transfers. Treated by vacuum gas plasma. Some users may face difficulties with physical interactions between surface and the droplet, e.g. droplets of specific sizes that become flat due to the hydrophilic nature of the treated surface. With a nontreated product this problem is eliminated. NUNC produces both nontreated – less hydrophilic and nunclon delta – hydrophilic IVF plates

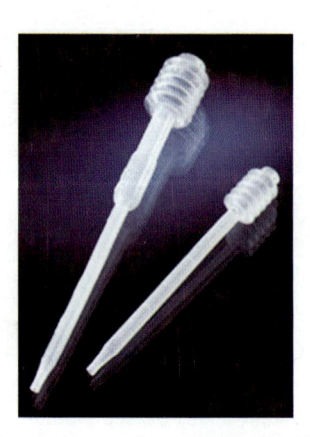

Fig. 9.25: Plastic Pipettes: For semi quantitative liquid handling made of polypropylene. Easy to handle, strong suction capacity, available in two sizes: 1.5 and 5 ml

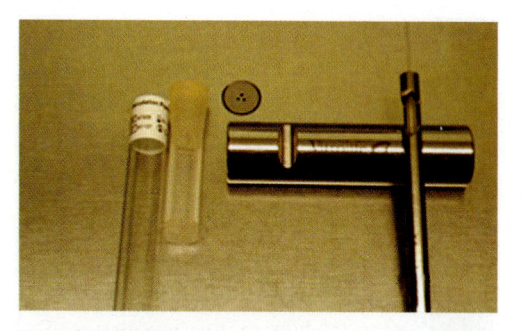

Fig. 9.26: Swemed glass pipettes and handle. The denudation pipettes are intended for removal of the cumulus cell layers of the oocyte. The transfer pipettes are intended for manipulation and transfer of oocytes, embryos and blastocysts, or to check for fertilization. The ready made individually packed denuding pipette diameter may vary from 130, 140, 170, 200, 275, 300 and 600 depending on the usage. 170 is good for OCC denuding for fertilization check. If the cumulus is tightly packed and does not to leave the oocyte easily, use of 140-size pipette does help. 170 is ideal for zygote/cleavage stage, embryo transfer to media droplets/during vitrification, etc. 300 is ideal for blastocyst transfers between media plates. 600 is recommended for OCC handling and manipulation

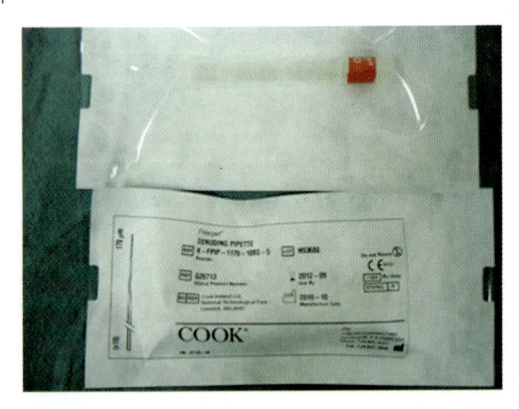

Fig. 9.27: Cook flexipets available in various sizes. Used for denuding cumulus mass from the oocyte prior to ICSI, to check fertilization, or for manipulation of oocytes, embryos, blastocysts and blastomeres.
- The flexible polycarbonate pipettes are designed for use with reusable pipetting handles/cook handle
- Supplied sterile; sold as individual vials - ten (10) per vial, or in boxes of five (5) vials - fifty (50 pipettes per box)

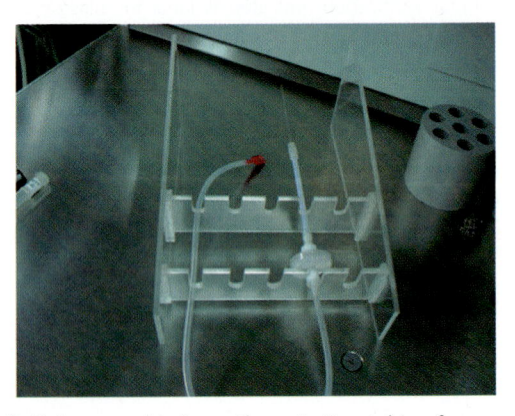

Fig. 9.28: Fully assembled mouth aspiration tubing for oocyte and embryo handling. Red mouthpiece and 0.2 µm filter can be easily appreciated

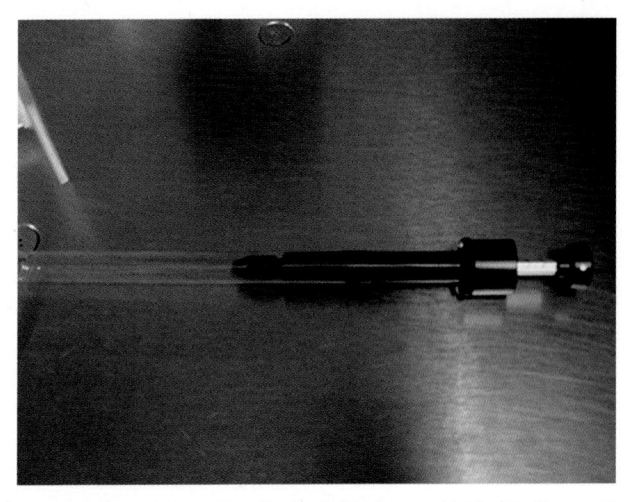

Fig. 9.29: *Micro pipette. Handle:* Available from midatlantic diagnostics, cook medical, swemed, etc. Used with flexipet pipettes for handling gametes and embryos. Aspiration volume can be preset from 0.25 microliters to 3.0 microliters. Provides the fine control necessary for oocyte, embryo and blastomere manipulation. It can be used to strip cumulus and corona cells from oocyte prior to ICSI procedures, easily removes the corona to assess the presence of pronuclei in conventional IVF and safely transfers embryos and oocytes through various media and solutions Unique dispenser packaging maintains sterility. The body is constructed from machined aluminum and the plunger from high quality stainless steel, making it very easy to keep the unit clean and sanitary

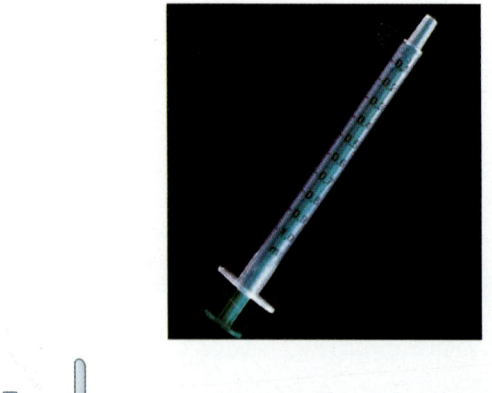

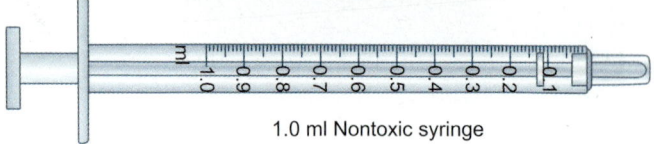

Fig. 9.30: Nontoxic two-piece syringe contains no rubber. We use it for embryo transfer and embryo reduction procedures

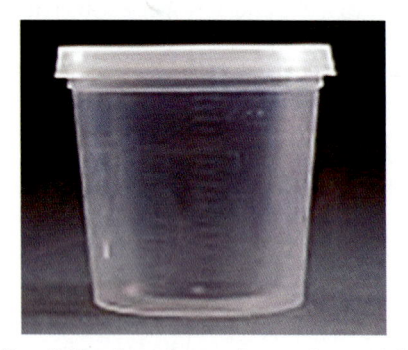

Fig. 9.31: 4 1/2 oz (110 ml) sterile sample container with lid. Disposable polypropylene containers provide secure sample containment. Molded in graduations for easy measurement. Graduated in ounces and milliliters; from ½ oz. to 4½ oz. in ¼ oz. increments, and from 20 ml to 110 ml in 10 ml increments. Inert and chemically resistant to commonly used laboratory reagents at room temperature. Sterilized by gamma irradiation

REFERENCES

1. IVF Manual. Recommended use of G5 Series™ Eds Gardner DK. Edition 2, May 2008.
2. Gardner DK, Reed L, Linck D, Sheehan C, Lane M. Quality control in human *in vitro* fertilization. Semin Reprod Med. 2005;23(4):319-24.
3. Gardner DK, Lane M, Embryo culture systems. Handbook of *in Vitro* Fertilisation (Second edn.), Eds. Trounson AO and Gardner DK, CRC Press, Boca Raton. 1990;205-64.
4. Davidson A, Vermesh M, Lobo RA, Paulson RJ. Mouse embryo culture as quality control for human *in vitro* fertilisation: the one-cell versus the two-cell model. Fertil. Steril. 1998;49: 516-21.
5. Lane M, Gardner DK. Differential regulation of mouse embryo development and viability by amino acids. Reprod Fertil. 1997;109: 153-64.

Chapter 10

Andrology and Beyond

Pankaj Talwar, Kuldeep Jain

SEMEN PREPARATION FOR IVF

Introduction

Sperm preparation is carried out in order to remove the seminal plasma, dead spermatozoa, and other cells, as well as to select the best spermatozoa.

The choice of sperm preparation method is based on patient history and previous semen analysis as well as an examination of the present sample. Another consideration is whether the fertilization will be performed by IVF or ICSI, as more spermatozoa are needed for IVF insemination.

Prior to being used for IUI, IVF and ICSI, motile sperm cells are separated from the seminal plasma, dead sperm cells and other cells. This can be done by different procedures.

The preparation methods select sperm based on their motility, ideally selecting only live sperm, or on their density thus selecting only mature sperms. If the sperm count and motility are adequate, migration (swim-up) is suitable. If semen quality is poor and includes large numbers of other cells, density gradient centrifugation is preferred. Recovery of sperm is more effective using the gradient centrifugation method rather than using the swim-up procedure, with respect to total yield. However, in some instances percent motility can be higher in sperm prepared by swim-up.[1]

The initial sperm separation methods recommended one or two washing procedures with subsequent resuspension of the spermatozoa or swim-up from the pellet. Latter, more sophisticated methods were developed to obtain sufficient amounts of motile, functionally competent spermatozoa for IVF. The aim was to universal method for all types of semen sample having improved sperm functions and reduced detrimental effects from reactive oxygen species.

Essentials of Sperm Preparation[2,3]

1. The sperm preparation should be performed in a clean aseptic work area. Nontoxic, nonpowdered gloves and protective eyeglasses should be worn while handling semen samples.
2. All samples should be collected in appropriate sterile, nontoxic jars. It is recommended that the semen sample be collected not more than one hour before preparation. The semen sample should be protected from cold and heat.
3. All laboratory procedures, including a thorough identification protocol of the patient should be followed.
4. The first portion of the ejaculate contains most of the spermatozoa (high fraction) while the rest of the ejaculate mostly consists of secretion from the seminal vesicle (low fraction). It is therefore of the utmost importance that the first drops of the ejaculate are collected in the test tube provided for sperm collection.
5. Time from ejaculation to the beginning of sperm preparation should not exceed 60 minutes.
6. A normal semen sample liquefies within 30-60 minutes after ejaculation.
7. Incubating sperm in the seminal plasma for too long will reduce recovery of motile sperm and render the

sperm unable to undergo the alterations that make them capable of fertilization.
8. It is not recommended to centrifuge raw semen as potential toxic round cells and dead spermatozoa will concentrate around the motile spermatozoa.
9. For viscous semen samples, sperm preparation medium can be mixed with the semen sample prior to the sperm preparation.

Nomenclature—Semen Variables (WHO)

The common terms we use while preparing sample are enumerated below.[2]

1. WHO Parameters 2010

Parameter	Lower reference limit
Semen volume (ml)	1.5 (1.4-1.7)
Total sperm number (10^6 per ejaculate)	39 (33-46)
Sperm concentration (10^6 per ml)	15 (12-16)
Total motility (PR + NP, %)	40 (38-42)
Progressive motility (PR, %)	32 (31-34)
Vitality (live spermatozoa, %)	58 (55-63)
Sperm morphology (normal forms, %)	4 (3.0 – 4.0)
Other consensus threshold values	
pH	≥ 7.2
Peroxidase-positive leukocytes (10^6 per ml)	< 1.0
MAR test (motile spermatozoa with bound particles, %)	< 50
Immunobead test (motile spermatozoa with bound particles, %)	< 50
Seminal zinc (μmol/ejaculate)	≥ 2.4

Seminal fructose (µmol/ejaculate)	≥ 13
Seminal neutral glucosidase (mU/ejaculate)	≥ 20

2. Comparative analysis of the WHO report: Analyzing the values of WHO values (1999) and WHO values (2010)

Volume: The WHO manual 1999 states 2 ml or more as normal whereas WHO 2010 states even 1.5 ml of ejaculate is within the normal limits.

Sperm count/ejaculate: It is same 40 mill/ejaculate (WHO 1999) v/s 39 million/ejaculate (WHO 2010).

Sperm concentration/ml: 20 mill/ml (WHO 1999) v/s 15 mill/ml (WHO 2010).

Total motility: 50% or more (WHO 1999) v/s 40% (WHO 2010).

Progressive motility: 25% or more (WHO 1999) v/s 32% (WHO 2010).

Morphology (Normal %): 15% normal (WHO 1999) v/s 4% (WHO 2010).

Vitality (live spermatozoa, %): 50% or more live, i.e. excluding the dye (WHO 1999) v/s 58% (WHO 2010)

WBCs: Less than 1 million (WHO 1999) v/s <1 million (WHO 2010).

pH: 7.2 or more in WHO (1999, 2010).

In conclusion, we can say that parameters like sperm count/ejaculate, pH, vitality and the number of WBCs in ejaculate is the same in both the WHO manuals.

Sperm concentration (/ml) of 15 million is considered as normal so also is total motility of 40%, which clearly indicates that the values have been relaxed than the WHO 1991.

Major difference is seen in the percent of normal morphology of sperms from 15% in WHO 1999 to as low as 4% in WHO 2010.

This clearly indicates that the values of most of the semen parameters are relaxed in the WHO manual 2010.

3. Advantages: With the WHO manual (2010), the number of males falling within the normal range of semen parameters will clearly increase and it is definitely an encouraging news to the couples trying to conceive naturally or with help of assisted reproductive techniques.

From the old quantifying criterions of semen volume and sperm count, the focus has shifted to more specific criterions like morphology, progressive sperm motility and vitality.

Reduce the incidence of male infertility in general population.

Enormous psychological trauma to the male when labeled with infertility will lessen and probably he would able to take control of the painful treatment better.

Relieve financial burden on the infertile couple.

Unwanted side effects of the drugs on the patients are avoided, as less number of male infertility cases would be identified.

4. Disadvantages: WHO parameters are having very low limit for the markers of fertility. 5th percentile looks very convincing but clinical apprehensions persists.

Morphology is the major parameter, which has been altered.

Study carried out in European countries, Australia and USA. Majority of the Afro-Asian countries are under-represented.

Third world countries do not have andrology facilities as in Europe, nor qualified manpower to carry out the test in quality controlled laboratories. This may alter the outcome while considering the values of sperm morphology, which is specific in the outcome in infertility cases.

5. Confusion
Morphology: Plays an important role in deciding for ICSI. 4% normal morphology creates a scare in the mind about the outcome if ICSI is not carried out.

Motility: Fall of motility from 50 to 40% is again conflicting. We are scared to do normal insemination and prefer ICSI in cases with semen count of 15 million with 40% active sperms only.

In short, the new semen parameters have to be taken with pinch of salt till the time as we embryologists have worked forfew years and are reassured that our results are not falling.

To summarize the WHO 2010 needs re-evaluation in the clinical settings before adopting them fully at ART centers.

6. Future: Semen parameters are being relaxed with passing years. More emphasis is being laid on the intrinsic factors then the quantifying factors. We would soon be able to achieve fertilization both *in vivo* and in *vitro* with lower values of semen parameters, thus increasing the chances of fertility .The incidence of male infertility will also reduce at some extent.

Techniques of Semen Preparation
Swim-up and Wash

1. This method is commonly used on semen samples with normal sperm count/motility and selects the spermatozoa based on motility, ideally selecting only live sperm.

2. Aseptic technique should be used and semen should be processed within one hour of collection.
3. Allow approximately 20 minutes for liquefaction of semen. If the sample does not liquefy, you may need to pass it through a 23-gauge needle or a nontoxic sterile narrow Pasteur pipette.
4. Make a microscopic assessment of the sperm sample to confirm the optimal method for processing the sperm.
5. Flushing medium/sperm preparation media (MediCult), gamete buffer (Cook), sperm rinse (Vitrolife) is used for the initial swim-up. Warm the (sperm preparation/sperm rinse medium) to 37°C and equilibrate in a 6% CO_2 incubator for a minimum of 4 hours prior to use. Other media have to be only warmed, as they are HEPES based.
6. Gently underlay (300 µl) of fully liquefied semen under 0.5 ml of equilibrated flushing medium/sperm preparation media (MediCult), gamete buffer (Cook), sperm rinse (Vitrolife) in round bottom 5 ml tubes.
7. Place tubes in a test tube rack so that the tubes are at 60° angle to the horizontal. Place the rack in the CO_2 incubator. The test tubes are incubated at 37°C for 30–60 minutes to allow the spermatozoa to swim-up from the liquefied semen. Confirmation that sperm have successfully swum-up into the overlaying culture medium is reflected by an increase in turbidity. If the culture medium appears clear, then more time may be needed to allow spermatozoa the opportunity to swim out of the pellet.
8. Remove the rack after 20 to 60 minutes and remove the medium above the semen sample (approximately 250 µl of supernatant is removed).
9. Add 4.0 ml of equilibrated Universal medium (MediCult), fertilization medium (cook), G-IVF™

PLUS (Vitrolife) to the aspirated sample and centrifuge at 600 g for 10 minutes.
10. Remove the supernatant and resuspend the pellet in a small volume of equilibrated Universal medium (MediCult), fertilization medium (Cook), G-IVF™ PLUS (Vitrolife).
11. Count sperm and calculate the concentration.
12. Adjust as required. Store in a 6% CO_2 incubator at 37°C until required.

The principle of this conventional wash and swim-up method is based on the active movement of spermatozoa from the cell pellet into an overlaying medium. Typically, the incubation time is 60 minutes. This technique has a recovery of a very high percentage (>90%) of motile sperm in the absence of contaminating dead or immotile spermatozoa, nongerm cells, and debris. The efficiency of the technique is based on the surface area of the cell pellet and the initial sperm motility in the ejaculate. The yield of motile spermatozoa is limited by the concept of pellet formation. Many layers of cells in the pellet may not allow healthy motile spermatozoa in the lower levels of the pellet to reach the interface with the culture medium layer. In addition, a significant decrease in the percentage of normally chromatin-condensed spermatozoa has been reported after the swim-up procedure.

Density Gradient Centrifugation Method

This typical methodology for the density gradient centrifugation comprises of continuous[4] or discontinuous gradients.[5] In the continuous gradient technique, there is a gradual increase in density from the top of the gradient to its bottom, whereas the layers of a discontinuous gradient show clear boundaries between each other. The ejaculate is placed on top of the density media and is then centrifuged for 15 to 30 minutes. During this procedure, all cells reach the semen sediment. Highly active and motile spermatozoa move actively in the direction of the sedimentation gradient and can therefore penetrate the boundary quicker than less motile and or immotile cells. Thus we find that highly motile sperm cells are enriched in the soft pellet at the bottom. This method can be used to wash all samples of sperm regardless of quality.

Colloidal gradient is a solution stabilized with suprasperm (MediCult), sperm gradient (K-SISG) (Cook), SpermGrad™ (Vitrolife) covalently bound hydrophilic silane coated, colloidal silica particles in an isotonic balanced salt solution. By preparing different dilutions of, solutions of different densities are obtained. Layering these solutions of different densities carefully in a centrifuge tube creates a density gradient. Cells and other particles with different buoyant densities will sediment until they reach a solution with higher density. Centrifugation accelerates this sedimentation. We Commonly use, a two-step gradient of 90% and 45% SpermGrad™. Since mature sperm with tightly packed DNA have a higher density than 90% SpermGrad™, they sediment through this layer and are found at the bottom of the tube, whereas other cells, including immature and dead sperm, stop sedimenting at the 90% or 45% interface. SpermGrad™ is to be diluted in G-IVF™ PLUS for 90% and 45% gradients. G-IVF™ PLUS must be equilibrated at +37°C and 6% CO_2 before use. The final suspension of the pellet after the procedure is done in Universal medium (MediCult), fertilization medium (Cook), G-IVF™ PLUS (Vitrolife).

Procedure of sperm preparation by double density gradient media (Vitrolife):

1. Mix SpermGrad™ with supplemented G-IVF™ PLUS in separate tubes to obtain 90% and 45% stock solutions. For 90% stock solution, mix 9.0 ml SpermGrad™ with 1.0 ml supplemented G-IVF™. For 45% stock solution, mix 4.5 ml SpermGrad™ with 5.5 ml supplemented G-IVF™. Mix the solutions thoroughly and store in sterile nontoxic tubes or sterile tissue culture flasks. Label and refrigerate until use.
2. Always use a sterile nontoxic pipette to aliquot amounts needed for individual sperm preparations. Stock solutions should be labeled with the date and kept for recommended time frames. Before use, allow the solutions to warm to ambient temperature and allow them to equilibrate in 6% CO_2 to attain correct pH.
3. The density gradient should be layered in 2 to 4 sterile and rinsed conical nontoxic centrifuge tubes (depending on the volume of the semen sample) marked with patient ID.
4. Pipette 1.5 ml of 90% solution into the tube first and then slowly pipette 1.5 ml of 45% solution on top of it. Finally, 1.0 ml of the semen is gently layered on the top.
5. Make up 2 to 4 gradient tubes. Up to 2 ml of semen can be layered on top of the gradient.
6. If the semen sample is of normal quality reduce the semen volume. Adding too much semen will result in poor separation.
7. The tubes are then centrifuged for 10 to 20 minutes at 300 to 600 g.
8. Remove the two top layers and take care not to leave any residue' on the tube wall.

9. Transfer the sperm pellets with as little of the 90% solution as possible to a sterile conical rinsed tube with 5 ml of equilibrated supplemented G-IVF PLUS and centrifuge for 10 minutes at 300–600 g.
10. Aspirate and discard the supernatants and repeat the wash. After the second wash, combine pellets and resuspended in 1 ml of equilibrated supplemented G-IVF™ PLUS.
11. Dilute the washed sample with equilibrated supplemented G-IVF™ PLUS to a final concentration of 75,000 to 200000 motile sperm/ml.
12. Alternatively: Add equilibrated sperm suspension to equilibrated dishes with the oocytes already present. It is recommended to inseminate in a volume of 0.5 to 1.0 ml without oil overlay. If oil overlay is used, droplets of at least 100 μl volumes are recommended.

Advantage of the density gradient method is the recovery of a higher percentage of morphologically normal spermatozoa than found in conventional swim-up or glass wool filtration. This method harvests spermatozoa from ejaculates with a very low sperm density, sperms can be separated with good yields, round cells and dead sperms are eliminated to a large extent and reactive oxygen species are significantly reduced in the semen sample.

The technique has also been shown to yield sperm populations with better DNA quality and chromatin packaging.[6,7] Further, preliminary reports suggest that specimens known to be contaminated with sexually transmissible viruses can effectively be "cleaned up" using density gradient centrifugation and the isolated spermatozoa can be used for therapy with exceptionally low risk for horizontal disease transmission.[8]

One disadvantage of density gradient centrifugation is that the density gradient medium is a bit more expensive than either of the swim-up techniques, and there is a potential risk of endotoxins from the gradient constituents.

Double Wash and Swim-Up

This method is commonly used on semen samples with normal sperm count/motility and selects the spermatozoa based on motility, ideally selecting only live sperm.

1. Semen sample is mixed with 4 ml of Flushing medium (MediCult), gamete buffer (Cook), sperm rinse (Vitrolife) after the sample is liquefied.
2. The sample and the media mixture are now transferred to the 15 ml round conical tube (Falcon) and the sample is centrifuged for 10 minutes at 1500 RPM. This step insures that the sample is mixed with the media and the dead sperms and leukocytes and debris are separated.
3. Now the supernatant is discarded and the pellet resuspended in 2 ml of Universal medium (MediCult), fertilization medium (cook) or sperm rinse medium (Vitrolife). Pellet is gently and thoroughly mixed with the above media and transferred to the 5 ml conical tube (Falcon).
4. The sample is now spun for 5 minutes at 1500 RPM in a centrifuge machine.
5. The supernatant is discarded and approximately 700 microliters of Universal medium (MediCult), fertilization medium (Cook), G-IVF™ PLUS (Vitrolife) overlaid on the pellet.
6. The 5 ml (Falcon) tube is placed in rack and kept in the CO_2 incubator at 37°C for 20 minutes at an angle for the final swim-up. Swim-up from an intact sperm pellet requires that centrifugation speeds be such that the final pellet is loosely compacted. If we get a tight pellet the sperms may not swim-up from it leading

to lower yield. The consistency of the pellet may be verified by gently and slowly tilting the test tube and observing whether the pellet tilts or not. If we have to resuspend the sperm pellet, then extreme care must be taken to ensure that no mixing occurs when overlaying the non-compacted pellet with the culture medium.

7. Remember to keep the cap loose so that the sample can be easily equilibrated (exchange of CO_2 can take place).
8. After 20 minutes the swim-up is removed and placed in a fresh 5 ml tube for minimum 15 minutes for equilibration. The efficiency of the sperm swim-up is based not only on the initial sperm motility in the ejaculate, but also on the size, level of compaction, and exposed surface area of the final pellet.
9. Meanwhile perform the semen count and insemination may be carried out within 2 hours of removing the final swim-up.
10. This technique remains my favorite and has given us persistently good results. It is easy to perform and reproduce.

Advantages of this method are that it is the simplest and the least expensive to perform with recovery of a high percentage of motile sperm and absence of other cells and debris. The swim-up method also results in significant improvement in the rates of acrosome reaction, hypo-osmotic swelling (HOS), and nuclear maturity.

A disadvantage of the swim-up from washed pellet is the low overall recovery of motile spermatozoa. Motile spermatozoa trapped at the bottom of the pellet may never be able to reach the interface with the culture medium. A noncompacted, soft pellet may lead to immotile spermatozoa, leukocytes, squamous epithelial cells, or noncellular debris in the swim-up. This technique also may cause a sudden burst of ROS produced by the damaged sperms. The Reactive oxygen species were found to impair the functional competence of normal spermatozoa in the same suspension and lead to impairment in impaired capacity for sperm–oocyte fusion.

Peculiar Conditions

Obstructive Azoospermia: Epididymal and Testicular Sperm

Epididymal sperm: Epididymal sperm can be obtained by MESA (microscopic epididymal aspiration) or PESA (percutaneous epididymal sperm aspiration) by using 21 'g' butterfly needle to aspirate fluid.[6]

- If large number of sperms are obtained, they can be processed by swim-up or buoyant density gradient. Density gradient is preferred.
- If only few sperm are found, the sample is washed and centrifuged with fresh media and resuspended in minimal volume of media.

A drop is put in ICSI injection dish under oil and sperms are picked up using injection pipette.

Testicular sperms: Testicular sperms can be obtained by TESE (Testicular sperm extraction-open method) or by TESA (Testicular sperm aspiration) using butterfly needle.[7]

Specimen obtained is crushed between two slides or by fine scissors or by a fine needle.[8,9]

Further processing is similar as for epididymal sperm depending on number of sperms obtained. If no motile sperm are present, sperm are suspended in a fresh drop and observed under phase contrast optics of inverted microscope for occasional twitching of tail and are harvested for ICSI. Alternatively, sperms are put in a hypo-osmotic solution drop and observed for curling of tail suggestive of viability. Such sperms are picked up and washed in fresh media drop before used for ICSI.

Retrograde Ejaculation

In cases of retrograde ejaculation, alkalization of urine is carried out by alkalizers 48 to 72 hours before the procedure. Before ejaculation, bladder is catheterized and emptied. Approximately 20 ml of media is instilled in the bladder. After ejaculation, bladder is emptied immediately and sample centrifuged. Pellet is resuspended in fresh media and processed on buoyant gradient for IVF or ICSI.

Erectile dysfunction: In cases of significant erectile dysfunction, use of sildenafil and abstinence may help. In severe cases vibratory stimulus may be used. In very severe cases, or those with spinal cord injury, electroejaculation under general anesthesia can help obtain samples.

Basis of Centrifugation

Two important factors which have a relevant impact on the outcome of the centrifugation procedure are the temperature and centrifugation speed during the semen preparation. Unfortunately all the centrifuge machines locally available do not have temperature control or G force regulation.[9]

1. *g-force:* The exact indication of g-force helps the ideal sperm pellet formation by subjecting the sperm to an exact and precise amount of g–force. Now a days centrifugation speeds are never reported in RPM as those numbers are not useful for any one wanting to reproduce the method. (Being dependent Rotor radius). The existing dependency on RPM can be eliminated by on screen g-force selection by using spermfuge centrifuge machine (manufactured by Shivani scientific India)

The g-force of your centrifuge can be calculated using this formula:

$g = 1.118 \times r \times rpm^2$ or

$rpm = \text{Square root}\{g/(1.118 \times r)\}$

r = radius of centrifuge in mm

Rpm = rotations per minute/1000

Example 1

r = 100 mm, rpm = 1800 rotations per minute

$g = 1.118 \times 100 \times 3.24 = 362$ g

Example 2

R = 100 mm, g = 350 g,

rpm = SQR $\{350/(1.118 \times 100)\}$ = 1.77 rpm = 1770 rotations per minute

---

Tips while centrifuging the sample and handling the pellet

1. Balance centrifuge with a tube filled with the same volume of water
2. Do not centrifuge for more than 20 minutes, as abnormal sperms may also accumulate at the bottom, lowering percentage of motile sperms
3. Do not break the spin when removing the tube from the centrifuge
4. Do not disturb the pellet. If pellet is disturbed recentrifuge for afew minutes longer until pellet is reformed
5. If sperm count is low, a clearly defined pellet may not be present. In that case remove all but 0.8 ml of the medium.

---

2. *Temperature:* Maintenance of this critical temperature throughout the entire sperm processing procedure helps the sperm maintain their peak motility and enhanced linearity.

Spermfuge is an improvised centrifuge, dedicated totally for elevating the total motile sperm recovery from the parent semen sample, by controlling/maintaining the main parameter of "temperature" thus aimed at enhancing the

ART results. The instrument has been designed to regulate and subsequently maintain the "critical" inner chamber temperature before, after and during centrifugation. The two of the most vital parameters which act as a yardstick to gauge the effectiveness of an ideal sperm wash.

The Spermfuge has been designed after taking into consideration detailed cellular physiological demands, locomotion kinetics and pooling together ideal suggestions, opinions, ideas and propositions of numerous andrologists and embryologists and other professionals in the field of human reproduction.

The Spermfuge with its temperature controlled chamber (room temperature to 42°C), programmable microprocessor based controls, multiple tube selection, accurate g-force selection, independent centrifugation and/or heating selection and other added advantages make it an ideal state of the art instrument for use in an ART laboratory.

Improvement of Motility and Sperm Function

Many chemicals and chemically defined pharmacological substances like progesterone, adenosine analogs have been proposed to stimulate human sperm functions. Caffeine, pentoxifylline and 2-deoxyadenosine are substances that were used to stimulate motility. Recent approaches to stimulate spermatozoa include bicarbonate, metal chelators or platelet-activating factor (PAF). Few of these methodologies used for improving the sperm of the semen are discussed below.

Pentoxifylline

Pentoxifylline is a nonspecific inhibitor of phosphodi-esterase that has stimulatory effects on sperm motility and motion characteristics like sperm velocity or hyper-activity. The stimulatory effect is attributed to increased intracellular levels of cAMP via inhibition of its breakdown by cAMP phosphodiesterase. Pentoxifylline is also reported to enhance the acrosome reaction[10] presumably by increasing the levels of cAMP.

The results of pentoxifylline treatment in assisted reproduction are equivocal. Depending on the conditions, especially the time of stimulation relative to the capacitative state of the spermatozoa and the concentration of pentoxifylline in the medium, overstimulation can result in a premature acrosome reaction. Thus, pentoxifylline is not used routinely in the ART. There are trends towards use of pentoxifylline in the preparation of epididymal and testicular sperm for IVF/ICSI.

Spermatozoa retrieved from the testis are immature physiologically than epididymal or ejaculated spermatozoa. Treatment of immotile or very poorly motile fresh cryopreserved testicular spermatozoa with pentoxifylline very frequently simulates some form of motion, from twitching to nonprogressive motility. This helps us in sperm selection for ICSI. The combination of these two attributes lends greater assurance that the DNA has not been made more vulnerable to the deleterious effects of ROS.

Platelet-Activating Factor

Platelet-activating factor (PAF) is a biologically active phospholipid thought to be a cellular mediator in regulating spermatozoal function of many different species, including human. PAF has been reported to have positive effects on motility, capacitation, acrosome reaction, and oocyte fusion.[11,12] The positive effect of PAF on sperm function has led to its use in assisted reproduction. Roudebush et al.[13] reported that pregnancy rates in IUI cycles were significantly increased after the spermatozoa from normozoospermic males were prepared with a medium containing PAF.

Hypo-osmotic Swelling Test (HOS)

Sperm motility is an important indicator of viability, especially when performing ICSI. when the testicular/epidiymal/ejaculated sperms are immotile the assessment of viability becomes critical. Hypo-osmotic swelling test (HOS). This is a simple vitality test based on the semipermeability of the intact and physiologically functional plasma membrane which causes spermatozoa to swell under hypo-osmotic conditions, when an influx of water results in an expansion of cell volume.[14]

When setting up a dish for the ICSI procedure, a small (5 µL) drop of HOS solution is placed near the PVP drop and two extra drops of culture medium are placed nearby. A small volume of sperm suspension is placed in one of the extra drops. When spermatozoa are located, they are picked up in the ICSI micropipette and placed in the HOS solution. Immediately after contact with the hypo-osmotic medium, the tails of some spermatozoa will begin to coil or swell. Tail swelling or curling indicates that the cell is viable. The spermatozoon is then picked up in the ICSI micropipette and placed in the other extra drop of medium in order to wash off excess hypo-osmotic medium from both the micropipette and the spermatozoon. The spermatozoon is then placed in the PVP drop in order to proceed with ICSI.

The Ideal Sperm Separation Technique Should

 i. Be fast, easy to perform and cost-effective.
 ii. Isolate as much motile spermatozoa as possible.
 iii. Does not cause sperm membrane damage of the sperm cells.
 iv. Eliminate dead spermatozoa and other cells, including leukocytes and bacteria.

v. Eliminates and does not generate toxic substances like reactive oxygen species (ROS).

Till date we don't have any ideal method of sperm preparation and we have to select the available method from the various options available depending upon the semen sample

The choice and application of the appropriate sperm preparation technique can be a major contributor in influencing the quality of sperms used for IVF. Ejaculates from infertile/subfertile males commonly have the potential for producing ROS, which are known to compromise sperm function and damage DNA. Therefore, it is imperative that the laboratory technician selects a technique that will directly separate functional and highly motile spermatozoa from all that remains. Density gradient centrifugation is the ideal and most effective method for semen preparation.

Thus, depending on the initial sperm parameters, the direct swim-up from semen can safely and effectively be used for semen preparation. We have to remember that final outcome of IVF depends upon the quality of semen preparation, thus this critical step should never be ignored.

Tips
- A flexible approach is required in order to obtain a suitable sample for IVF and ICSI
- Preprocedural detailed evaluation is very important and helps in deciding the method to be adopted
- A trial preparation may be carried out before the actual procedure to select appropriate semen preparation method especially in cases with variable previous reports
- Problem of wide variation in two seminal sample can be handled by obtaining a second sample after sometime and pooling the sample
- If recovery is not satisfactory in spite of appropriate method used, conversion to ICSI should be considered without any hesitation.

Appendix to Semen Preparation

Method (Figs 10.1A to E)

1. *Pelleting and swim-up method:* The method is good for normal semen parameters, with low volume or viscous samples. All preparations to be done under laminar flow at 37°C with aseptic precaution. Initial semen analysis to be done after liquefaction before starting the procedure in the following steps.
   - Mix equal volumes (1.5-2 ml) of semen with prewarmed Hepes buffered HTF media in 5 ml round bottom Falcon tube. If volume of semen is high, more tubes should be used.
   - Centrifuge at 1500 rpm for 10 minutes.

   > Practical Tip—Gently shake the pellet if it is too tight.

   - Carefully remove supernatant without disturbing the pellet.
   - Gently overlay 1 ml fresh HTF culture media over the pellet without disturbing the interface.

   Tips
   - Adjust the time according to motility of initial sample
   - Keeping the tube at a slant of 45 to 60 degrees creates a greater surface area of medium over the pellet and hence a better recovery of motile sperms.

   - Incubate for 30-45 minutes in CO_2 incubator with cap loosen.
   - Carefully remove supernatant from all tubes in a clean 5 ml round bottom falcon tube.
   - Centrifuge for 5 minutes at 1400 rpm.
   - Remove supernatant leaving 3 ml at the bottom.
   - Shake gently. Asses for count and motility.

228 | *Protocols in Clinical Embryology and ART*

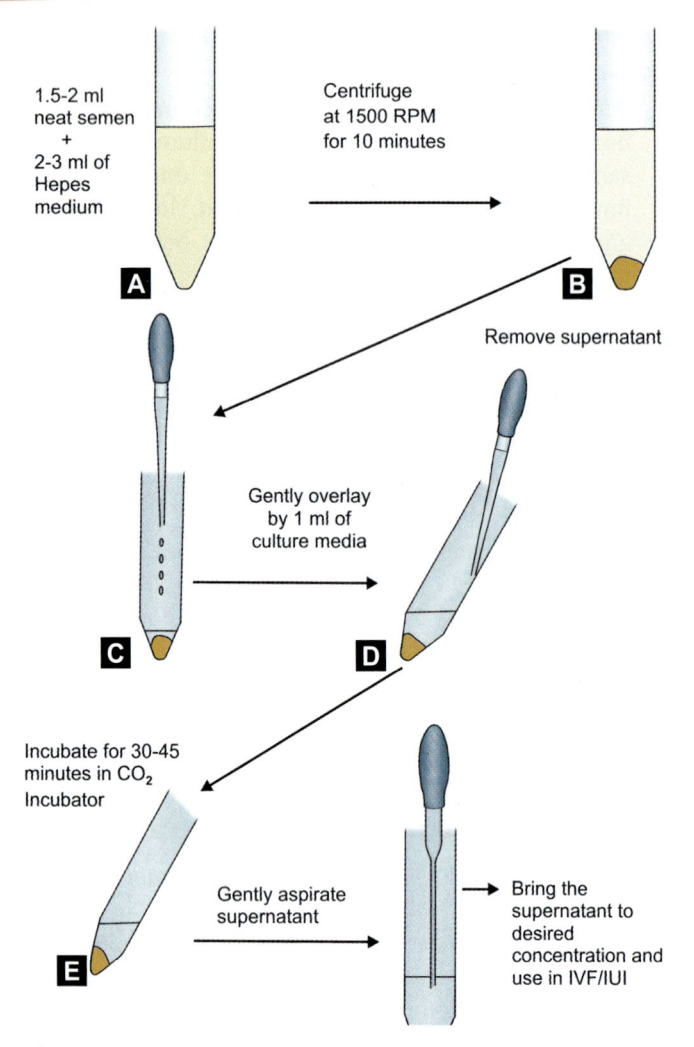

Figs 10.1A to E: Wash and swim-up method

Andrology and Beyond

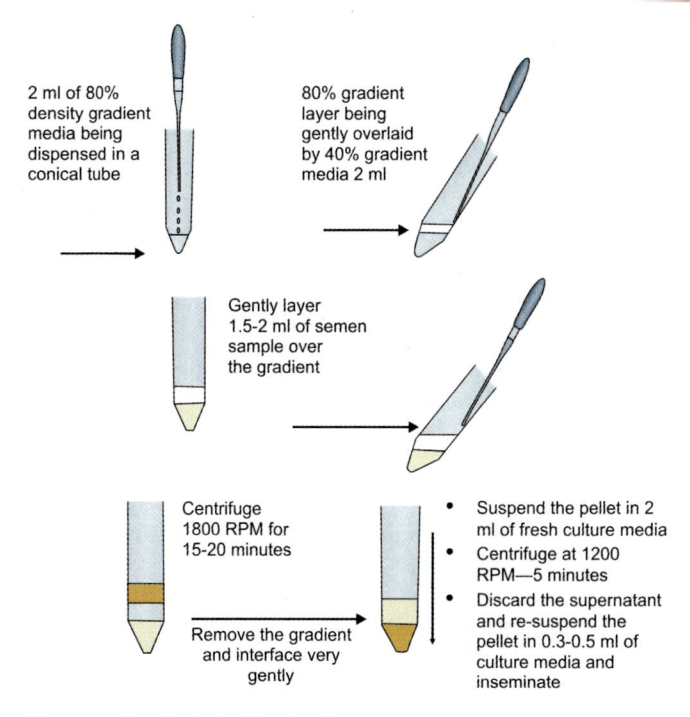

Fig. 10.2: Gradient double density

- Keep the tube in CO_2 incubator till used for insemination with Cap loosen.
2. *Two step gradient (80/40):* 100% gradient can be diluted to prepare 80% and 40% gradients or prepared solutions can be used.

    80%: 8 ml gradient solution + 2 ml culture media (Fig. 10.2).

    40%: 4 ml gradient solution + 6 ml culture media.

- Pipette 2 ml of 80% gradient followed by 2 ml 40% gradient in the conical test tube. Top it with 1.5 to 2 ml of liquefied semen sample
  (Tips: Volume can be adjusted according to quality of semen)
  Centrifuge at 1800 rpm for 15 to 20 minutes depending on quality of semen.
- Cell debris and immotile/abnormal sperms accumulate at interface and motile sperms settle at bottom pellet.
- Gently recover the pellet and resuspend the pellet in 1 ml of fresh medium.
- Resuspended pellet centrifuged at 1200 rpm × 5 min.
- Remove the supernatant.
- Resuspend the pellet in 0.3 ml of media and use for the procedure.

OOCYTE ASSESSMENT

The mature oocyte is the largest cell of the human body with diameter of 100 to 120 micro m, surrounded by a gelatinous, glycoprotein zona pelluida, and several layers of follicular cells forming the cumulus oophorus complex. The female gamete carries the 23 chromosomes at the time of fertilization. Preovulatory oocytes, collected from multiple follicles after ovarian stimulation have commenced the final stages of meiotic maturation, ranging from germinal vesicle breakdown (GVBD), metaphase I (MI), to metaphase (MII) oocytes.[1,2] Nuclear maturation occurs hand-in-hand with cytoplasmic maturation. Morphological and biochemical changes also occur in the egg vestments markedly in the zona pellucida (ZP), increasing receptivity to sperm binding and penetration. Germinal vesical breakdown (GVBD) heralds the resumption of meiosis and initiates the expansion of the cumulus during maturation. This usually occurs immediately following hCG administration or in the culture medium prior to insemination (IVF) or sperm injection (ICSI) The process might be completed after insemination with washed sperm during IVF.

After the oocyte is denuded of cumulus cells before ICSI, it is possible to precisely identify the mature metaphase 2 oocyte, which has the first polar body (PB1) at the animal pole (AP) (Table 10.1 and 10.2).

Table 10.1
Oocyte maturity

Stage of maturity	Description—morphological	Clinical significance
The fully mature oocyte	An expanded cumulus and radiating CR around the ZP. A polar body (PB1) in the PVS at the animal pole. A clear, homogenous ooplasm with even distribution of organelles. A barrel-shaped, anastral MII spindle beneath PB1. One to three layers of CG beneath the oolemma.	The MII oocyte is ovulated around day 14 in the natural cycle
The maturing, metaphase I oocyte	No polar body. No germinal vesicle. An expanding cumulus and corona cells. A metaphase I spindle with homologous chromosomes. One or two layers of CG beneath oolemma.	This stage is transient, there being no interphase

Contd...

Contd...

Stage of maturity	Description—morphological	Clinical significance
The immature oocyte at prophase I	No polar body (LM) A GV or nucleus with a dense nucleolus. A compact, unexpanded cumulus and corona. A discontinuous layer of CG beneath oolemma. An agranular cortex with Golgi membranes that secrete CG.	Oocytes about to mature will show an eccentrically located GV at one pole
The immature Oocytes during GVBD	A disappearing GV or nucleus. Breakdown of the nuclear envelope Condensation of chromosomes. Formation of a spindle with microtubules. Uncoupling of cell junctions between CR cells and oocyte.	This stage heralds the resumption of meiosis after its arrest at the GV stage.

Table 10.2
Grading of cumulus–oocyte complexes

Cumulus–oocyte complexes (COCs)	Cumulus morphology
Cumulus mass (CM)	• 3 or fewer layers of cumulus cells (CM0).
	• More than 3 but fewer than 10 layers of cumulus cells (CM1).
	• 10 or more layers of cumulus cells (CM2).
Cumulus expansion (CE)	• Tight, dense cells (CE0). • Moderate expansion of cells (CE1). • Fully expanded cells (CE2).
Contact (CO) between cumulus cells and oocyte	• Naked (CO0). • Partially naked CO1). • Fully enclosed (CO2). • Fully Enclosed and part of • follicle wall (CO3).

INSEMINATION PROTOCOLS IN ART

Introduction

In vitro fertilization requires oocyte to be inseminated with sperms in culture media and incubated for a few hours to allow fertilization to take place. Subsequent to this, fertilized oocytes are denuded, washed and cultured in another dish.

Time of Insemination

Oocyte fertilization is performed ideally within 2 to 4 hours after oocyte recovery. This time is essential not only for the stabilization of the oocyte and its equilibration with the *in vitro* environment but also helps in final maturation of few of the immature oocytes to metaphase 2 stage.

> *Note:* Delayed insemination is avoided, as the quality of sperms will decrease exponentially with passage of time because they are always swimming and metabolizing glucose, releasing reactive oxygen species and toxic metabolites, which will reduce the fertilization rate.

Sperm Concentration

The optimum sperm concentration is approximately 80,000 to 100,000 progressively motile sperm for each oocyte in the inseminate, provided that there is no other major male factor involvement.

Media for Sperm Preparation and Insemination

The medias used for sperm preparation and insemination should have high levels of glucose as it is used by spermatozoa as the main energy source. Glucose improves sperm capacity and motility and also participates in sperm-oocyte fusion.

Various commercial medias used for final swim-up and fertilization used at our center are as per Table 10.3.

Table 10.3
Media used in IVF

Commercial company	Sperm washing media	Final swim-up media	Fertilization/ insemination media
Vitrolife	Sperm rinse	G-IVF PLUS	G-IVF PLUS
Cook	Gamete buffer/ Sydney IVF Sperm Medium	Sydney IVF Fertilization Medium/Sydney IVF Sperm Medium	Sydney IVF Fertilization Medium
MediCult	Flushing media	Universal IVF media	Universal IVF media

MediCult (flushing media) and Sydney—Cook (Gamete buffer) are HEPES based media and thus do not require CO_2 equilibration. All other media used in this procedure have to be equilibrate for minimum of 6 hr in CO_2 conditions before use (Table 10.3).

Protocols for Insemination and Embryo Culture (Figs 10.3A and B)

There are essentially two culture systems to choose from for insemination and culture of gametes and embryos:[1]

A. Large volumes (0.5 ml – 1.0 ml) in wells, with or without oil (Fig. 10.3)
B. Small volumes droplets (50 micro L – 100 micro L) under oil.

Culture of embryos in micro-drops of culture medium under an oil overlay is the favored and effective method of embryo culture. Decreasing the incubation volume significantly increases embryo viability as seen with an increase in blastocyst development. Embryos are known to secrete autocrine and chemotactic factors and their Incubation in large volumes will dilute autocrine factor(s) produced by the developing embryos. It has been noted that cleavage rate and blastocyst formation

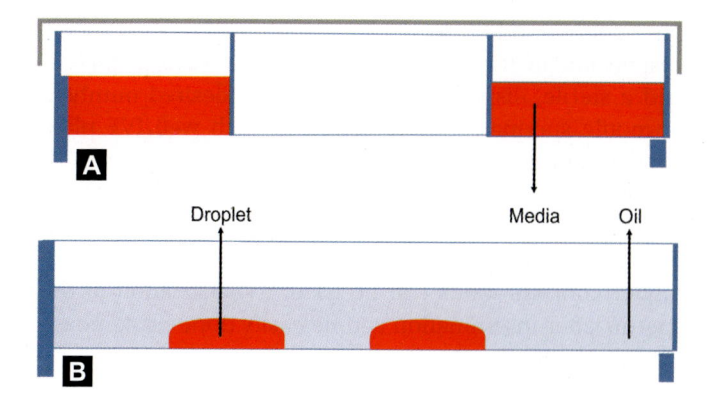

Figs 10.3A and B: (A) 0.5-1 ml wells with or without liquid paraffin overlays; (B) 10-100 µl microdroplats covered with liquid paraffin

increase when embryos are grown in groups (up to 8-10) and in reduced volumes of micro droplets (around 20-30 µl each).

Methods of Insemination

Insemination

Ideally, insemination should be carried out in a controlled environment chamber. But if one is not available then a heated stage should be used and insemination done under steroozoom microscope visualization.

Insemination is usually carried out 38-40 hours post hCG, i.e. 3-4 hours after oocyte recovery. Average fertilization rates of 70% should be expected. If these results are not achieved then the embryologist should reconcile and all laboratory procedures be reviewed.

Sperm preparation: The sperm preparation should be counted accurately and should be at a concentrations of $8-10 \times 10^6$ motile sperm per ml. This way small volume of swim-up is inseminated, minimizing changes to the final volume.

Insemination: Add the calculated volume of washed sperm suspension to the oocytes using a 20 µl -200 µl pipette and a sterile, disposable tip so that the desired numbers of motile spermatozoa are added to each well/IVF plate containing the oocytes.

The inseminate volume should be calculated so that a final sperm concentration (usually 100000/egg is achieved). Polyspermy may be prevented although some studies feel higher concentrations can be used.[18] Visualization of the sperms after insemination can be easily done using phase contrast optics.

> Always add the inseminate away from the eggs so that the sperms can gradually swim-up to the eggs attracted by the chemotactic factors.

Incubation

Return the dish to the incubator until either the fertilization check (16-18 hour Postinsemination) or until a shorter incubation time is reached (minimum of two hours).

There are various methods for insemination recommended depending upon media volume, culture dish used, personal choice of embryologist or incubator space.

- *35 mm plate:* We at our center inseminate 6 to 8 eggs in a 35 mm IVF plate. OCC's are placed in 2 ml of bicarbonate-based media and covered with 1.5 ml of oil. After 2 hr of stabilization in CO_2 conditions, semen sample is added. We add 2-3 drops of semen sample under vision. It is ensured that final swim-up sperm concentration is approximately 15 to 20 million/ml.
- *Single well dish:* If the final swim-up is low, say 8-10 million then we inseminate the OCC (max 6 number)

in a single well dish under oil. Here 6 eggs are placed in 500 microliters of bicarbonate-based media under oil. 2 to 3 drops of swim-up is inseminated in the media. In such a situation the denudation has to be carried out quickly as eggs are clustered together and sometimes difficult to denude due to limited space in a single well as compared with the 35 mm plate.

- *Micro-Droplet method:* The insemination can be carried out by droplet insemination method. Here we make 100-150 microliter drops (8-10 in number) in a 35 mm or 60 mm plate and cover they with oil and equilibrate in CO_2 incubator for 4 to 6 hr. One oocyte complex is placed per microdrop and plate is equilibrated for one hour. Now the semen inseminate, few microliters the inseminate in the microdrop.[17]
- *Four well dish:* Few embryologist carry out insemination in the 4 well plate. 4-6 Occ's are placed in 400 microliters of bicarbonate media in one well and covered with oil. Insemination is carried out with few microliters of inseminate in desired concentration after necessary dilution.

Role of Oil Overlay

Oil overlay of media is cumbersome but has many added advantages.

1. Prevents the evaporation of media in the incubator, thus reducing the unwanted effects of increased osmolality.
2. Reduces changes in pH caused due to handling the embryos plates outside the incubator, during denudation and observation.
3. Creates a breathing nonpermeable window between the oil droplet and exterior which may trap unwanted particles in air and volatile organic compounds.

Paraffin oil is chosen for its viscosity and its high purity.

> *Recommendation:*
> - Oil should be ideally stored in the dark and in glass bottles as oil can leach styrene from plastic containers
> - Pharmaceutical grade light paraffin oil, sterilized by filtration using a 0.22 µm pore size sterile filter is to be used.

The disadvantages of an open system is that more medium is required and both temperature and pH shift quickly once dishes are removed from the incubator.

> *Precaution:* Be aware that while oil will have slower out gassing times for the medium it also results in slower regassing.

Temperature and pH change does not happen as fast using oil, but the disadvantage of oil is that it must be tested for embryo toxicity, washed and filtered to ensure that it is nontoxic.

DENUDATION

IVF inseminated oocytes should be checked for fertilization 16 to 20 hours postinsemination. Denudation is performed in an environmental chamber under steroozoom microscope on a warm stage. Denudation is performed in the insemination plates with a 170 micro pippette by aspirating in and out the conceptus till the OCC is clear of surrounding cummulus cells. Work as quickly as possible as the oocyte is outside the incubator. Avoid mouth aspiration set as it can cause contamination. Rarely with unregulated mouth suction pressure eggs may be aspirated in the tubing and get lost.

There are 2 methods of denudation, which are followed worldwide, and choosing one is entirely a matter of personal choice. One is the conventional method where standard time of 16 to 18 hours of sperm exposure to the oocyte has been a laboratory benchmark for many years. The second method is a short insemination method for 2 hours. Recent evidence suggests that the production of reactive of reactive oxygen species by excess sperm exposure may be detrimental to subsequent embryo development. The principle of this technique is that the oocyte cumulus complexes are fertilized within minutes of insemination. If we prolong the contact period of oocytes and the sperms large number of sperms coats the oocytes and form spermatozoal shell along the oocyte complex and release of reactive oxygen species may affect the metabolism of the oocytes. Prolonged insemination this also creates lots of debris in the insemination plates leading to difficult denudation done after 18 hours.

This is the reason also for recommendation of never adding more than 100,000 sperms per egg in the culture plate. This will also avoids polyspermy. Insemination time as short as one hour has been shown not to be detrimental to fertilization rates. A recent study showed ultrashort exposure of 30 seconds to be better than conventional method.[15]

However, there are studies which do not agree to short incubation.[16]

Short Denudation Method

If a short insemination is used then the sperm and oocytes are incubated in for two hours before they are denuded gently and moved to fresh culture plate. These are incubated for 14 to 16 hours and then denuded again. The main disadvantage of this technique is repeated exposure of the conceptus to atmospheric conditions. The embryologist should be quick in carrying out this procedure and temptation to completely denude the complexes should be avoided. The protocol followed at our center is follows:

Step 1. Dish preparation: Same as standard method.

Step 2. Insemination: Here semen preparation must be gently mixed so that the entire surface of the cumulus mass is exposed to sperm

Step 3. Incubation: Return the dish to the incubator until shorter incubation time is reached (minimum of two hours).

Step 4. Early denudation: Carry out denudation in the original insemination plates. After two hours of incubation, the sperm have "loosened" the cumulus cells which are stripped off using a Cook 300 µm Flexipet.

> *Caution:* Only strip off as much cumulus as comes off easily, don't completely denude the oocyte.

Step 5. Washing of OCC: Wash the partially denuded complexes in the single well plate with 500 µl, G-IVF Plus/Sydney Fertilization/universal media prepared 6 hr prior to the procedure and covered with oil, which has been equilibrated overnight.

Step 6. Incubate in culture dish: Incubate the conceptus in 35 mm falcon plate with 6-8, 80-100 µl droplets of G-IVF Plus/Sydney Fertilization/universal media covered with mineral oil and equilibrated under CO_2 conditions overnight.[19]

Step 7. Denudation: Same as standard method.

Step 8. Assessment of fertilization: Same as standard method.

Step 9. Washing denuded oocytes: Same as standard method.

Step 10. Transfer to culture dish: Same as standard method.

> *Caution:*
> - Use appropriate size flexipet to avoid damage to the zona pellucida
> - Always work under oil overlay to maintain pH and temperature for longer periods
> - Never denude more than 6 oocytes at a time to avoid exposure of the eggs to the atmosphere for a longer period.

ASSESSMENT OF FERTILIZATION (FIGS 10.4 to 10.18)

Embryos should be assessed once every day, preferably at same times (morning) so that the rate of development can be noted.

> *Tips for handling embryos.*
> - *Size of pipette tip:* It is important to use a pipette containing a tip with a diameter that is slightly larger than that of the embryo to avoid damage. For example, for embryos on day 1 to 3, a pipette tip of 150 to 200 µm would suffice. Using the appropriate size tip minimizes the volumes of culture medium moved with each embryo, which typically should be less than one microliter
> - *Incubation of dishes:* Dishes must gas in the incubator for a minimum of 4 h (this is the minimal measured time for the media to reach the correct pH under oil).

Fertilization Assessment on Day 1 (Table 10.4)

Assessment of fertilization is done by visualizing the pronuclei after denudation.

Using the flexipet roll presumptive zygote and view under maximum magnification on the stereozoom microscope (~40 X). Adjust the illumination to enable maximum contrast. On higher magnification (minimum 200X) on an inverted microscope with Nomarski or Hoffman optics, record the number of:
- Pronuclei
- Polar bodies
- Presence of a germinal vesicle.

It is difficult to be accurate in the assessment of fertilization if lower magnifications are used.

Grouping of scored zygotes: Score all zygotes and group them together for culture in equilibrated cleavage medium before incubation. Only embryos derived from normally

Table 10.4

Grading of PN—pronuclear scoring system developed by Scott et al.

Z score	Morphological description	Clinical significance
Z1	Equal PN Equal number and size of nucleoli (ranging between 3 and 7) All nucleoli aligned at the pronuclear junction in both PN	
Z2	Equal PN Equal number and size of nucleoli (ranging between 3 and 7) Nucleoli unaligned in both PN	Scores of Z1 and Z2 considered morphologically normal zygotes
Z3	Equal PN Equal number and even and/or uneven size of nucleoli (ranging between 3 and 7) Nucleoli aligned at the pronuclear junction in one PN and unaligned in the other PN	
Z4	Unequal or separated or not centrally located PN	

PN—Pronuclei

fertilized oocytes (2 PN) should be considered for embryo culture and transfer.

> *Note:* Nonfertilized or degenerated oocytes, oocytes with only 1 PN, and oocytes with more than 2 PN should be removed from culture.

Washing Denuded Oocytes

As a general rule, the zygotes are washed in 500 microliters of prewarmed and equilibrated G1 PLUS media in a single well or

Andrology and Beyond | 243

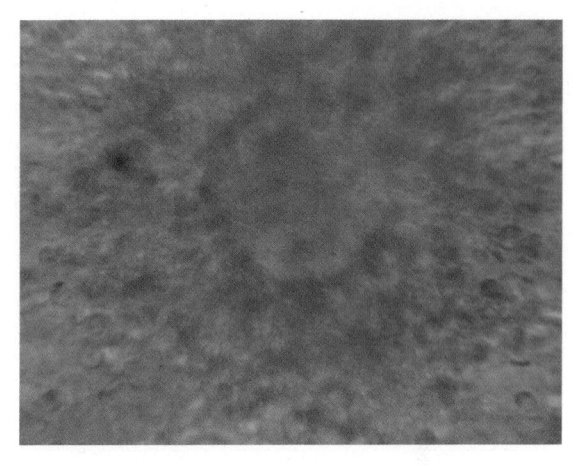

Fig. 10.4: Freshly aspirated oocyte cumulus oophorous complex. The oocyte is seen in the center with well-expanded granulosa cells

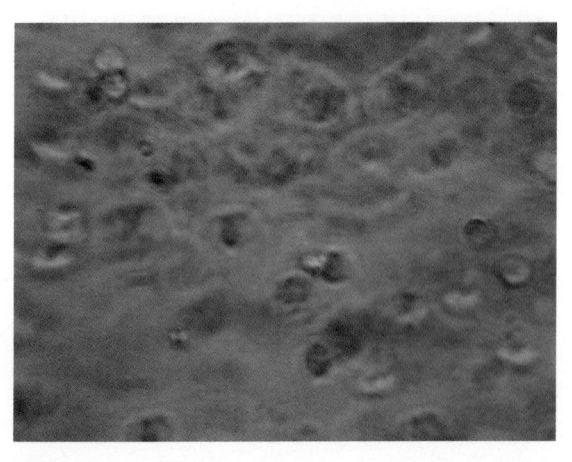

Fig. 10.5: Well expanded granulosa cell complex under 300X magnification

244 | *Protocols in Clinical Embryology and ART*

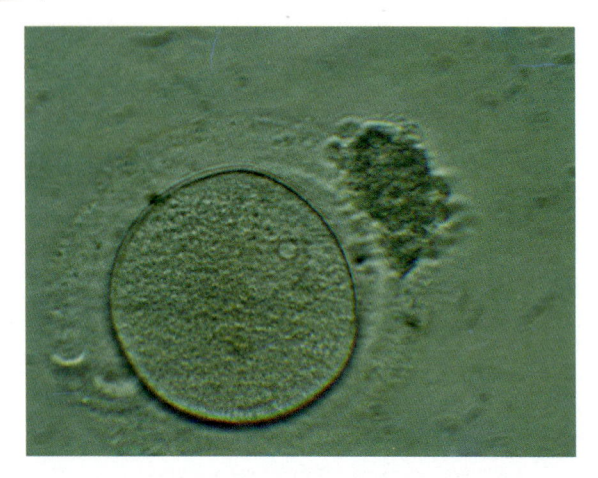

Fig. 10.6: Germinal vesicle seen after denudation for ICSI. It is seen at 1 o'clock position as dark area

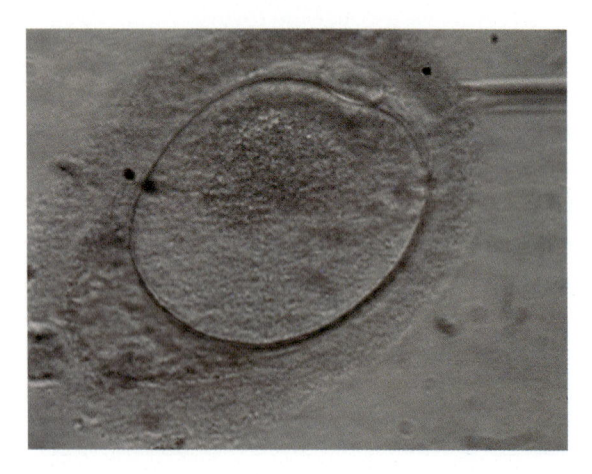

Fig. 10.7: An oblong cell with well-defined polar body seen during ICSI. Polar body is at 1 o'clock position

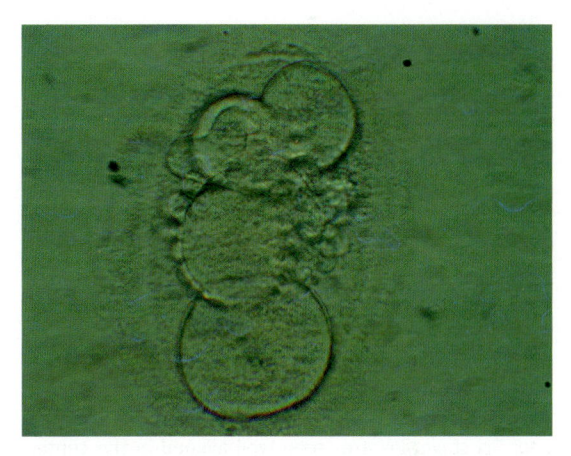

Fig. 10.8: An oblong embryo with 4 blastomeres after regular ICSI and denudation. Blastomeres are of irregular shape and number. 20-30% fragments are visualized

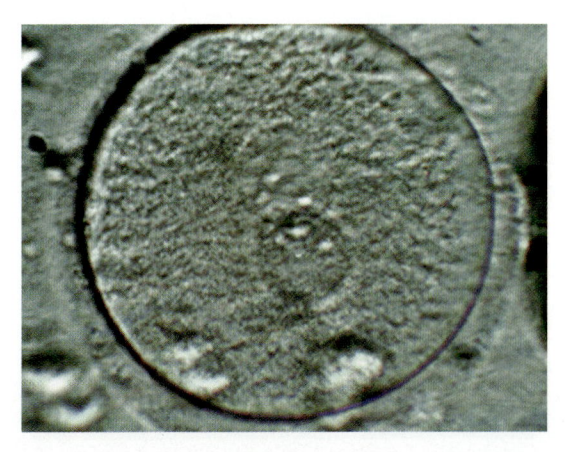

Fig. 10.9: PN stage. Two pronucleus are seen in the center of the conceptus. Polar body is at the 5 o'clock position. NPB are seen arranged in opposed manner

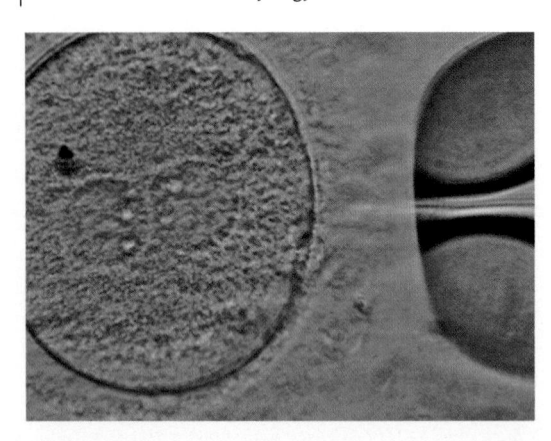

Fig. 10.10: PN stage. PN are seen well aligned in the center of the conceptus. Polar body is seen at 3 o'clock position. NPBs are aligned in the well apposed manner. Mitochondrial clearing is noted along the edges of the PN

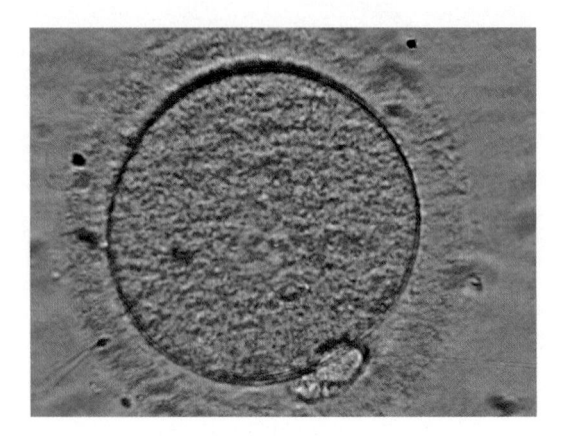

Fig. 10.11: A conceptus seen after the denudation. Two polar bodies are seen at the 5 o'clock position. Doubtful PN bodies are seen in the center. This conceptus degenerated

Andrology and Beyond | **247**

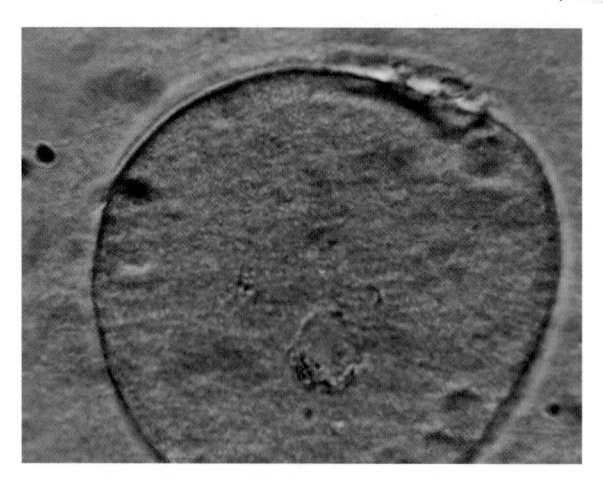

Fig. 10.12: A metaphase 2 oocyte with vacuole in the center. Polar body is seen at 1 o'clock position

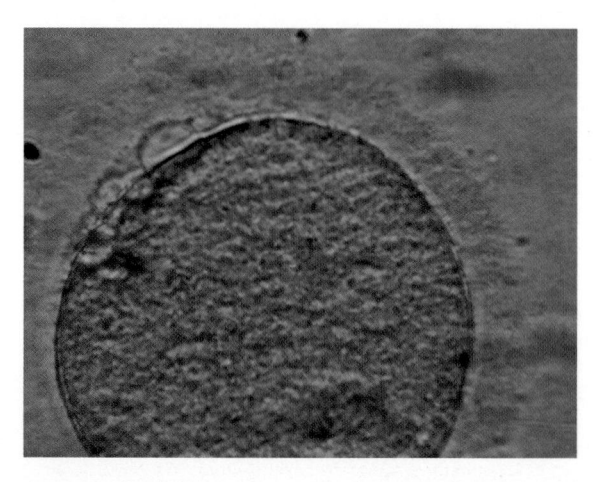

Fig. 10.13: A fertilized oocyte with fragmented polar body at 11 o'clock position

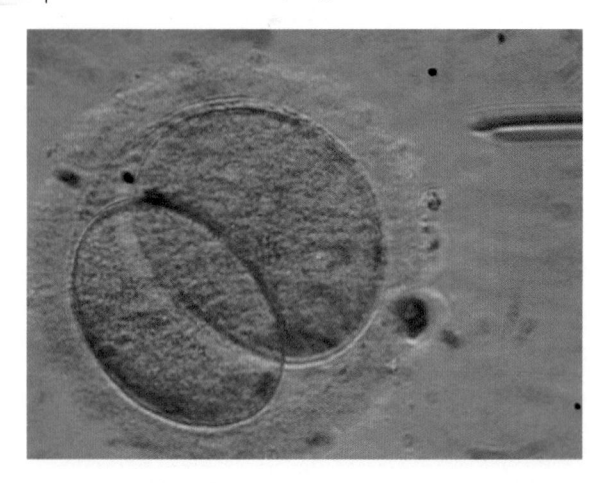

Fig. 10.14: A 2 cell embryo without any polar body. The egg has had an parthenogenetic activation and was arrested thereafter

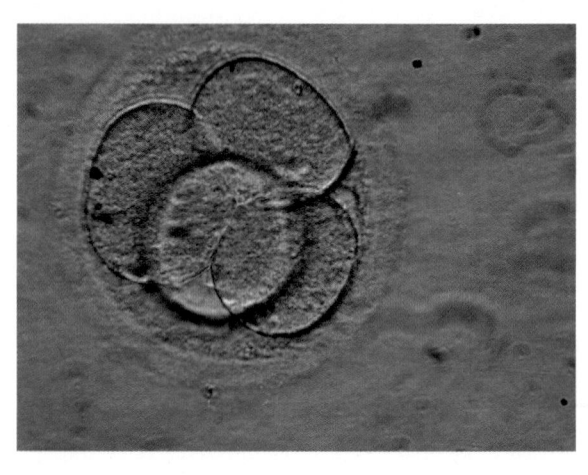

Fig. 10.15: A grade 1, 4 cell embryo. Regular blastomeres with no fragmentation are visualized

Andrology and Beyond | **249**

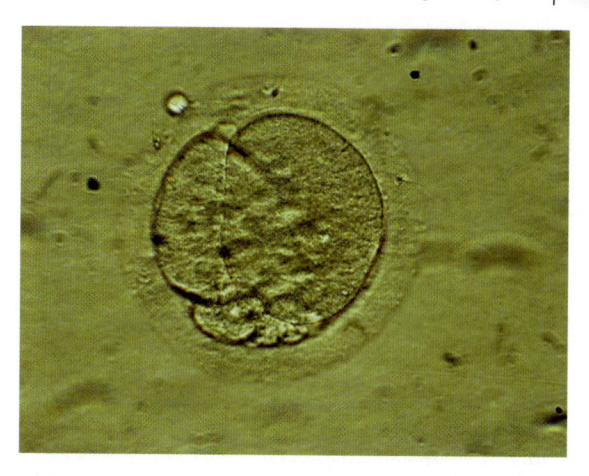

Fig. 10.16: A 2-cell embryo at 48 hours. Both the blastomers are of unequal size. Fragments are unequal in size and are crowded at 5 o'clock position

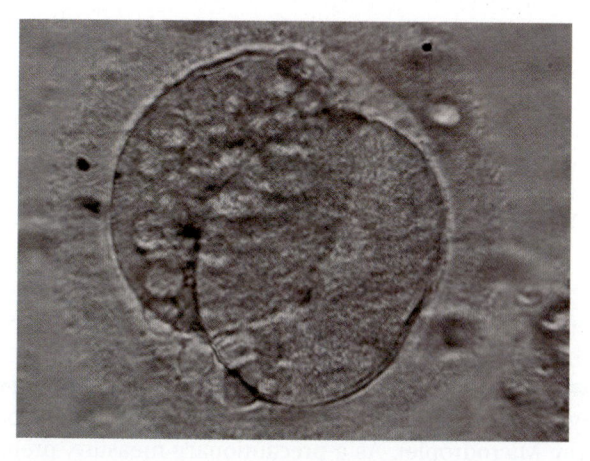

Fig. 10.17: A 2-cell embryo with 20% fragmentation seen. Fragments are of similar shape and size and are arranged in the regular pattern

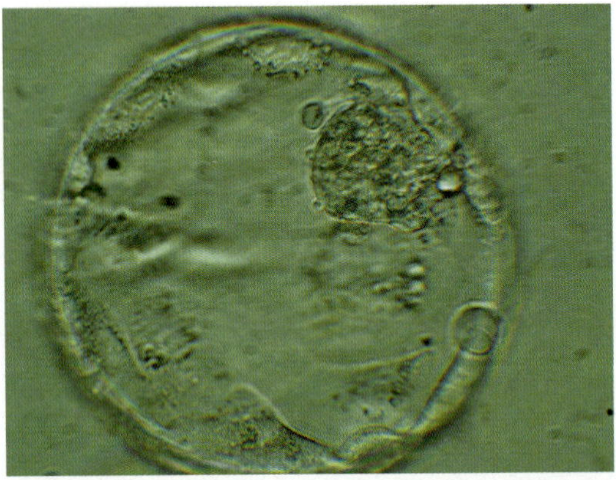

Fig. 10.18: A well expanded blastocyst seen. Cavity is well expanded. ICM is not healthy and situated at 2 o'clock position. Regular trophectoderm is visualized

4 well dish before transferring them in 50 µL microdrops to avoid cell contamination. The plates are prepared 6 hours prior to the procedure. Washing entails picking up the embryos 2 to 3 times in a minimal volume of the culture media and moving them around within the 100 µL droplet few times before transferring them to microdroplets.

Transfer to Culture Dish

Fertilized oocytes are transferred to fresh culture dish. Place up to 5 PN's in each 50 µL drop of equilibrated supplemented G-1 PLUS. Five is the maximum number of embryos that should be cultured in each drop due to the nutrient requirements. Culture of more than 5 embryos may result in a significant depletion of the nutrient pool in the Microdroplet. As a precautionary measure, prepare two culture dishes if the patient has more than 10 embryos. Return the dish to the incubator immediately.

Embryo Assessment on Day 2 (Table 10.5)

1. Approximately 24 hours after the fertilization check (40 m–48 hours postinsemination) the embryos are assessed again for:
   - Embryo transfer
   - Cryopreservation of the spare embryo's
   - Extended culture.

   The embryos can be regrouped if so desired.

2. Generally, for both day 2 and 3 day transfers, embryos only need to be cultured in G1/cleavage/universal medium. If the culture is to be extended to day 4 or 5 then the embryos must be placed in equilibrated G2/blastocyst medium on day 3.

Note: More extensive washing will reduce the risk of transferring medium from the old dish to the fresh one.

Table 10.5
Embryo grading

Grade of cleaving embryos	Morphological findings	Clinical significance
1	Blastomeres of equal size and no cytoplasmic fragmentation	Grades 1 and 2 have a greater potential of establishing a clinical pregnancy
2	Blastomeres of equal size and minor cytoplasmic fragmentation (<10%)	
3	Blastomeres of equal or unequal size and significant fragmentation (>10%)	
4	Few blastomeres of any size and severe fragmentation (>50%)	

The highest score is characterized by:
- 4 cell stage with symmetrical alignment of blastomeres.
- Blastomeres "fill out" the zona pellucida
- Equal size blastomeres with homogeneous cytoplasm and distinct plasma membrane with one nucleus in each blastomeres
- No multinuclear cells seen
- No fragments or a maximum of 20% fragments visualized
- Normal and even zona pellucida.

4. Place dish onto warming stage and check 2 PN embryos for stage of division. Using a Flexpet, roll the embryo and view under maximum magnification on the stereozoom microscope.
5. Embryos are assessed according to number of blastomeres; regularity of degree of cytoplasmic fragmentation and cleavage rate. The embryos should be at the 4-cell stage of development.
6. Embryos that are chosen for transfer are placed into a fresh dish of equilibrated media (Cleavage medium) G2 PLUS/ISM media.

Embryos for cryopreservation: Remaining embryos can be cryopreserved using the cryopreservation kit for cleavage stage embryos.

Embryos for culture to day 3: If embryos are to be cultured to day 3, they can be left in the same medium or transferred into fresh, equilibrated cleavage G2 PLUS/ISM media for incubation overnight.

Embryo Assessment on Day 3

At 66 to 74 hours postinsemination, the embryos should be again assessed for either embryo transfer, cryopreservation

or extended culture (to day 5-6). The embryos should be at the 6 to 8 cell stage of development on day 3. Embryos are assessed according to
- Number of blastomeres
- Degree of cytoplasmic fragmentation
- Cleavage rate.

Embryos for transfer: The embryos that are chosen for transfer are selected and placed in a fresh dish of equilibrated EmbryoGlue® or in equilibrated G2 PLUS (Vitrolife)/cleavage (COOK)/ISM 1 (MediCult).

Embryos for cryopreservation: Remaining embryos can be cryopreserved using the cryopreservation kit for cleavage stage embryos.

Embryos for day 5 culture: If embryos are to be cultured to day 5, wash all cleaving embryos in fresh and equilibrated blastocyst medium. Embryos can be transferred to pre-equilibrated for further culture to the blastocyst stage. ({G2 PLUS (Vitrolife)/blastocyst (COOK)/blastocyst (MediCult)})

Blastocyst culture does not improve embryo quality of poor day 2 and day 3 embryos, but improves embryo selection for transfer - beneficial especially in case of single embryo transfer.

Embryo Assessment on Day 5 (Blastocyst Culture) (Tables 10.6 to 10.8)

On day 5, embryos should be evaluated and one or two top scoring blastocysts selected for transfer. Move the selected blastocyst(s) in G-2 PLUS (Vitrolife) or equivalent media and leave at +37°C and 6% CO_2 for 10 to 30 minutes before transfer.

Precaution: Manipulation of blastocysts requires the use of a capillary with bore size of 275–300 μ.

Table 10.6

Blastocyst grading: cavity

Grade	Stage	Morphological findings
0	Morula or lesser stage	No blastocoel cavity seen
1	Early blastocyst	Blastocoel less than half the volume of the embryo
2	Blastocyst	Blastocoel ≥ half of the volume of the embryo
3	Full blastocyst	Blastocoel completely fills the embryo
4	Expanded blastocyst	Zona thinning and overall increase in size
5	Hatching blastocyst	Trophectoderm has started to herniate through the zona
6	Hatched blastocyst	Blastocyst has completely escaped from the zona

Table 10.7

Blastocyst grading: somatic criterion: blastocysts graded at stage 3 to 6 onward

	Inner cell mass (ICM)	Trophectoderm grading
A	Tightly packed, several cells	Many cells forming a tightly knit epithelium
B	Loosely grouped, several cells	Few cells
C	Very few cells	Very few cells forming a loose epithelium.

Good quality spare blastocysts not being transferred can be cryopreserved.

Note: Should an embryo not have formed a blastocyst by day 5, it should be cultured in a fresh drop of equilibrated supplemented G-2 PLUS (Vitrolife) for 24 hours and assessed on day 6.

Table 10.8
Morphological features of normal embryos and blastocyst

Normal cleavage stage embryos	Normal blastocysts on day 5/6	Hatching blastocysts on day 6/7
Rounded equal-sized blastomeres, except when cells are dividing.	Distinct trophoblast, ICM and blastocoel	A fully expanded trophoblast and blastocoel
Blastomeres with well-defined outlines or cell membranes.	Well-defined, compact ICM with many cells and cell junctions	A thinned-out zona
Cells with centralized, single nuclei, or metaphases	Trophoblast forming a continuous, flat epithelium with cell junctions	Evidence of early hatching–trophoblast emerging at one pole
No fragments or show minimal fragmentation (10%).	A large fluid-filled blastocoel, when expanded	Plump 'zona-breaker' (trophoblast) cells at hatching point
	Few cleavage stage fragments in the blastocoel and PVS	

CONCLUSION

Oocyte and embryo classification as a matter of course are based on morphological characteristics. Evaluation and classification by morphology alone, however, may be subjective and may not foretell success. In the past decade, systems have evolved that, in addition to morphological criteria, incorporate cleavage rate to forecast embryo survival and subsequent implantation. Lately, components of follicular fluid and culture media are being evaluated for their prognostic value and embryo quality may be predicted better.

Classification systems currently in place differ greatly between clinics. An accurate, standardized oocyte and embryo classification system could improve interaction among embryologists, and improve the quality and outcome of ART procedures by improving our understanding of distinctiveness influencing pre-embryo attributes.

REFERENCES

1. IVF Manual. Recommended use of G5 Series ™ by Gardner. Edition 2, May 2008.
2. Tips and Tricks Media for Assisted Reproduction 2007. Møllehaven 12, DK-4040 Jyllinge, Denmark.
3. A complete guide to cook culture media Copyright May 2004. William A. COOK Australia PTY LTD.
4. Bolton VN, Braude PR. Preparation of human spermatozoa for in vitro fertilization by isopycnic centrifugation on self-generating density gradients. Arch Androl. 1984;13:167-176.
5. Pousette A, Akerlöf E, Rosenborg L, Fredricsson B. Increase in progressive motility and improved morphology of human spermatozoa following their migration through Percoll gradients. Int J Androl.1986; 9:1-13.
6. Tomlinson MJ, Moffatt O, Manicardi GC, Bizzaro D, Afnan M, Sakkas D. Interrelationships between seminal parameters and sperm nuclear DNA damage before and after density gradient centrifugation: implications for assisted conception. Hum Reprod. 2001;16:2160.
7. Morrell JM, Moffatt O, Sakkas D, et al. Reduced senescence and retained nuclear DNA integrity in human spermatozoa prepared by density gradient centrifugation. J Assist Reprod Genet. 2004;21:217.
8. Politch JA, Xu C, Tucker L, Anderson DJ. Separation of human immunodeficiency virus type 1 from motile sperm by the double tube gradient method versus other methods. Fertil Steril. 2004;81:440.
9. Jeulin C, Serres C, Jouannet P. The effects of centrifugation, various synthetic media and temperature on the motility and vitality Reprod Nutr Dev. 1982;22(1A):81-91

10. Tesarik J, Mendoza C, Carrera A. Effects of phosphodiesterase inhibitors caffeine and pentoxifylline on spontaneous and stimulus-induced acrosome reaction in human sperm. Fertil Steril. 1992;58:1185.
11. Sengoku K, Tamate K, Takaoka Y, Ishikawa M. Effects of platelet-activating factor on human sperm function. Hum Reprod. 1993;8:1443.
12. Krausz C, Gervasi G, Forti G, Baldi E. Effect of platelet-activating factor on motility and acrosome reaction of human spermatozoa. Hum Reprod. 1994;9:471.
13. Roudebush WE, Telede AA, Kert HI, Mitchell-Leef D, Elsner CW, Massey JB. Platelet-activating factor significantly enhances intrauterine insemination pregnancy rates in non-male factor infertility. Fertil Steril. 2004;81:52.
14. WHO Laboratory Manual for the Examination of Human Semen and Sperm–Cervical Mucus Interaction (4th edn.) Cambridge: Cambridge University Press. 1999.p.1:29.
15. Bungum M, Bungum L, Humaidan P.A prospective study, using sibling oocytes, examining the effect of 30 seconds versus 90 minutes gamete co-incubation in IVF. Hum Reprod. 2006;21(2):518-23.
16. Barraud-Lange V, Sifer C, Pocaté K, Ziyyat A, Martin-Pont B, Porcher R, Hugues JN, Wolf P. Short gamete co-incubation during *in vitro* fertilization decreases the fertilization rate and does not improve embryo quality: a prospective auto controlled study. J Assist Reprod Genet. 2008;25(7):305-10.
17. Fiorentino A, Magli MC, Fortini D, Feliciani E, Ferraretti AP, Dale B, Gianaroli L. Sperm:oocyte ratios in an in vitro fertilization (IVF) program. J Assist Reprod Genet. 1994;11(2):97-103.
18. Uhler ML, Buyalos RP. The effect of varying inseminating sperm concentration in male factor and non-male factor infertility during *in vitro* fertilization. Int J Fertil Menopausal Stud. 1995;40(6):322-8.
19. IVF Manual. Recommended use of G5 Series ™ by Gardner. Edition 2, May 2008.

Chapter 11

Intracytoplasm Sperm Injection and Troubleshooting

Pankaj Talwar

INTRODUCTION

The intracytoplasmic sperm injection (ICSI) process involves the placement of a single spermatozoon directly into the ooplasm of the denuded mature oocyte, thus circumventing the zona pellucida and the plasma membrane. The fact that ICSI technology can result in higher fertilization and pregnancy rates irrespective of sperm numbers makes it an attractive micromanipulation procedure.

INDICATIONS FOR ICSI

1. Oligoasthenospermia.
2. Azoospermic men where spermatozoa are surgically retrieved from the testes or epipidymis.
3. Occytes from a poor harvest should also undergo ICSI as denudation guides us about the oocyte maturity and has prognostic significance.
4. Preimplantation genetic diagnosis (PGD).
5. Repeated fertilization failure with IVF.

ICSI MEDIA

Types of Media Needed for ICSI

Media needed for ICSI procedure are:
1. *ICSI medium:* A buffer system, supplemented with antibiotics, proteins and an energy source. Fertilization, MOPS/HEPES medium may be used.

2. *Denudation medium:* Similar to ICSI medium but supplemented with hyaluronidase in desired concentration. Used for oocyte denudation, during ICSI.
3. *PVP* is used to slow down sperm progression and facilitate the ICSI procedure. This is a viscous medium, containing polyvinyl pyrolidone.
4. Embryo culture media to culture injected oocytes.

Handling

- These media are best stored in a refrigerator at 4–8°C and aliquoted for use as required within the expiry period as per the manufacture's recommendation.
- Prewarm all media to 37°C in an incubator before use. The media vials once warmed should not be refrigerated again.
- All culture media for embryo cultures are to be equilibrated in CO_2 atmosphere overnight except PVP and hydase medium.

Note: Carbon dioxide equilibration of the PVP and hyaluronidase media is not recommended by most manufacturers, except with Cook's hyaluronidase media, which requires overnight equilibration in CO_2 atmosphere.

PIPETTES (FIGS 11.1 TO 11.3)

Pipettes are of two types:
1. Holding Pipette
2. Injecting Pipette

The holding and injecting pipettes, which are to be fixed on the micromanipulator, are both made from borosilicate glass capillary tubes. A spike is present on the injection pipette for nontraumatic injection of the sperms into the oocyte. Both pipettes are bent, 1 mm from the tip at an

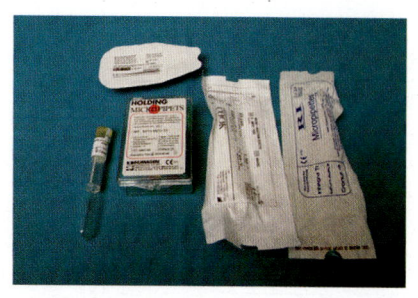

Intracytoplasm Sperm Injection and Troubleshooting | **261**

Fig. 11.1: Glass ICSI pipettes. These are commercially available in sterile packs. The tip is bent at an angle for the alignment of the pipettes. Pipettes are produced with available angles of 20°, 30°, and 35°. Injecting pipettes have outer diameter (OD) of 7 µm and inner diameter (ID) of 5 µm. Holding pipettes possess a flame-polished interface for holding the oocyte. The smooth surface couples with a 20 µm inner diameter and 110 µm outer diameters to grip oocytes safely and solidly during ICSI procedures

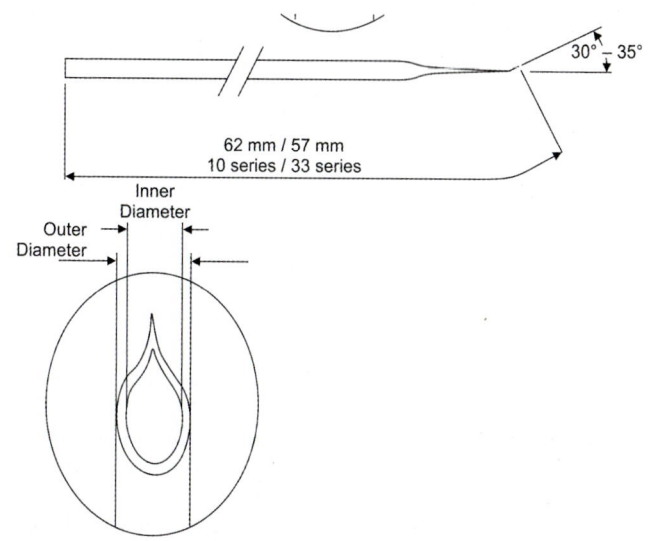

Fig. 11.2A: Injecting pipette

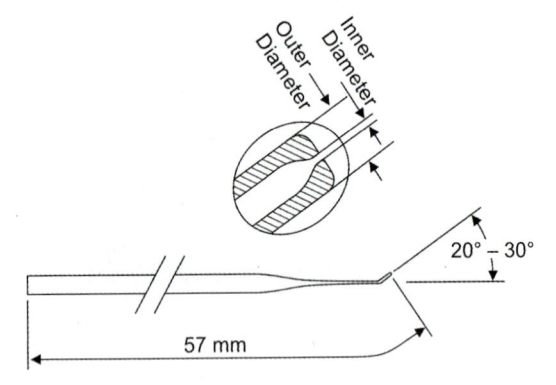

Fig. 11.2B: Holding pipette

Figs 11.2A and B: The construction (line figure) of holding and injecting pipette

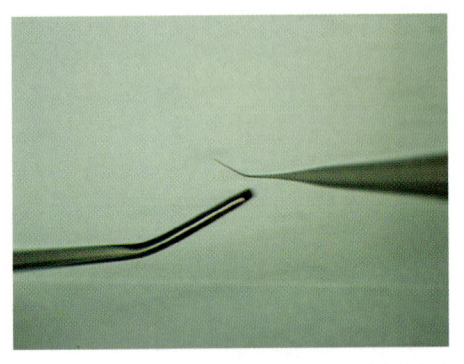

Fig. 11.3: ICSI holding (left) and injecting Pipettes (Right). Angulations' at the tips are clearly seen. Once the micropipettes have been fitted to the tool holders and attached to the universal joints, their alignment can be checked and adjusted. Fairly accurate alignment of the holding pipette can be achieved by eye, but precise alignment requires the aid of an inverted microscope. Alignment of an injection pipette depends almost entirely upon the use of the microscope because it is extremely difficult to see the angle by naked eye

Intracytoplasm Sperm Injection and Troubleshooting | **263**

angle of approximately 35°, to enable injection procedure to be performed with the tips positioned horizontally in a falcon ICSI dish.

PREPARATION OF ICSI DISHES (FIGS 11.4 TO 11.9)

- *Time of preparation:* The preparation of the microinjection dishes is done before oocyte denudation. This step takes 30 minutes, as it is essential for the media droplets to warm to desired temperature.
- *Preparation of microinjection droplets:* For ICSI procedure, small droplets (10–15 µl) of medium and PVP, are placed into a microinjection dish (Falcon 1006 ICSI dishes) and overlaid with pre-equilibrated mineral oil at 37°C. These dishes are then placed in the incubator for equilibration.

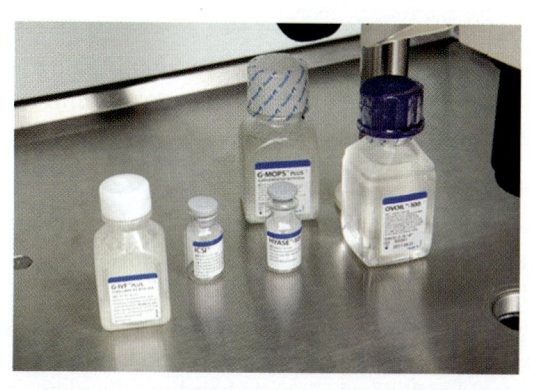

Fig. 11.4: The media required for ICSI. We use Vitrolife range of medias comprising of G-IVF PLUS, MOPS PLUS, OVOIL, ICSI (Polyvinylpyrrolidone—PVP) and Hyase (hyaluronidase)

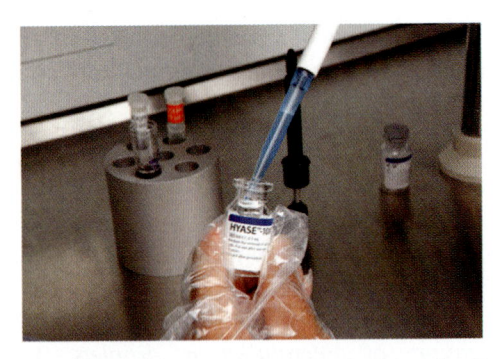

Fig. 11.5: HYASE™ (hyaluronidase) is used to facilitate the dispersal of the cumulus mass and corona. HYASE™ is concentrated 10 times and should be diluted 1:10 with supplemented MOPS™ PLUS, Exposure to HYASE™ for longer than 30 seconds may damage the oocyte by overdigestion of the zona pellucida

> *Note:* The most important consideration when preparing dishes for microinjection is that the droplets of medium should be small so that they stick to the bottom of the plate and are therefore are more stable and covered completely with oil.

- *Denudation plate (Fig. 11.6):* Hyaluronic acid and ICSI media are required for the preparation 35 mm or single well dishes may be used.

Precautions

1. Each droplet must be labeled and numbered so that there is no confusion while working under the microscope.
2. The distance between each droplet should be adequate, so that they do not coalesce with each other.
3. To avoid spilling of oil while handling the plate, droplet should be small so that they are easily covered with minimal quantity of oil.

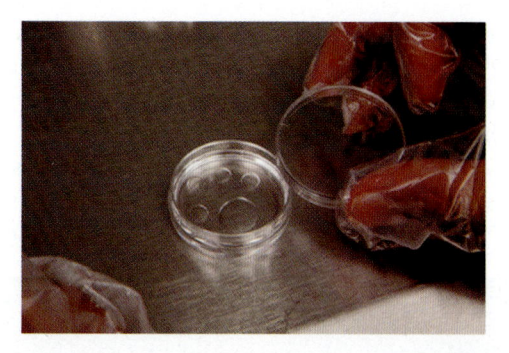

Fig. 11.6: Denudation plate. 100 μl drop of hyase at 6 o'clock position is made. Around this drop 4–5 drops of G-IVF media are made to wash the oocytes. Exposure to HYASE[TM] for too long or rough handling as well as exposure to subphysiological pH and temperatures may also damage the oocyte. The diameter of the pipette should be slightly larger than that of the oocyte (approximately 130–175 μm)

- *Choice of the buffered media:* The choice of the buffered media for the microinjection droplets will depend upon the experience of the ICSI operator.
  - If the operator is experienced then, manipulation may be performed in microdroplets of bicarbonate buffered media. With this media the operator has approximately 5–10 minutes to conduct the microinjection before the pH is altered.
  - If the operator needs more time due to inexperience MOPS/HEPES buffered flushing media may be used. Here the operator has nearly 15–20 minutes per dish with 4–6 denuded oocytes.
- *Placement of PVP droplet:* Droplet of PVP in which spermatozoa are manipulated is fundamental to the

procedure and should be located easily and quickly. PVP droplet is placed centrally as a longitudinal line with small droplets of buffered media placed around them at a close distance.

- *Droplet for sperm reservoir:* Sometimes when the semen sample is oligospermic or sperms have been surgically extracted a larger droplet

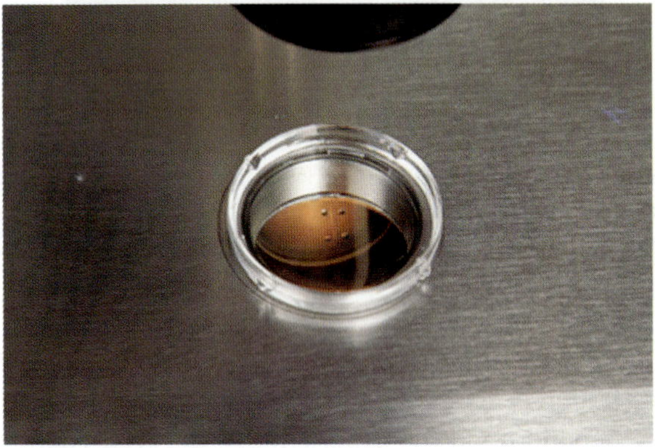

Fig. 11.7: PVP Plate. Falcon Petri Dish (1006) is used. Thin central line is made with the PVP. Four 10 µl droplets are made of G-MOPS for oocyte injection. These are then covered with the Oil. Polyvinylpyrrolidone (PVP) is commonly used in ICSI because of its viscous properties. It slows the motility of the sperm and makes it easier to "catch" the sperm, allowing immobilization of the sperm and "slashing" of the tail before injection. PVP also allows for controlled injection of the sperm by slowing down the speed of the injection fluid. This helps to stabilize the microinjection procedure and minimize the volume of fluid that is injected into the oocyte. It is advisable not to overfill the dish with oil as this can lead to spillage, which can result in coating of the underside and sides of the dish with oil. The oil may spill over and coat the lens of the objective. Now the ICSI dish may be placed in the incubator at 37°C for 30 minutes for temperature equilibration

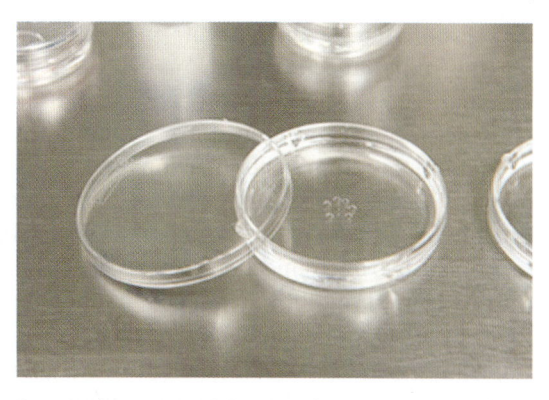

Fig. 11.8: PVP Plate. Central droplet of PVP surrounded by G-MOPS plus Droplets for microinjection. PVP is very viscous and difficult to handle with narrow pipettes. I use the wider end of 140 micrometer or nontoxic sterile pipette tip to make the droplets or central streak of PVP

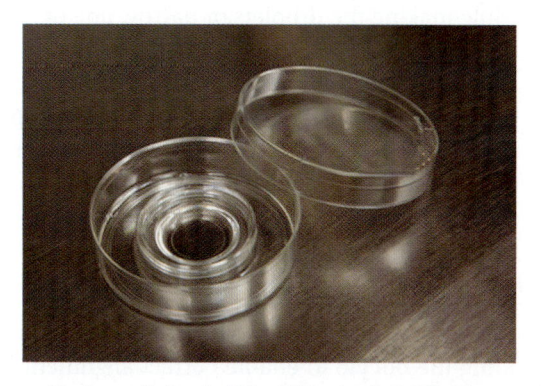

Fig. 11.9: Single well Petri dish. 500 µl of G-IVF Plus media is dispensed and covered with same amount of oil. Injected oocytes are placed in this dish for further assessment and Culture. 100 µl droplet is made in the outer well at (11 o'clock) position to rinse the microinjected eggs before placing them into the G-IVF in the inner well

of buffered media (20 µl) may be made in the microinjection dish as a reservoir for spermatozoa. Sperms are aspirated from this 'sperm drop' and moved to the PVP droplet for manipulation prior to injection.

- *Number of dishes to be prepared:* If more than five mature oocytes are to be injected, it will be essential to prepare two microinjection dishes so that while one dish is being used for microinjection, the other can be kept warm and equilibrated inside an incubator.
- *Pipettes:* Cook/Swemed/Midatlantic 140 microns pipette is preferred to make buffered media microinjection droplets. To dispense PVP, which is very dense and viscous, falcon polystyrene pipette's (3 ml) may be used. Small micropipette tips may be used for the same. This gives complete accuracy while making the droplets or narrow line of the PVP media.
- *Oil overlay:* Equilibrated and warm oil is now pipetted over them until the drops are completely covered. This can be confirmed by examining the interface between the medium and oil under stereozoom microscope.

DENUDATION

Hyaluronidase is used to remove the cumulus cells surrounding the oocyte to enable correct alignment of the oocyte with respect to polar body prior to sperm injection.

Steps of Denudation During ICSI (Figs 11.10 to 11.12)

- *Timing of denudation:* Oocytes are denuded an hour or two after their retrieval and ICSI may be conducted immediately after cumulus removal.

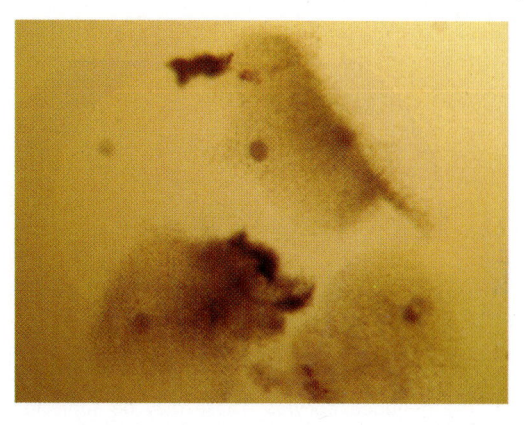

Intracytoplasm Sperm Injection and Troubleshooting

Fig. 11.10: Freshly aspirated oocyte cumulus complex. We always equilibrate the eggs in incubator for 2 hours before their denudation for ICSI

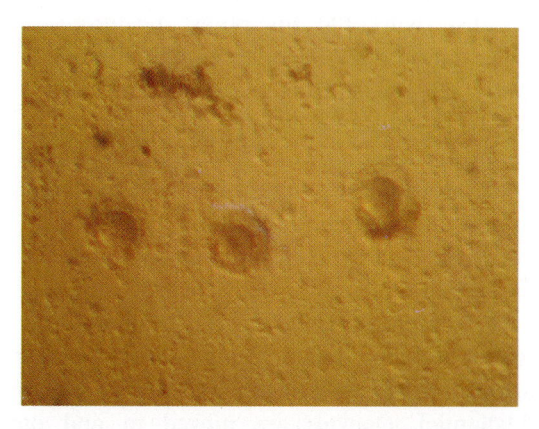

Fig. 11.11: For ICSI the oocytes will need to have their cumulus mass and corona removed. This process is called denudation. This process may be performed either using the large volume method without oil, using multi-wells and dishes or the droplet method under oil. HYASE™ (hyaluronidase) is used to facilitate the dispersal of the cumulus mass and corona

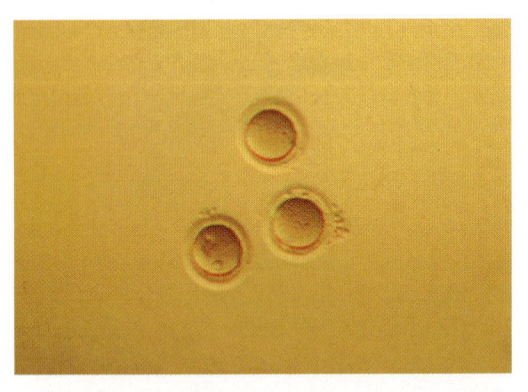

Fig. 11.12: The denuded oocytes. These may be subjected to ICSI immediately after the process of denudation

- *Equilibration of hyaluronic acid:* Allow the single well dish with 400 microliters hyaluronic acid at concentration of 80 IU/ml to equilibrate to 37°C.
- *Pipettes:* Before starting the procedure keep 140/170 microns pipettes preheated and ready.
- *Making hyaluronidase and wash droplet:* Droplet of 100 µl of hyaluronidase solution media is made. 3-4 wash droplets are made with bicarbonate media.
- *Transfer of oocytes in hyaluronidase droplet:* Using an appropriate pipette, transfer between 1 and 5 cumulus oocyte complex (COC) into the hyaluronidase for 20 seconds and then denude using a series of progressively narrower Flexipets (170 µm, 140 µm) (cook/swemed/midatlantic). Oocytes are moved in and out very gradually and repeatedly until most of the cumulus cells are loosened and the zona pellucida is clearly seen.
- *Washing of oocyte:* As each oocyte is denuded it should be moved through the series of wash wells with bicarbonate media to remove the excess hyaluronidase.

Intracytoplasm Sperm Injection and Troubleshooting

These are finally collected together in the clean drop of bicarbonate buffered media and incubated till they are loaded in the injection dish.

Steps of Sperm Immobilization

↓

Load the sperms to the periphery of central PVP droplet streak after adequate dilution (1 µl with a concentration of 10 million sperm)

↓

Load the denuded oocytes in the bicarbonate media droplet

↓

To immobilize spermatozoa, localize the sperm near the edge/ of the PVP drop and bring both the tail of the sperm and the injecting pipette in sharp focus

↓

After aligning the injection pipette perpendicular to the tail, the sperm is immobilized with a swift moment of the pipette from left to right thus severing the tail of the sperm against the bottom of the dish with a quick and deliberate movement

↓

Spermatozoon aspirated into the injection pipette, tail first, by slowly turning the injector anticlockwise

↓

Once aspirated, stop movement by turning injector clockwise. Confirm that the movement of the spermatozoon along the injection pipette is completely under control before proceeding to manipulate the oocyte

---

Precautions
1. The oocyte cumulus complexes should be placed into the hyaluronidase for not more than 30–40 seconds.
2. Avoid excessive or rough handling of the oocytes as they are quite fragile and can be susceptible to lyses if aspirated too vigorously.
3. Do not use too thin a pipette as zona pellucida can be damaged.
4. Avoid creation of air bubbles as the denuded oocytes may stick to bubbles and get lost. This phenomenon is common and is called the parachute effect.

MANIPULATION OF SPERMATOZOA

> *Sperm immobilization. Points to remember...*
> 1. It is better to load less sperms than many, as higher concentration will make the visualization and immobilization of the sperms difficult.
> 2. To locate and manipulate spermatozoa in the PVP drop, it is preferable to switch to a 20x objective lens and refocus upon the injection pipette.
> 3. If the concentration of the sperms is very low as in case of surgically retrieved sample, load the sample in the buffered media drop from where sperms are selected and transferred to the PVP drop for micromanipulation.[1-3]
> 4. It is absolutely vital to damage the plasmalemma of the spermatozoon and to immobilize it before the injection to allow the release of a sperm cytosolic factor, which activates the oocyte. This has been shown to markedly enhance fertilization rates following ICSI.[4-6]
> 5. Immobilization should be done at the edge as the most motile, and the therefore probably the most viable sperms, are found at the periphery of the droplet.
> 6. Immobilization should be done in a single stroke as if repeated again and again the tail becomes sticky and there will be difficulty while aspirating in the injecting pipette.
> 7. Kinking or curling of the tail confirms immobilization.

MANIPULATION OF OOCYTES

1. Oocytes must be examined under stereozoom microscope to look at polar body, ooplasm, zona pellucida and oolemma and confirm the oocyte is at metaphase II.
2. Transfer the oocytes to the media drops.
3. Manipulate oocytes by blowing and sucking the oocyte with the holding pipette and using the injecting needle

in the X, Y, Z axis to rotate it such that the polar body is at 6 or 12'o clock as it ensures that the injection pipette does not penetrate the oocyte closer to where the spindle is presumed to lie.
4. Before holding the egg bring the oolemma and the holding pipette tip in focus at one time.
5. Very mild negative pressure in the holding pipette is used so as not to deform or suck oocyte during the procedure.

Manipulation of oocyte. Points to remember...
1. It is essential to have a heated stage/platform on the micromanipulator while manipulating oocytes.
2. Smaller aperture in the heated stage of the micromanipulator is preferred as there is more efficient heating of the ICSI dish and less thermal damage of the spindle apparatus of the oocytes.
3. The immature oocytes (GV & MI) should not be injected, as they will not fertilize.
4. Very mild negative pressure is used, as zona pellucida and oolemma is very sensitive to mechanical stress and excessive pressure, which can damage the cytoskeleton of the oocyte. At the same time negative pressure should be adequate to hold the oocyte during the injection procedure.
5. Coronal cells attached to the oocyte, can be used as a means of attaching the oocyte to the holding pipette with the advantage that superior and gentle suction may be applied, with less risk of damaging and distorting the oolemma.

MICROINJECTION OF OOCYTES WITH MATURE SPERMATOZOA (FIGS 11.13 TO 11.20)

1. *Positioning the injection needle:* The injection pipette tip is brought adjacent to the zona pellucida at the midline of the oocyte, taking care to keep both the tip and the oolemma focused.

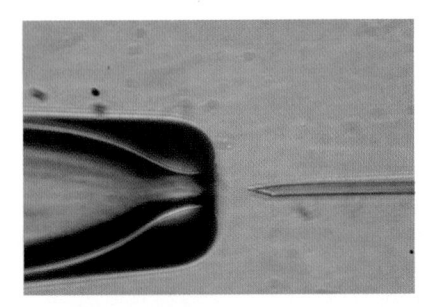

Fig. 11.13: Final alignments of the pipette. The alignment methodologies of the holding and injection pipettes differ. Holding pipette is aligned without tilt in the horizontal plane, as it has to aligned flat on the bottom of the dish to aspirate the denuded Oocyte. On the other hand the injection pipette needs to be tilted downwards towards its tip in the horizontal plane, so that the tail of the spermatozoon can be slashed and easily aspirated. Thus the, final alignment of the injection pipette is recognized by it touching the bottom of the dish

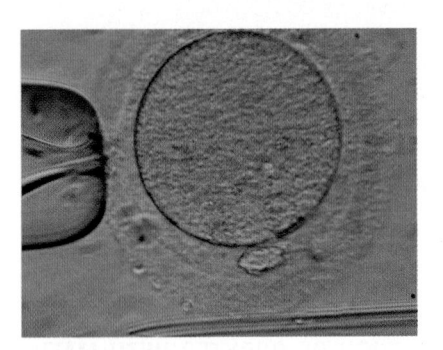

Fig. 11.14: After the spermatozoon has been immobilized and aspirated into the injection pipette, and the oocyte has been held by the holding pipette with the PB at either 6 or 12 o'clock, injection of the spermatozoon may be done. The use of slight negative pressure or even just capillary action should be all that is required to attach the oocyte gently but firmly to the holding pipette. On the other hand, the oocyte should not be held so loosely that it becomes detached from the holding pipette when withdrawing the injection pipette from the oocyte

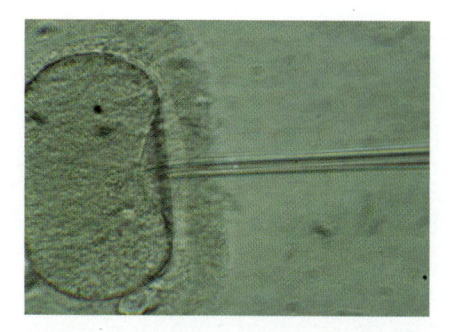

Intracytoplasm Sperm Injection and Troubleshooting | **275**

Fig. 11.15: The injection pipette may then be advanced carefully in a straight line towards the oocyte to penetrate the ZP. Enter the egg from the geometric center horizontally with minimum shake. Observe the pattern of indentation that it creates

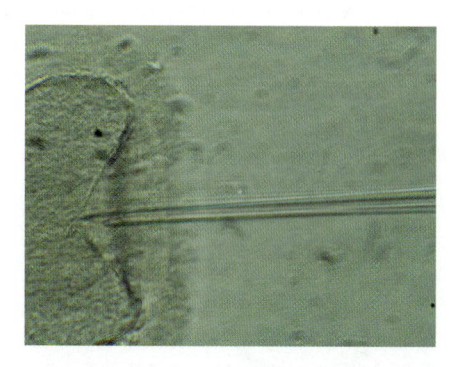

Fig. 11.16: A deep indentation is created in the oolemma with the injecting pipette and acute funnel is obtained. Please do not push the injection pipette much more than halfway into the oocyte, as to avoid piercing the oolemma on the opposite side. Ooplasm is now aspirated into the injection pipette by slowly turning the injector screw in an anticlockwise direction. Initially, the flow of ooplasm into the injection pipette will be slow as it is impeded by the intact oolemma. Latter with increasing negative suction the oolemma will rupture to allow a sudden free flow of ooplasm in the injecting pipette. Immediately halt the influx of ooplasm into the injection pipette by quickly reversing the negative pressure

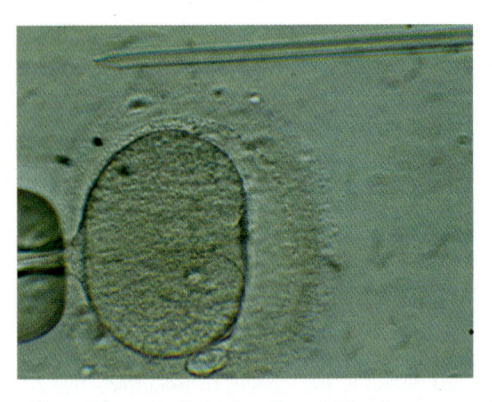

Fig. 11.17: The oolemma funnel will quickly disappear after the withdrawal of the injecting pipette. Earlier the egg attains the original state healthier it is, as funneling is the indirect evidence of elasticity of the oolemma

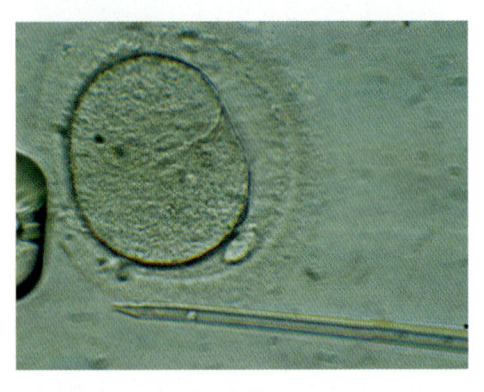

Fig. 11.18: The Oocyte is now released from the holding pipette by turning the injector screw clockwise. A gentle knock by the injecting pipette may help in final release of the egg from the holding pipette. The egg is now shifted to the single well dish containing G-IVF-Plus media

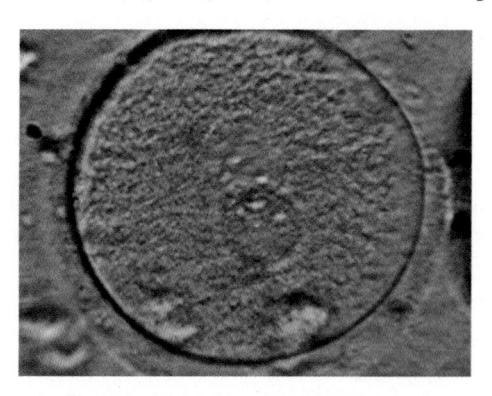

Intracytoplasm Sperm Injection and Troubleshooting | **277**

Fig. 11.19: Post ICSI PN as observed after 18 hours

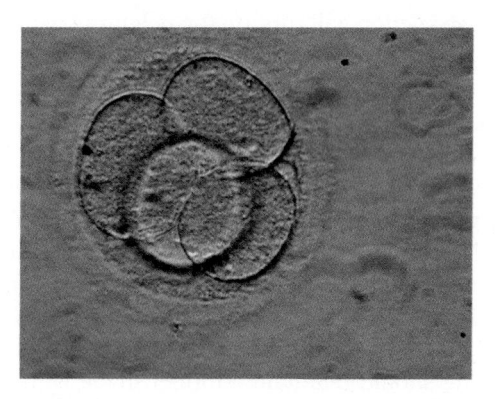

Fig. 11.20: Grade 1,4-cell embryo as observed after 44 hours

2. *Positioning sperm to tip of needle:* Gradually turn the injector syringe clockwise to move the spermatozoon towards the tip of the injection pipette. As the sperm moves towards the pipette tip apply anticlockwise force to stabilize the sperm movement, taking care that the sperm is not expelled.

3. *Injecting the oocyte:* The injection pipette with loaded sperm is advanced cautiously in a straight line towards the oocyte to perforate the zona pellucida at the approximate midline of the geometrical curvature. As the injecting needle perforates the zona pellucida and the oolemma, usually, the oolemma remains intact due to its inherent strength and elasticity being wrapped around the injecting pipette.
4. *Aspiration of ooplasm:* Ooplasm may now be aspirated into the injection pipette by slowly turning the suction syringe in the anticlockwise direction. To begin with, the aspiration of ooplasm into the injection pipette will be slow as it is impeded by the intact oolemma. Persistent negative suction will rupture the oolemma with sudden free flow of ooplasm. At this juncture, it is important to halt the influx of ooplasm into the injection pipette by quickly reversing the negative pressure being created by the injector syringe.
5. *Deposition of sperm:* Now by slowly turning the injector syringe in a clockwise direction replace the ooplasm that has been aspirated, along with the immobilized sperm, into the oocyte. Quickly withdraw the injection pipette from the oocyte. After the pipette is removed, the breach area is observed, and the order of the opening should maintain a funnel shape with a vertex into the egg.[7] Immediate rupture of the oolemma without any aspiration has been associated with lower oocyte survival rates.
6. *Releasing injected oocyte:* Now we can gently release the negative suction of the holding pipette by clockwise movement of the suction syringe and release the egg.
7. *Washing oocytes:* Other oocytes are injected in a similar fashion, before washing them all in a bicarbonate-buffered medium for culture.

8. *Assessment of fertilization:* The oocytes are assessed for fertilization next day by the presence of two PN and two polar bodies on the following day (Figs 11.18 and 11.19). Nonfertilized, degenerated oocytes and oocytes with more than 2 PN or less than 2 PN should be removed from culture. After assessment, the zygotes should be rinsed in equilibrated supplemented G-1^{TM}/G-1^{TM} PLUS and then transferred to a new dish with equilibrated supplemented G-1^{TM}/G-1^{TM} PLUS for culture (Fig. 11.20).

Microinjection of oocytes. Points to remember….

1. Both oolemma and injection pipette tip should be in focus concurrently, as it ensures that the injection pipette correctly pierce the oocyte at its midline.
2. With fine control it is possible to stabilize the movement of the sperm at the tip of the injection pipette.
3. If the oolemma fails to rupture despite aspiration, we try to perforate the membrane by employing a very rapid jabbing movement of the injection pipette into the oocyte. While giving a jab, contact with the opposite segment of the oolemma must be avoided. In case this fails, it is better to compromise by depositing the spermatozoon into the perivitelline space rather than subjecting it to more excessive manipulation, which might well result in its demise.
4. Deliberate attempt is made to deposit the spermatozoa towards the center of the oocyte as this not only confirms the placement but also ensures that proper funnel is created during the placement of the sperm.
5. Injection pipette should be quickly withdrawn from the oocyte after release of sperm to avoid minimal deposition of PVP in the cytoplasm.
6. If equipment may develop an error or the pipettes malfunctions, the oocytes are transferred to the media dish and put in incubator till the problem is resolved.

DIFFICULT ICSI CASES

An abnormal sperm sample can present difficulties during the procedure. For example, sperm suspensions prepared from testicular biopsies as well as severe cases of oligoasthenoteratospermia usually exhibit very low count, low and sluggish motility, and presence of debris and other cells. Frozen thawed epididymal sperm may also be problematic. Only a small fraction of the sperm may survive and the surviving sperm may exhibit a very low progressive movement or no movement at all. A third example of a difficult ICSI case is sperm obtained by Electro-ejaculation. In this case, the sperm count can be very high and the motility very low. In addition there are other cells and debris also present in the sample.

CONCLUSION

The intracytoplasmic sperm injection (ICSI) bypasses the ZP and the oolemma. The ability of ICSI to achieve higher fertilization and pregnancy rates regardless of sperm characteristics makes it the most prevailing micromanipulation procedure with which to treat male factor infertility.

REFERENCES

1. Palermo GD, Cohen J, Alikani M, Adler A, Rosenwaks Z. Intracytoplasmic sperm injection: a novel treatment for all forms of male factor infertility. Fertil Steril. 1995;63:1231-40.
2. Palermo GD, Cohen J, Rosenwaks Z. Intracytoplasmic sperm injection: a powerful tool to overcome fertilization failure. Fertil Steril. 1996;65: 899-908.
3. Palermo GD, Schlegel PN, Hariprashad JJ, et al. Fertilization and pregnancy outcome with intracyto-plasmic sperm injection for azoospermic men. Hum Reprod. 1999;14:741-8.

4. Dozortzev D, Rybouchkin A, De Sutter P, Quian C, Dhont M. Human oocyte activation following intra-cytoplasmic sperm injection; the role of the sperm cell. Hum Reprod. 1995;10:403-7.
5. Palermo GD, Joris H, Derde MP, et al. Sperm characteristics and outcome of human assisted fertilization by subzonal insemination and intracytoplasmic sperm injection. Fertil Steril. 1993;63:1231-40.
6. Fishel S, Lisi F, Rinaldi L, et al. Systematic examination of immobilizing spermatozoa before intracytoplasmic sperm injection in the human. Hum Reprod. 1995;10:497-500.
7. Palermo G, Alikani M, Bertoli M, et al. Oolemma characteristics in relation to survival and fertilization patterns of oocytes treated by ICSI. Hum Reprod. 1996;11:172-6.

Chapter 12

Gamete Cryopreservation

Pankaj Talwar

OOCYTE CRYOPRESERVATION

OOCYTE FREEZING

Introduction

The recent option of integration of oocyte cryopreservation into the standard IVF program has clearly improved the medical care for women at risk of losing ovarian function.[1] Recent advances in embryology techniques, fertilization, use of intracytoplasmic sperm injection (ICSI), and standardization of cryoprotectants, have made oocyte cryopreservation a practical application. The metaphase-II oocyte is extremely fragile due to its:
- Large size and low surface area
- Large water content
- Scattered spindle apparatus is easily damaged by intracellular ice formation during the freezing or thawing process.
- Human oocyte cryopreservation is performed either using conventional slow-rate freezing or vitrification. Techniques with conventional freezing, cells are cooled to a very low temperatures slowly, minimizing intracellular ice crystal formation, and at the same

time low molarity cryoprotectants are used which reduce the unwanted influences of increased solute concentrations. On the other hand vitrification, a nonequilibrium approach to cryopreservation utilizes high concentrations of cryoprotectants that solidify without forming ice crystals which is a major cause of intracellular cryodamage. The vitrified solution may be considered as an extremely viscous, glassy and supercooled liquid. During vitrification the oocytes are dehydrated by short exposure to a high molarity cryoprotectant before plunging the gametes directly into liquid nitrogen.

Indications

1. Cancer patients about to undergo chemotherapy or pelvic irradiation.[1]
2. Young women undergoing ovarian surgery for benign disease.
3. Single women with a strong family history of premature ovarian failure.
4. Healthy women, who desire to postpone pregnancy for unavoidable reasons.
5. Patients who are opposed to embryo cryopreservation for religious or ethical reasons.
6. Women whose partners are unable to produce semen specimens on the day of oocyte retrieval.[2,3]

Essential Principles of Controlled Rate Cooling

1. Initial exposure of the eggs to low cryoprotectant concentrations, which are associated with minimal toxicity. This step is performed at the room temperature when the oocyte is still metabolizing.

2. The oocytes are exposed to increasing cryoprotectant concentrations while still working at room temperature.
3. They are then cooled up to –8°C.
4. At the temperature of –8°C, ice crystals are induced in the cryostraw solution by inducing seeding, a small crystal of ice that allows extracellular water molecules to undergo crystallization. This ice formation releases latent heat of fusion, which may suddenly heat up the straw contents, which have been gradually cooled. Thus, the cryostraws are held at –8°C for period of 10 minutes, to allow equilibration and stabilization of the gametes.
5. After equilibration, the temperature is gradually decreased to a final temperature of –30°C bringing about 3 main changes:
    i. As the oocytes are gradually cooled to subzero temperatures due to osmotic effect and extracellular ice formation, there is gradual increase in concentration of cryoprotectants in the extracellular and intracellular compartment.
    ii. The cellular metabolism also decreases as eggs are cooled gradually aiding in the reduced toxicity and cryodamage to oocytes due to these supra-physiological concentrations of cryoprotectants in the cryosolution.
    iii. The very slow rate of cooling (0.3°C per minute) allows gradual diffusion into the oocyte of additional permeating cryoprotectant while maintaining equilibrium with the extracellular space.
6. At the final temperature of –30°C, PROH still is well above its freezing temperature but its concentration has increased considerably. The metabolic rate of the

oocyte now is quite slow, further limiting the toxicity of the increasing concentrations of the cryoprotectants.
7. The oocytes are then quickly cooled to –150°C.
8. The cryostraw now is plunged into liquid nitrogen, and the remaining nonsolidified solution is converted to a glassy, vitrified state.

Essential Principles of Thawing

During thawing, a rapid transition of temperature is preferred to prevent re-crystallization of water with the potential for ice-crystal damage. Here, caution must be taken to avoid osmotic shock from the permeating cryoprotectant, which now is at a very high concentration in the intracellular space. Therefore, additional non-permeating cryoprotectant is used. As the permeating cryoprotectant gradually diffuses out of the oocyte, the concentration of the non-permeating cryoprotectant gradually is decreased, until the oocyte is equilibrated in the bicarbonated culture medium.

Evaluation of Oocyte Quality

The oocytes may be graded before or after denudation and it's morphological maturity should be recorded, for latter outcame and reference.

Oocyte-denudation—To do or not?

Removal of the cumulus mass before oocyte freeing is always a matter of debate. However, advantages are:
1. Differences in the layers of cells surrounding the oocyte would be a source of variability that could affect the reproducibility of the method used.
2. Presence of cumulus cells makes grading of the oocytes difficult thus leading to storage of oocyte cumulus complexes of varied maturity.

3. An expanded cumulus mass may influence the exchange of water and CPAs and thereby ultimately have an effect on the whole cryopreservation procedure.
4. After freezing- thawing cycle, a higher survival rate was observed in the cumulus-free group (69% vs 48%).[4]

For oocyte cryopreservation, we prefer to carry out the denudation as it improves the permeability of the oocytes to cryoprotectants and leads to better outcome.

Factors Affecting the Clinical Efficiency of Oocyte Cryopreservation

Freeze thaw cycle may lead to:
1. *Zonal hardening:* There may be alterations to the zona pellucida microarchitecture, making it harder and thus reducing the fertilization rate.[5]
2. *Premature release of cortical granules:* This may increase the risk of polyspermy.
3. *Disruption of meiotic spindle:* The microtubular spindle must configure itself correctly to achieve accurate chromosome segregation and thus preventing aneuploidies.[6] Injury to the meiotic spindle might increase the risk of aneuploidy in the conceptus. Oocytes have very high water content and have scattered microspindle apparatus holding the chromosomes. This makes the oocytes particularly vulnerable to exposure to low temperature during the freezing process. Many studies have raised concerns about aneuploidies after observing disruption of the spindle apparatus during oocyte freezing.[7] Spindles are realigned and reconstructed after few hours of oocyte warming.[8]
4. *Injuries to the ooplasm organelles:* Injuries to the ooplasm organelles due to the formation of intracellular ice crystals and sudden changes in the oocyte volume due

to the different osmotic pressures between intracellular and extracellular solutions may also lead to poor oocyte recovery post thaw.

Cryopreservation of Immature Oocytes at Prophase I (GV Stage)

Cryopreservation of immature oocytes at prophase I (GV stage) has also been proposed as an alternative to standard oocyte cryopreservation as it was thought that these oocytes were less sensitive to cryoinjury, as they lack spindle and have different membrane permeability, however no advantage was seen. In fact, this technique requires oocyte *in vitro* maturation after thawing and has been related to an increased incidence of chromosomal abnormalities.

Recent Advances in Cryopreservation Media

1. *Calcium free media:* Vitrifying oocytes in calcium-free media reduced zona hardening, increased subsequent fertilization, and did not adversely affect embryonic development to the blastocyst stage.[9]
2. *Choline:* Substitution of sodium by choline in the oocyte cryopreservation media appears to improve cryopreservation outcome.[10]
3. *Trehalose:* A recent innovation in oocyte freezing involves the use of the sugar trehalose as a cryoprotectant.[11]
4. *Sucrose concentration:* Increasing the sucrose concentration to 0.2 mol/l to 0.3 mol/l in the freezing solution it was possible to improve dramatically the survival rate up to 80%.[12]

Procedure of Oocyte Slow Freezing (Table 12.1)

Table 12.1
Oocyte freezing protocol

i. The Cook Oocyte Cryopreservation Kit is a three-step cryopreservation kit for the freezing of MII oocytes containing HEPES buffered salt solutions using propanediol and sucrose as cryoprotectants.
   - *Vial 1:* Cryobuffer supplemented with 0.75 mol/l propanediol,
   - *Vial 2:* Cryobuffer supplemented with 1.5 mol/l propanediol,
   - *Vial 3:* Cryobuffer supplemented with 1.5 mol/l propanediol and 0.2 Mol/l sucrose
   - All Oocytes must be completely denuded of cumulus and coronal cells
   - The freezing solutions should be warmed to room temperature (~20° C) before use.
   - All dehydration steps must be performed at room temperature (~20°C).

ii. Method
   - Label sufficient number of cryostraws with the specific patient information
   - Dispense 0.4 ml of freeze solution 1 into well 1 of a 4 well dish, dispense freeze solution 2 and 3 into the corresponding wells of the 4 well dishes and label accordingly. Allow solution to equilibrate to room temperature (20°C).
   - Transfer oocyte(s) to freeze solution 1, and incubate for 7 minutes, 30 seconds.
   - Transfer oocyte(s) with a minimum volume of freeze solution 1 into well 2, containing freeze solution 2 and mix thoroughly. Incubate for 7 minutes, 30 seconds.
   - Transfer oocyte(s) with a minimum volume of freeze solution 2 into well 3, containing freeze solution 3 and mixed thoroughly. Incubate for 5 minutes.
   - Using freeze solution 3, in well 3, as the loading solution, load the oocyte(s) into the labeled straw

Contd...

Contd...

- Aspirate a 20 mm column of freeze solution 3 into the straw followed by 10 mm of air, 30 mm of freeze solution 3 with oocytes followed by 10 mm column of air 20 mm column of FS 3 and 10 mm column of air in the end.
- The first column of the freeze media will seal the plug, stopping all further movement in the straw. Seal the open end of the straw plug, seal-ease putty (Becton Dickinson).
- The straws are placed into a controlled rate-freezing machine and the prescribed freezing program is used.

iii. Controlled rate freezing program for oocytes
  - Decrease temperature from +20°C to –8°C with a rate of –2°C/min
  - "Hold" at –8°C for 10 min
  - Perform manual seeding at 3 minutes into the "hold" ramp
  - Decrease temperature from –8°C to –30°C with a rate of –0.3°C/min
  - Decrease temperature from –30°C to –150°C with a rate of –50°C/min
  - Hold at –150°C for 10 min
  - Transfer into LN_2 for long-term storage
  - Seeding is achieved by touching a cold forceps to the upper meniscus of oocyte column to initiate planned crystallization.

Procedure of Oocyte thawing (Table 12.2)

Table 12.2

Constituents of Media

i. The Cook oocyte thawing kit is a four-step thawing system for MII oocytes containing a HEPES buffered salt solution with propanediol and sucrose as cryoprotectants.
   Vial 1: Cryobuffer supplemented with 1.0 mol/l propanediol and 0.3 mol/L sucrose.

Contd...

Contd...

Vial 2: Cryobuffer supplemented with 0.5 mol/l propanediol and 0.3 mol1/l sucrose

Vial 3: Cryobuffer supplemented with 0.3 mol/l propanediol and 0.3 mol1/l sucrose,

Vial 4: Cryobuffer.

- The thawing solution should be warmed to room temperature (~20°C) before use
- All rehydration steps must be performed at room temperature
- Prepare a culture dish containing Cook Cleavage medium for culture of the oocyte post thaw and equilibrate in a 6% CO_2 incubator at 37°C
- Prepare all necessary items to perform ICSI.

ii. Method
- Dispense 0.4 ml of thaw solution 1 in well 1 of a 4 well dish and 0.4 ml of solution 2 and 3 into the corresponding wells of a 4 well dish and label according. Allow solution to equilibrate to room temperature (~20°C) for 30 minutes.
- Label a single wall petri dish and dispense 400 microliter of thaw solution 4 (for final incubation). Warm the dish to room temperature (~20°C)
- Remove the straw containing oocytes from the liquid nitrogen
- The straw is warmed in air at room temperature (~20°C) for 30 seconds
- Transfer the straw(s) to a 30°C water bath for 40 seconds
- Remove the straw(s) and dry with a tissue
- Cut the sealant end off the straw, fit a syringe and then cut the other end the straw, if sealed or remove the straw plug
- Under a dissecting microscope, expel the contents of the straw into a Petri dish
- Incubate the oocyte(s) sequentially through the thawing solution
  TS1 RT, 5 min
  TS2 RT, 5 min
  TS3 RT, 10 min
  TS4 RT, 10 min and 10 min at 37°C

Contd...

Contd...

- Take care to minimize the volume of solution used for transferring the oocyte(s) and mix thoroughly.
- Finally, transfer the oocyte(s) to a dish containing pre-equilibrated Cook cleavage medium and return to a 6% CO_2 incubator at 37°C for 60 minutes prior to ICSI.

OOCYTE VITRIFICATION AND THAWING

Vitrification Simplified (Figs 12.1 to 12.7)

a. It is a recommended to use a container that is suitable for storing and holding the liquid nitrogen (LN_2). We use styrofoam box for storing the liquid nitrogen for the procedure. It is also recommended to use sterile LN_2 to avoid risk of contamination.

b. The recommended maximum load of the McGill Cryoleaf™ is 2 to 3 Oocytes.

c. In the process of vitrification, we are working with cryoprotectants of very high molarities. Prolonged exposure may lead to damage to the cells. Thus, we have to work with very small volumes and at speed. Never attempt vitrification till you are a accomplished embryologist because though the technique may look very simple but it may cause damage to live embryos due to our lack of training.

d. Below we will describe the technique of vitrification using medicult vitrification media using cryoleaf as the carrier. We use medicult vitrification cooling pack. Media in the freeze pack are HEPES buffered and pH-stable so that all steps can be performed outside the incubator and at room temperature.

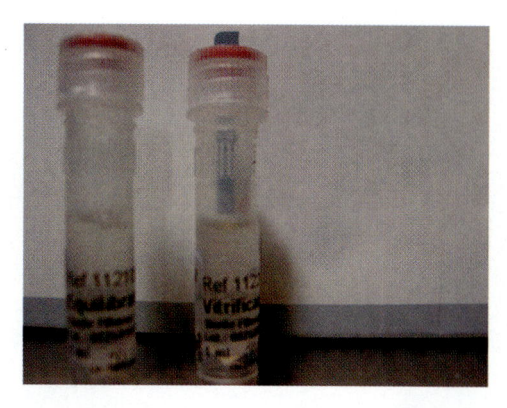

Fig. 12.1: I Freeze oocytes using medicult vitrification kit which consist of McGill Cryoleaf,™ equilibration and vitrification media. The vitrification media contains ethylene glycol and 1, 2-propanediol in HTF medium, in increasing concentrations. Dispense 500 µl of EM and VM in well 1 and well 2 of four well dish and equilibrate them at room temperature for 30 minutes

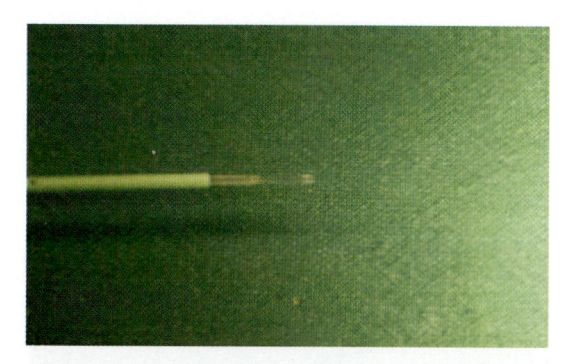

Fig. 12.2: Close up of the tip of cryoleaf. The loading surface of the cryoleaf is flat and embryos are placed on its tip in minimal volume of vitrification solution. Maximum of 2–3 oocytes loaded on the cryoleaf at one time. We Label the cryoleaf sleeve and cryoleaf before the procedure

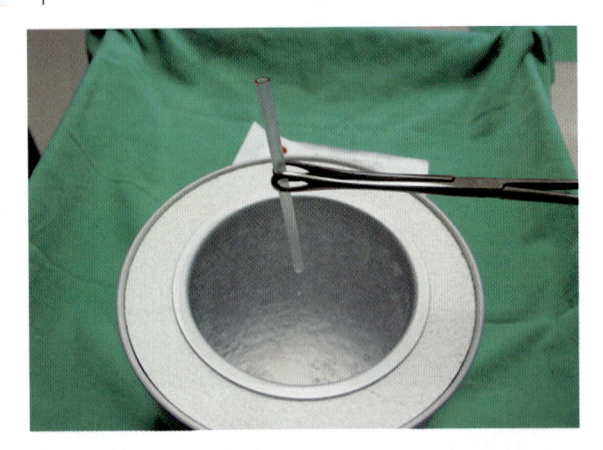

Fig. 12.3: Labeled outer cover of the cryoleaf is held with the forceps and plunged in the liquid nitrogen. Ensure that the whole sleeve is completely immersed and filled with LN_2. The loaded cryoleaf is finally placed in this outer sleave before final storage

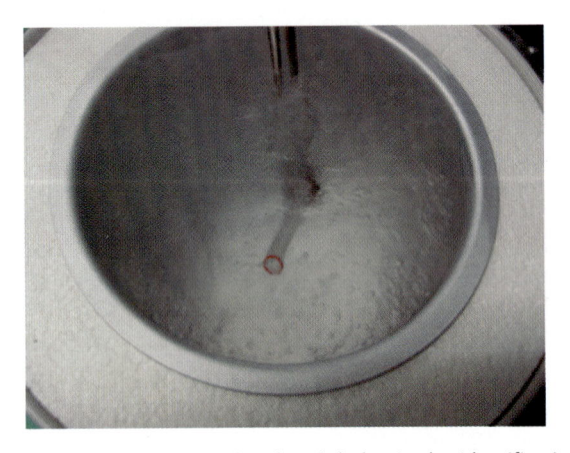

Fig. 12.4: The red circle on the sheath helps in the identification of the upper edge of the leaf cover

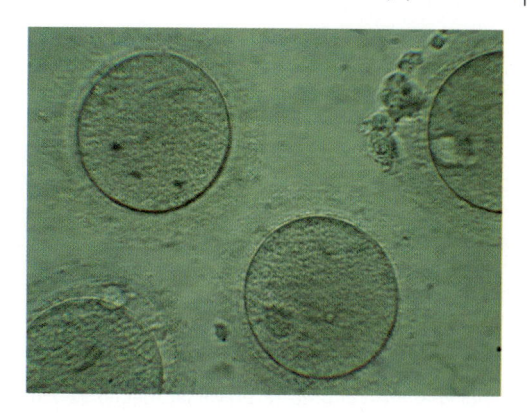

Fig. 12.5: Oocytes are denuded using hyaluronic acid. Any commercial brand may be used in concentration of 80 IU/ml. some embryologist prefer to used 40 IU/ml concentration. In the picture we can see Metaphase 2 denuded oocytes. Oocytes have regular oolemma with clear cytoplasm, Polar bodies are regular and nonfragmented

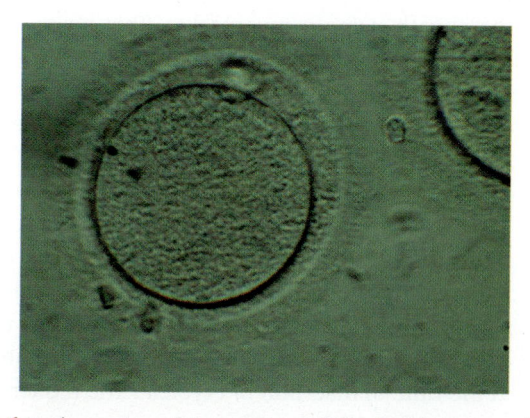

Fig. 12.6: A closer view of the oocyte at 200x. Regular zona pellucida is visualized with normal perivitelline space. Healthy polar body is also visualized

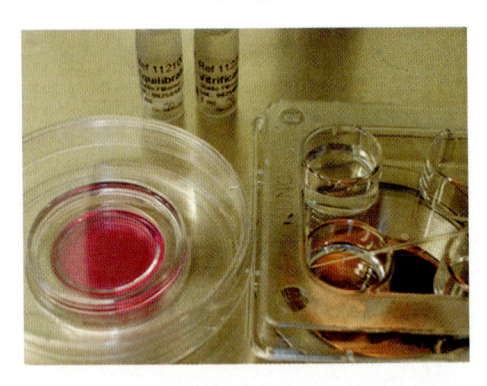

Fig. 12.7: Oocytes are cultured in universal media/G1 Plus/cleavage media for 1–2 hours after denudation. Rinse the pipette in the EM and spray small volume of EM over the embryos in single well culture media plate. Now we quickly transfer the oocytes to equilibration media (EM) for 5 minutes

1. Label the cryoleaf handle and the outer cover of the sheath using a cryomarker. This helps in easy identification during retrieval of the straws.
2. Equilibration media (EM) and vitrification media (VM) should be equilibrated at room temperature for at least 30 minutes. Dispense, vitrification media in a 4 well dish for the, procedure. Label the dish and write patients unique identification details. Enter the same in the cryobiology inventory book.
3. Labeled outer cover of the cryoleaf is now plunged in the liquid nitrogen so that temperature of the sheath reduces and it is filled with liquid nitrogen at the time of insertion of cryoleaf. The red circle on the sheath is the identification of the upper edge of the leaf cover.
4. Using the suitable pipette, transfer 2-3 denuded oocytes to the EM and let them equilibrate for

5 minutes (the oocytes initially shrink and then return to their former shape) (Figs 12.8 to 12.11).
5. Transfer the oocytes or embryos to VM, where they should remain for less than 1 minute (The oocytes now shrink again) (Fig. 12.12).
6. Quickly load the oocytes or embryos onto the McGill cryoleaf™ tip using the same pipette and as little VM as possible. The McGill Cryoleaf™ should stay dry during the process. Make sure to remove excess VM carefully and quickly using the pipette (Fig. 12.13).
7. Insert the McGill Cryoleaf™ with the oocytes or embryos directly into liquid nitrogen (LN_2) (Figs 12.14 to 12.16).
8. Carefully slide the protective sleeve (green) over the tip with the oocytes or embryos and it into place by turning. Take care that the McGill Cryoleaf™ remains immersed in LN_2 at all times.

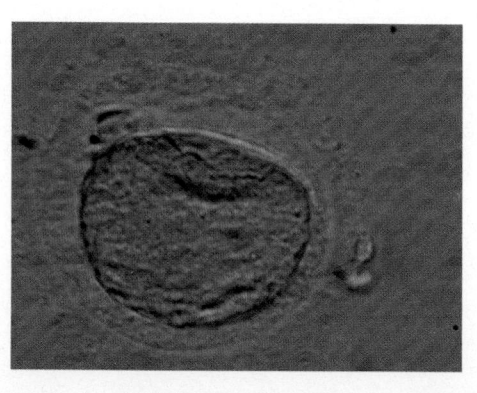

Fig. 12.8: Oocyte in equilibration media. We can visualize shrinking and irregularity of oolemma occurring immediately after contact of oocyte with the media. Infolding of the oolemma is seen. Intact polar pody is seen at 11 o'clock position

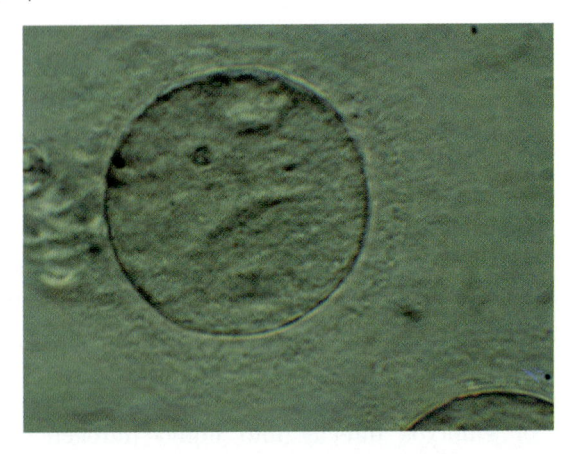

Fig. 12.9: After 3 minutes of contact period of EM and the oocyte, we can see the oolemma returning to the original state. The ooplasm looks healthy though some amount of crenations along the edges are still seen. Polar body is at 12 o'clock position and is nonfragmented

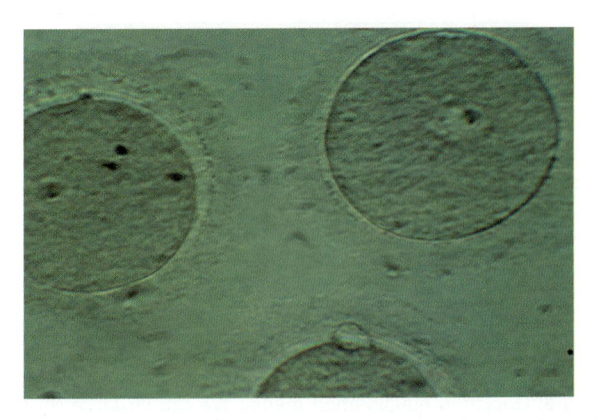

Fig. 12.10: Fully expanded oocytes. These have returned to the original state after the contact period of 4 minutes in EM

Gamete Cryopreservation

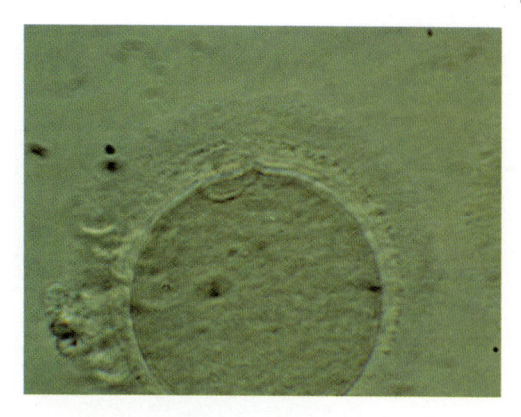

Fig. 12.11: A close-up view of the metaphase 2 oocyte. It has returned to the original shape and has had complete recovery. Polar body is seen at 11 o'clock position

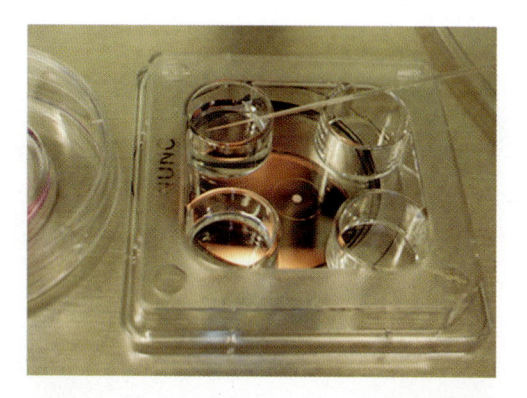

Fig. 12.12: Oocytes are now shifted to the vitrification media. Spray minimal volume of VM on oocytes in EM. These are now aspirated in minimal volume of EM and transferred to well 2 containing VM. Oocytes are to be handled very gently in vitrification media. From transfer of oocytes to the VM and to there loading on the cryo, leaf oocytes should not spend more than 60 seconds in VM

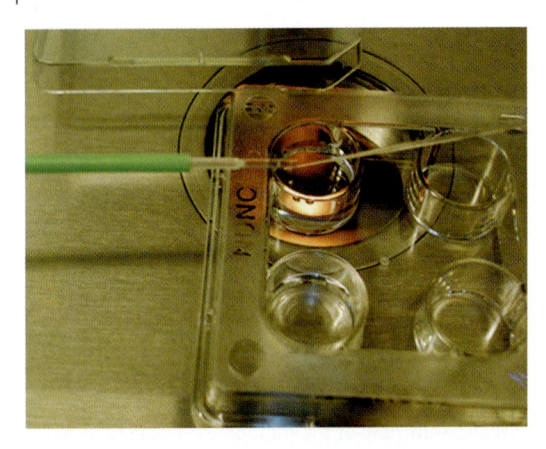

Fig. 12.13: This picture shows loading of the oocytes on the cryoleaf in minimal volume of vitrification media. This step should not take more than 10 seconds. Prolonged exposure to VM may lead to extreme dehydration of the oocyte and collapse of the gamete

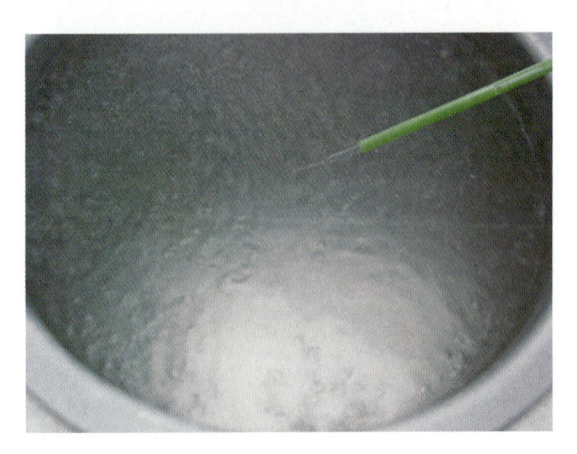

Fig. 12.14: Dip the cryoleaf with the oocytes directly into liquid nitrogen (LN_2) and slide the protective green sleeve over the loaded cryoleaf by unlocking and turning it clockwise

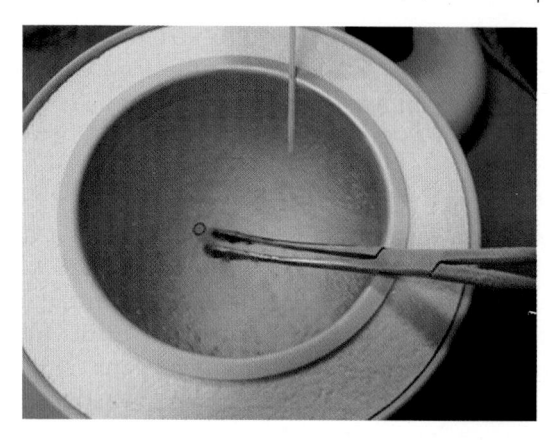

Fig. 12.15: Place the cryoleaf in the outer cover and press tightly

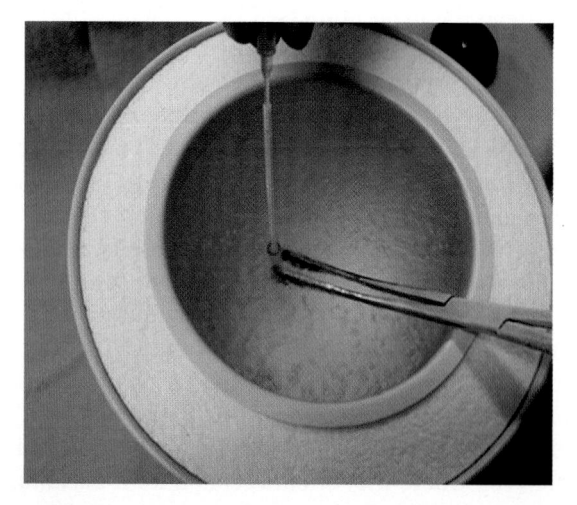

Fig. 12.16: Ensure that the leaf is dipped in liquid nitrogen throughout the procedure. Place the leaf in the cryocane and dip in liquid nitrogen till further required

9. Insert the McGill Cryoleaf™ into the outer cover and press tightly. Take care that the McGill Cryoleaf™ remains immersed in LN_2 at all times.
10. Transfer to storage container.

Steps of Oocyte Warming (Figs 12.17 to 12.27)

a. Label one single well dish and dispense in it half ml warming media (WM). Dispense dilution and washing media in the 4 well dish after suitable labeling. Prewarm the warming to 37°C while the other media (diluting and washing) are kept at room temperature.
b. Collect the McGill Cryoleaf™ from the storage container and place into bath of LN_2.
c. Using forceps, remove the outer cover from the McGill Cryoleaf™. Take care that all parts of the McGill Cryoleaf™ remain immersed in LN_2 at all times.
d. Unlock the outersheath of the cryoleaf and slide it upwards, exposing the cryoleaf tip. Ensure that the McGill Cryoleaf™ still remains immersed in LN_2. This manipulation can be performed easily if the foam box is filled almost entirely with liquid nitrogen. The container should be positioned close to the work station to avoid delay when transferring the Cryoleaf. The sterozoom microscope has to be focused to the center of the warming media dish under low magnification.
e. Take the McGill Cryoleaf™ out of the LN_2 and quickly transfer oocytes or embryos into warming media (0.5 ml at 37°C) in a single well dish. The oocytes will then loosen from the McGill Cryoleaf™ and be released into the WM, where they should remain for a maximum of 1 minute (at this point, the oocytes are still shrunken). Localize the oocytes and start counting for 60 seconds.

Follow all movements of oocytes continuously, as they become transparent during this stage of warming of the work and it is easy to lose them. Later, they will regain their normal appearance (Fig. 12.5).

f. Using a suitable pipette, spray Diluting Media-1 (DM1) over the oocytes in WM and transfer the oocytes into 400 microliter Diluting Media-1 in well 1 of the 4 well plate. Oocytes remain here for 3 minutes (at this point, the oocytes partially recover their shape). This step avoids osmotic shock to the oocytes. Oocytes are expanding now and are easily visible (Figs 12.6 to 12.9). Repeat the some step in (DM2) in well 2.

g. Transfer the oocytes into 400 microliter Washing Media in well 3 of 4 well dish. Wait for 3 minutes (at this point, the oocytes return completely to their original shapes). Time spent here may be extended to 5 minutes as this part of the procedure is primarily for the the equiliberation of the oocyte. Repeat the same step in (WM2), in well 4.

h. Transfer the oocytes into pre-equilibrated culture medium in single well falcon plate. Allow them to rest in the incubator for two hours before the ICSI is carried out.

SEMEN CRYOPRESERVATION

SPERM CRYOPRESERVATION

Introduction

Freezing and thawing techniques have been used to cryopreserve semen since 1776. Factors known to affect outcome of this delicate procedure depend upon the quality of the semen specimen, developmental stage at which sperms are being frozen, type of cryoprotectant being used and the freezing protocols.[13]

The atypical effects observed in frozen-thawed spermatozoa derive from the unique nature of the cell.

- The cells are relatively simple with a large surface area/volume ratio and have high permeability to water. This ensures rapid osmotic equilibrium in the presence of cryoprotectants.
- Sperms contain little cytoplasm and water and high protein content with a few organelles that are less susceptible to cryofreeze injury.
- The genetic material is highly condensed and is less prone to injury by cryoprotectants, unlike embryos.

Indications of Semen Cryopreservation

Sperm banking is semen cryopreservation, using well documented protocols for use of the same at a later date. Semen can be preserved for the use of the individual, himself (autologous sperm banking). Semen is also banked from fertile donors, after screening, for the purpose of third party reproduction (donor sperm banking). Adequate care is taken to do phenotypic/blood group matching in these cases. Matching physical characteristics and race of the partner, hair color, texture and eye color are mandatory. ICMR guidelines have to be strictly adhered to while doing donor semen banking by the semen banks.

Common Indications for Autologous Semen Banking

- Patients with malignancy, prior to surgery, chemotherapy or radiation therapy.[14,15]

- During performance of cold SSR (surgical sperm retrieval techniques), like testicular or epididymal aspiration of sperms.
- Soldiers/frequent travelers, before they go away for overseas assignments, or due to anticipated absence on day of insemination due to commitments of work.
- Anticipated performance anxiety on day of insemination.
- Semen retrieval by electroejaculation in men suffering from spinal cord injury.
- Men who work in places with risk of radiation hazard.
- Patients, before undergoing vasectomy may preserve semen as insurance to further fertility.

Indications for Donor Semen Banking

- Male factor infertility:
  Azoospermia, morphological abnormalities of the sperms.
  Hypergonadotropic hypogonadism.
  Partner is either impotent or has retrograde ejaculations (if sperm retrieval has failed).
- When the partner has been exposed to known toxins, such as lead, and agents with mutagenic potential.
- When male partner carries a genetic defect (Huntington's chorea, etc.).
- Rh incompatibility with isoimmunization.
- Single women donor insemination.
- Recurrent IVF failures/abortions.

Should Semen Sample be Prepared Before Freezing?

A satisfactory sample with good count and motility can be cryopreserved raw with aim to carry out IUI at latter date. On the other hand an oligospermic sample with round cells and debris should first be prepared and packaged for ICSI.

Outline of Cryoprotectants in Semen Cryopreservation

a. Biochemical and physical aspects of sperm cryopreservation.

Sperms subjected to cryopreservation and thawing can have:
- Reduced viability, motility, and fecundity
- Morphological damage to the membranes and acrosome is well documented
- Loss of the superoxide dismutase enzyme from the plasma membranes
- Loss of acrosomal integrity
- Increased plasma membrane permeability.

b. A variety of extenders (Cryoprotective media) exist for the cooling and cryopreservation of semen. The purpose of the extender is manifold. Contents of these media are:
  1. Nutrient
  2. Buffer solution
  3. A cryopreservant agent (Permeating and nonpermeating)
  4. An antibiotic
  5. Membrane stabilizer proteins/egg yolk.

Glycerol has remained the cryoprotectant of choice for preservation of spermatozoa for most species. Glycerol is superior to DMSO or ethylene glycol as a cryoprotectant. The addition of the cryoprotectant glycerol has been shown to increase the motile sperm cryosurvival to an average of 50 percent, well above the < 20 percent cryosurvival reported without addition of glycerol. The cryoprotectant dimethylosulfoxide (DMSO) was shown to be unsuitable for sperm cryopreservation as though it supported greater cryosurvival rates, it had lower post-thaw percent motility when compared to glycerol.

In order to improve cryosurvival rates, more complex dilutants, containing other mainly nonpermeable cryoprotective agents, such as glycine, zwitterions, citrate, and egg-yolk were developed. Among the earliest and best known extenders for human semen is glycerol egg-yolk citrate (GEYC). Commonly used human sperm preserving medium (HPSM) is a modified Tyrode's medium containing glycerol, sucrose, glucose, glycine as cryoprotective agents, human serum albumin as stabilizing agent and HEPES as the buffering agent. The other commonly used cryoprotective buffer is a zwitterion buffer system termed TESTCY. This contains TES, TRIS, sodium citrate, and egg yolk.

Specimen glycerolization: Glycerol is added, to neat semen/prepared semen in drop by drop fashion slowly over a period of 2–3 minutes, with subsequent mixing after each addition. This step is essential to reduce toxicity of the cryoprotectant. The glycerol is metabolized during the procedure with formation of neutral lipids. It is suggested that the metabolized glycerol may contribute to the plasma membrane of the sperm, increasing its stability, which may lead to improved post-thaw motility.

Packaging of Semen After Addition of Cryopreservative

There are various methods to pack the glycerated or extended semen sample during freezing. Common ones which are used are plastic straws sealed by a powder sealant or heat, glass ampoules, syringes or screw-capped cryovials (Table 12.3). Factors, which influence the decisions are:
- Volume of sample to be cryopreserved
- Ease of container labeling
- Handling, storage, recovery, and biocompatibility of the packaging material.

Table 12.3
Packaging of the semen sample

		Advantages	Disadvantages
Straws	Ionomeric resin CBS High Security (Cryo Bio System, Paris, France)	Straws are available in a variety of colors suitable for the easy identification of samples and many hundred's can be stored in plastic goblets in canisters within liquid nitrogen containers	1. Maximum capacity of approximately 0.5 ml only 2. Overfilled straws are prone to cracking and expelling the powder sealing plugs into the liquid nitrogen 3. Labeling and filling difficulties 4. A high surface/volume ratio which makes the sample very susceptible to warming shock damage resulting from exposure to ambient temperatures during handling
Cryovials	Polypropylene with screw caps	These are easy to fill and stores nearly 1.5 ml of the of semen plus cryoprotectant mixture	1. Storage on aluminum canes is not dependable as they lose their memory and cryovials may jump off the holder. 2. Screw-top vials do not maintain their seals. They have the potential of exploding upon thawing because liquid nitrogen trapped in the vials expand to many times its volume when it converts to gaseous nitrogen. 3. The low surface: volume ratio and thick wall of the cryovial increase the time required for samples to reach critical temperatures and thus increase the risk of damage from brief exposure to ambient temperatures
Glass vials	Glass	None over the other available cryocontainers.	Glass vials are very fragile thus there use is discouraged.

Cooling and Warming Rates

The outcome of sperm cryosurvival is related to the rate at which the cells are cooled and warmed.

Cooling rate: A relatively slow cooling rate allows excess intracellular water to diffuse out of the cells, resulting in extreme cell shrinkage, cell dehydration, and a high intracellular solute concentration. The risk of intracellular ice formation is not completely eliminated by slow cooling.

Warming rate: Sperm cooled at a slow rate should be warmed slowly. Rapid thawing may not allow enough time for the intracellular solutes to diffuse out of the cell, resulting in swelling and lysis of the cell due to the rapid influx of water.

The cooling rate determines the optimum thawing rate. In practice this means that a slow cooling rate (1°C/min) requires a similar (1°C/min) thawing rate, only achievable using a computer controlled freezer. As most clinical situations require a simpler protocol, a more rapid cooling rate (10°C/min) is compatible with a rapid thawing rate, achieved by removing straws from liquid nitrogen and placing them on the bench top at 22°C.

> The optimum warming rate depends on the prior cooling rate.

Step by Step Methodology in Semen Freezing

Freezing

Sperm cryopreservation is accomplished using liquid nitrogen vapours for controlled rate or noncontrolled rate, cooling (Tables 12.4 and 12.5). Comparisons of the controlled rate and non-controlled rate freezing have revealed no differences in sperm cryosurvival or post-thaw motility. Non-controlled rate freezing in liquid nitrogen vapor is simpler and less expensive.

Table 12.4
Methods of semen freezing

Methods	Principle	Storage
Vapor-phase cooling	1. The procedure is carried out manually. 2. LN_2 is always vaporizing due to its low boiling point and thus vapor phase that naturally exists around liquid nitrogen tank is utilized for desired cooling. 3. The cryovials/straws are placed at predetermined heights above liquid phase for predetermined periods so the desired cooling curve is attained.	Sample is stored either in the vapor phase in the LN_2 container or dipped in the LN_2 after gradual cooling.
Programmable freezing machine	1. Not essential for human sperm cryopreservation probably because such automated device is not needed for sperm freezing. 2. Sample is loaded in the straw or the vial. These are then cooled using a programmable machine and then dipped in liquid nitrogen.	Sample is Stored in the liquid phase.

Storage

Once specimens attain temperature of −80°C to −120°C, they are immediately plunged into liquid nitrogen (Table 12.5). After plunging, the vials are quickly transferred to pre-cooled, labeled plastic goblets, snapped onto a labeled aluminum cane. Straws should be oriented in the goblet so

Table 12.5
Constituents of media

Sperm cryopreservation Method using vapor phase cooling (Figs 12.28 to 12.34)	1. Ensure both the sample and sperm cryopreservation buffer (K-SISC) are at room temperature. 2. Mix two volumes of sperm cryopreservation buffer to 1 volume of sample. 3. Leave mixture for 10 minutes at room temperature. 4. Label straws with relevant information. 5. Load the sample into a freezing straw or cryovial and seal according to manufacturer's instructions.	
	Straws	*Cryovials*
Freezing using programmable freezer	Load straws into freezing machine and initiate freeze program for straws should have similar parameters to those are given below: • Start temperature is 20°C. • Cooling rate of 6°C/min until −80°C. • At −80°C plunge them into liquid nitrogen.	Load cryovials into freezing machine and initiate freeze program. The freeze program for cryovials should have similar parameters to those are given below: • Start temperature is 20°C. • Cooling rate of −0.5°C/ min to + 5.0°C. • At + 5.0°C cool at a rate of −1°C/ min to +4.0°C. • At + 4.0°C cool at rate of 2°C /min to + 3.0°C. • At +3.0°C cool at a rate of −4°C /min to + 2.0°C.

Contd...

Contd...

		- At +1.0°C cool at a rate of −10°C /min to −80.0°C. - At +80°C hold for 10 minutes. - Plunge into liquid nitrogen
Thawing	- Remove straws or cryovials from liquid nitrogen and place them at room temperature until thawing is complete. - Open the straws or cryo-tube and remove the thawed semen. - Dilute the semen with gamete buffer (1:1) to reduce the toxic effect of glycerol. - Quickly evaluate the survival of the sperm. Immediately prepare sperm by the density gradient method using sperm gradient or the swim-up.	

that identifying information can be read without completely withdrawing the straw from the goblet.

Aluminum canes are placed in predetermined locations within the cryostorage vessel. Specimen locations are recorded on the laboratory report.

How Long can Sperms be Stored

It is important to appreciate the length of time cryopreserved sperm may be stored.
- As long as the cells are maintained at −196°C, the only known potential for cell damage is degradation of deoxyribonucleic acid (DNA), caused by background radiation based on normal background radiation of

0.1 rads/year, it has been predicted that the male gamete should maintain its genetic integrity for over 200 years when stored at –196°C.
- At temperatures above –130°C, atoms, and molecules are able to move, thus leading to membrane instability
- Temperatures of –90°C and above allow ice crystal growth, and even short periods of exposure to such temperatures can cause lethal damage to cells.

Thawing

Thawing is accomplished by exposing the specimen container to water bath at room temperature or even under running tap water (Table 12.5). Once the sample is thawed, mix the sample well with a pipette, before sampling.

> Specimen should be processed immediately after post-thaw analysis to remove cryoprotectant.

Assessment of Post-thaw Fertility

The success of cryopreservation is measured by the number of motile spermatozoa recovered post-thaw. There is nearly 30 to 40% loss in motility in the thawed sample. These effects are due to ultrastructural damage to the bilayer plasma membrane, genetic component and acrosomal contents.

> Regardless of the cooling process, the ultimate quality control appraisal of sperm cryopreservation is the cryosurvival of the spermatozoa determined during thawing.

Cross-infection in the Semen Banks

There is a potential danger of cross-infection within the bank, so the samples must be handled and stored with paramount care.

Donor Screening Prior to Semen Banking

Fresh donor insemination is not recommended for the fear of transmission of common infective diseases. Donors should be tested for HIV 1 & 2, HTLV I & II antibodies, hepatitis B surface antigen, hepatitis B core antibody, hepatitis C, RPR, TP-PA, cytomegalovirus antibodies, *Chlamydia* and gonorrhea. As a donor may be in window period of an infection, it is necessary to repeat the examination for hepatitis B and HIV after an appropriate quarantine period of 180 days. If the history or physical examination indicates infection, the donor should be rejected and advised to seek appropriate medical advice.

Security and Maintenance

The straws or vials must be clearly labeled. Inventory control is of utmost importance. Every precaution must be taken to ensure that each straw or vial can be linked to the sperm source, date of cryopreservation and specimen number, canister/cane or rack/cryocan number.

Secure cryopreservation of semen requires regular maintenance of the equipment and refilling of liquid nitrogen in the cryocans. Liquid nitrogen evaporates very quickly or the cans can leak thus causing loss of precious samples. It is essential that the cryocans must have an inbuilt security system which can automatically get activated when the levels of liquid nitrogen are low or when unauthorized persons open the cryofreezing unit.

Cryopreservation of Epididymal Sperms

Epididymal spermatozoa can be retrieved either by microsurgery or by percutaneous needle puncture. These can be subsequently cryofreezed.[16,17] The frequent indication for epididymal aspiration is obstructive azoospermia and thus it is not uncommon for relatively large quantities of sperm to be obtained and subsequently used for IVF, or even intrauterine insemination (IUI).

Cryopreservation of Testicular Sperms

Testicular specimens are contaminated invariably with large amounts of red blood cells and testicular tissues; additional steps are needed to isolate a clean preparation of spermatozoa. In order to free the seminiferous tubule-bound spermatozoa, it is necessary to use either enzymatic digestants (collagenase) or mechanical methods. For the latter, testicular tissues in supportive culture medium is macerated using glass cover slips until a fine slurry of dissociated tissues is produced, and the resulting suspension can then be processed for therapeutic use. Excess testicular spermatozoa obtained in this manner can be frozen for future use in order to avoid further surgeries.

Cryopreservation of Sperm in Empty Human Zona Shell

Another method is cryopreservation of single human spermatozoa in empty human zona shell, which is established by Jacques Cohen. A hollow sphere remains when cellular material is removed from the zona. Because it can be seen and handled microscopically both before and after cryopreservation, it is an ideal capsule for freezing individual, and small groups of sperm cells.[18]

Vitrification Technique for Ultrarapid Freezing

Vitrification technique is used to perform ultrarapid freezing of human spermatozoa and can be successfully employed for freezing sample for ICSI. The technique involves directly plunging a copper cryoloop, loaded with a sperm suspension, into liquid nitrogen.[19]

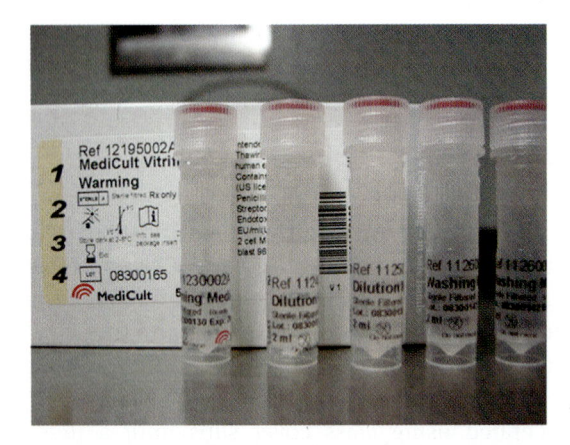

Fig. 12.17: MediCult vitrification warming medium pack consist of warming medium containing sucrose, two vials of diluent media with decreasing concentration of sucrose and two vials of washing medium with human serum albumin

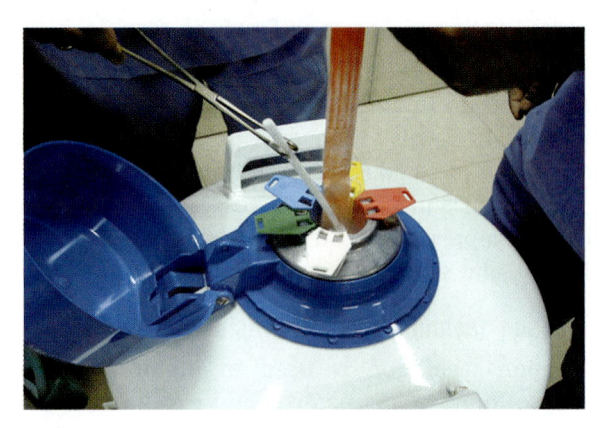

Fig. 12.18: Cryoleaf is being taken out of the cryocans at the time of warming. This should be done quickly and the cryoleaf immediately immersed in liquid nitrogen

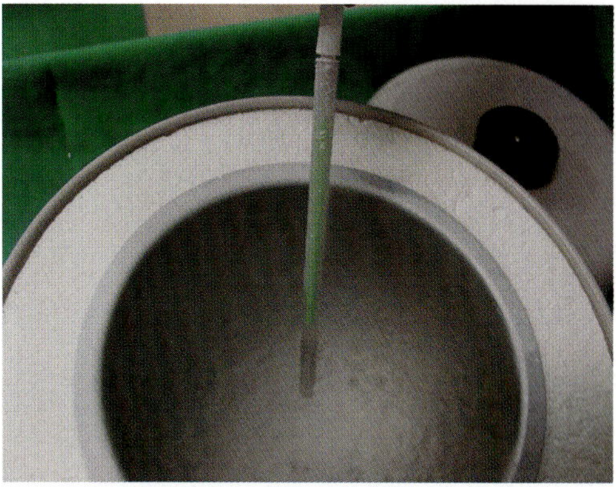

Fig. 12.19: Cryoleaf is immediately dipped in liquid nitrogen to avoid sudden thawing of the oocytes

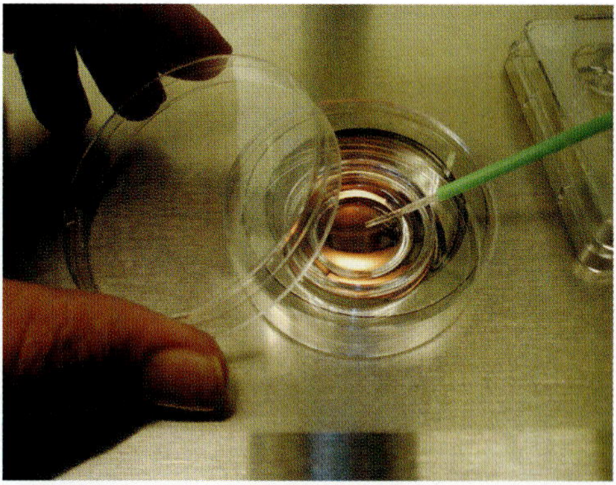

Fig. 12.20: Outer sheath of the cryoleaf is removed under liquid nitrogen. Green sleave is unlocked and the tip of cryoleaf containing the oocytes is dipped in the 400 microliter warming medium in a single well dish. Alternatively 100 microliter droplet could be made and warming carried out. The vitrification media are not recommened to be covered with oil as it will create contamination and coat the oocytes leading to delayed osmotic changes

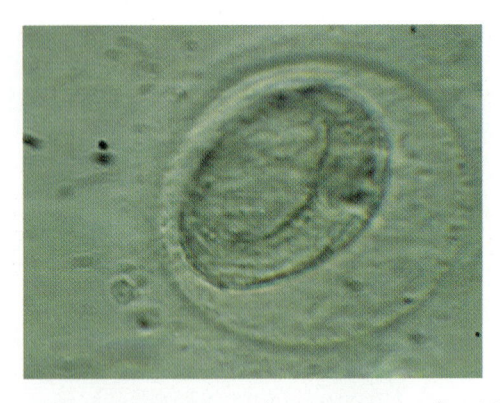

Fig. 12.21: Oocyte as seen in the warming media. Maximum contact period of the oocyte with warming media permitted is 1 min. Ooplasm here is contracted and oolemma is Wrinkled. Wide perivitelline space is observed and zona pellucida is intact. Infact the oocyte looks shrunken, hollow and scary

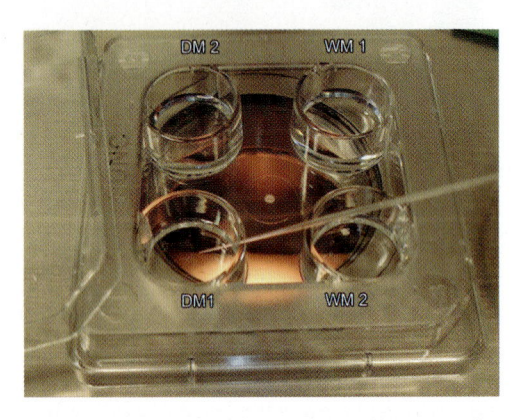

Fig. 12.22: Oocytes being transferred from diluent media 1 and 2 to washing media 1 and 2 as shown in the figure. Oocytes are kept in each media for 3 min each and then are finally transferred to the IVF media

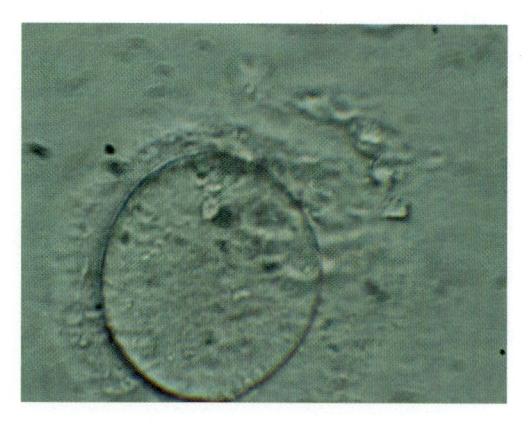

Fig. 12.23: Oocytes gradually recover in the diluting media 1. Maximum contact period permitted here is 3 minutes. Oocyte now is gradually expanding, looks normal and oolemma appears to be healthy. Polar body is seen at the 1 o'clock position

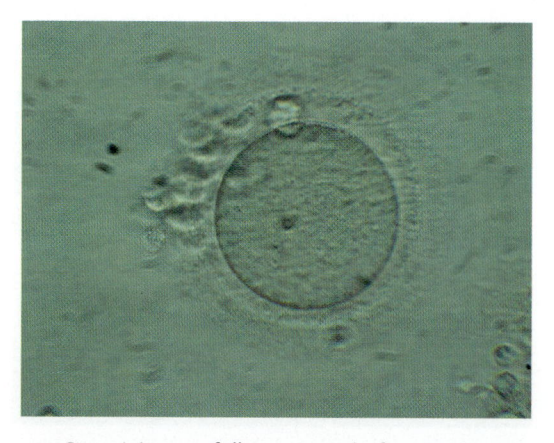

Fig. 12.24: Oocyte is now fully recovered after 3 minutes contact with the diluting media 2. It looks plump with distinct oolemma. Polar body and zona pellucida are intact

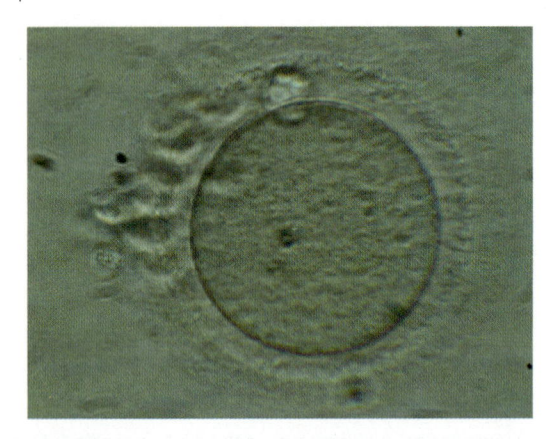

Fig. 12.25: Oocyte is further recovering in the washing media 1. Perivitelline space is decreasing and oolemma is expanding circumferentially. Zona pellucida is healthy and polar body is seen at 11 o'clock position

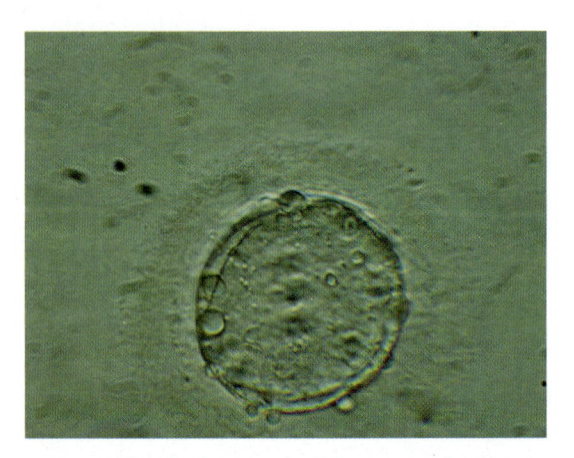

Fig. 12.26: Cryodamage to the oolemma. Plasma membrane blebs are well seen. Such oocytes do not recover during warming and are subsequently discarded

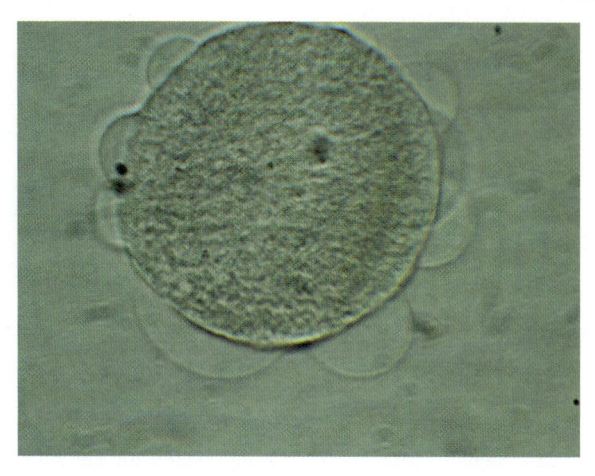

Fig. 12.27: Zona is fractured during the process of oocyte handling. Blebs in the oolemma are well-appreciated. Such oocytes degenerate/lyse during the warming procedure

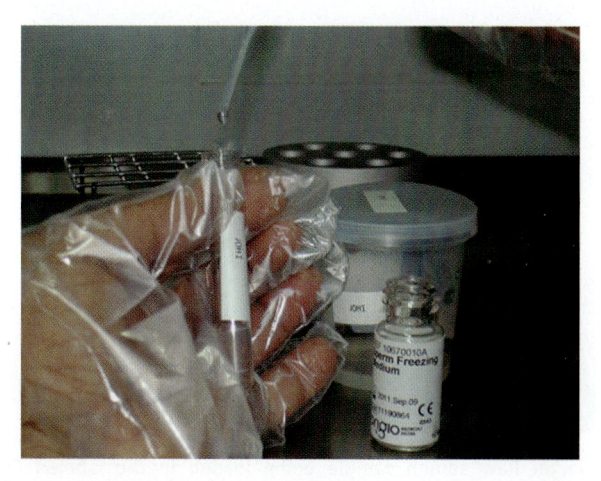

Fig. 12.28: Glycerolated semen being loaded in the cryovials

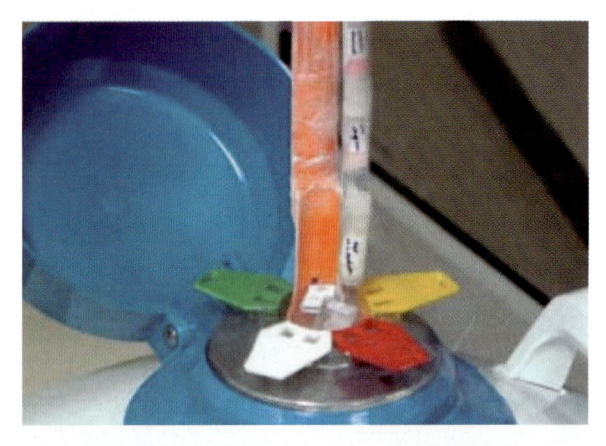

Fig. 12.29: Semen containing vials being loaded on the aluminum canes before being dipped in LN$_2$ in the cryocontainers

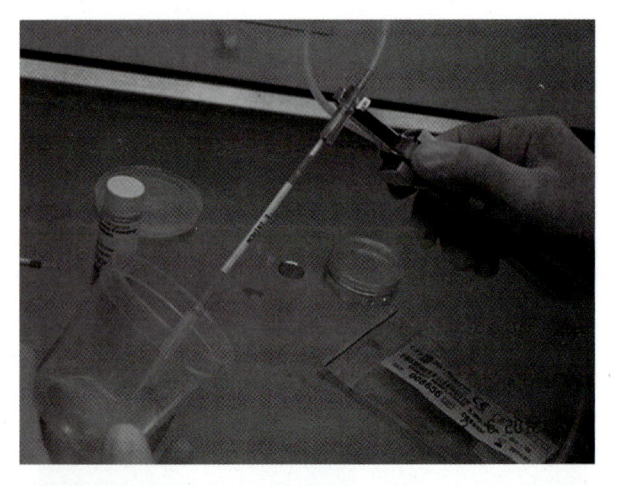

Fig. 12.30: Raw semen sample being loaded in the labeled CBS cryostraws using a manual aspirator

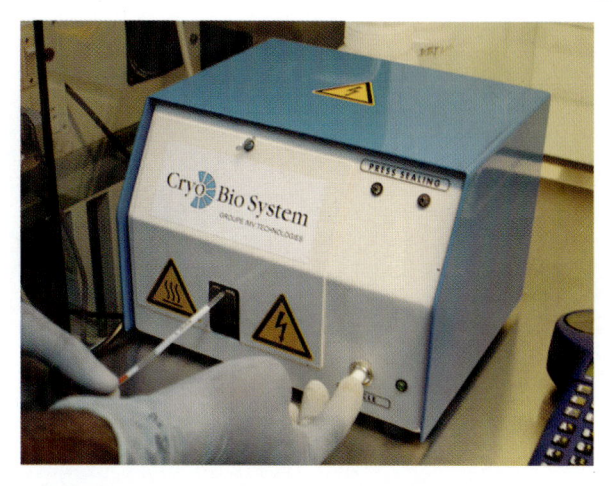

Fig. 12.31: Semen containing vials being loaded on the aluminum canes before cryofrozen

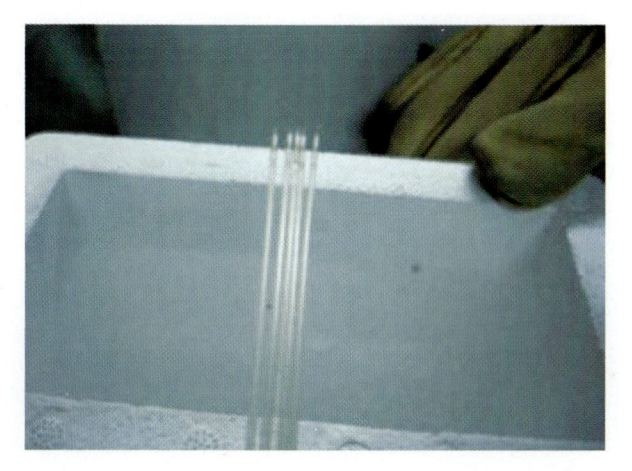

Fig. 12.32: Vapor phase cooling of the semen loaded straws

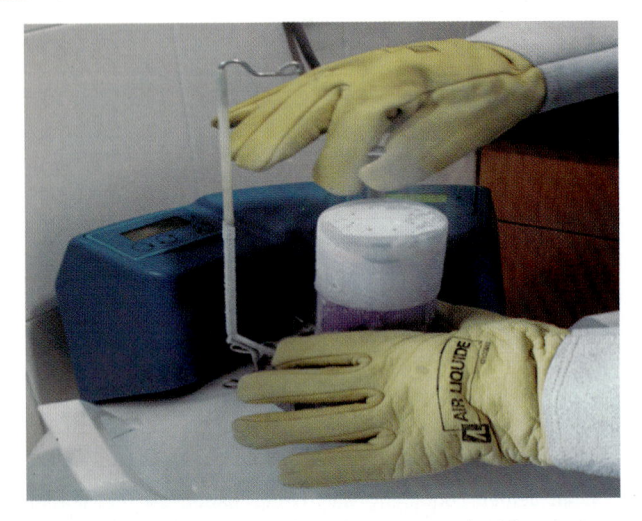

Fig. 12.33: Storage of goblets in liquid nitrogen tank with temperature and level alarms

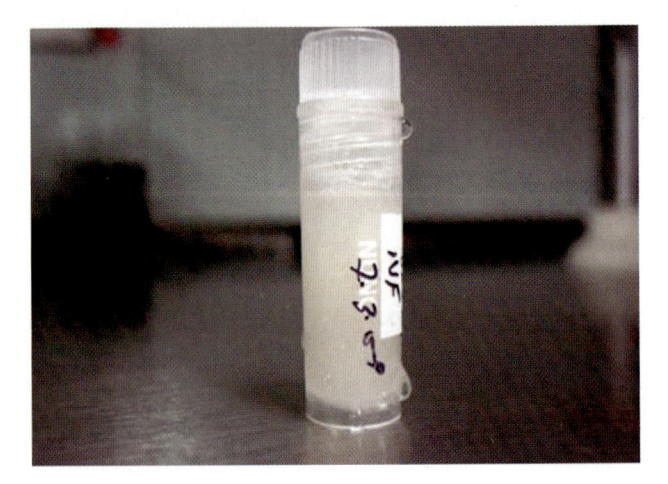

Fig. 12.34: Thawing of the semen containing vials at 37°C

CONCLUSION

Cryopreservation of human gametes expose them to numerous mechanical, thermal and chemicophysiological stresses, which can lead to compromised function of the gametes. We have come a long way since accidental discovery of glycerol as cryoprotectant for human sperms. The enigma of finding an ideal cryoprotectant would be the holy grail of the modern cryobiology. Gamete cryopreservation has become a widely accepted compendium of infertility treatment and in recent times mooted as having new role as fertility insurance.

REFERENCES

1. Kim SS. Fertility preservation in female cancer patients: current developments and future directions. Fertil Steril. 2006;85:1-11.
2. Shamonki MI, Oktay K. Oocyte and ovarian tissue cryopreservation: in- dications, techniques, and applications. Semin Reprod Med. 2005;23:266-76.
3. Lockwood G. Politics, ethics and economics: oocyte cryopreservation in the UK. Reprod Biomed Online. 2003;6:151-3.
4. Lassalle B, Testart J, Renard JP. Human embryo features that influence the success of cryopreservation with the use of 1,2 propanediol. Fertil Steril. 1985;44(5):645-51.
5. Schalkoff ME, Oskowitz SP, Powers RD. Ultrastructural observations of human and mouse oocytes treated with cryopreservatives. Biol Reprod 1989;40:379-93.
6. Stachecki JJ, Munne S, Cohen J. Spindle organization after cryo- preservation of mouse, human, and bovine oocytes. Reprod Biomed Online. 2004;8:664-77.
7. Almeida PA, Bolton VN. The effect of temperature fluctuations on the cytoskeletal organisation and chromosomal constitution of the human oocyte. Zygote. 1995;3:357-65.

8. Rienzi L, Martinez F, Ubaldi F, Minasi MG, Iacobelli M, Tesarik J, et al. Polscope analysis of meiotic spindle changes in living metaphase II human oocytes during the freezing and thawing procedures. Hum Reprod. 2004;19:655-9.
9. Larman MG, Sheehan CB, Gardner DK. Calcium-free vitrification reduces cryoprotectant-induced zona pellucida hardening and in- creases fertilization rates in mouse oocytes. Reproduction. 2006; 131:53-61.
10. Stachecki JJ, Cohen J, Willadsen SM. Cryopreservation of unfertilized mouse oocytes: the effect of replacing sodium with choline in the freezing medium. Cryobiology 1998;37:346-54.
11. Eroglu A, Toner M, Toth TL. Beneficial effect of microinjected trehalose on the cryosurvival of human oocytes. Fertil Steril. 2002;77:152-8.
12. Bianchi V, Coticchio G, Distratis V, et al. Differential sucrose concentration during dehydration (0.2 mol/L) and rehydration (0.3 mol/l) increases the implantation rate of frozen human oocytes. Reprod Biomed Online. 2007;14(1):64-71.
13. Hammerstedt RH, Graham JK, Nolan JP. Cryopreservation of mammalian sperm; what we ask them to survive. J Androl. 1990;11:73-88.
14. Saito K, Suzuki K, Iwasaki A, Yumura Y, Kubota Y. Sperm cryopreservation before cancer chemotherapy helps in the emotional battle against cancer. Cancer 2005;104(3):521-4.
15. Schmidt KL, Carlsen E, Andersen AN. Fertility treatment in male cancer survivors. Int J Androl. 2007;30(4):413-9.
16. Oates, RD, Lobel SM, Harris D, et al. Efficacy of intracytoplasmic sperm injection using intentionally cryopreserved epididymal sperm. Hum Reprod. 1996;11:133-8.
17. Elnaser TA, Rashwan H. Testicular sperm extraction and cryopreservation in patients with non-obstructive azoospermia prior to ovarian stimulation for ICSI. Middle East Fertil Soc J. 2004;9:128-35.

18. Cohen J, Garrisi GJ, Congedo-Ferrara TA, Kieck KA, Schimmel TW, Scott RT. Cryopreservation of single human spermatozoa. Hum Reprod. 1997;12:994-1001.
19. Isachenko V, Isachenko E, Katkov II, Montag M, Dessole S, Nawroth F, Van Der Ven H. Cryoprotectant-free cryopreservation of human spermatozoa by vitrification and freezing in vapor: effect on motility, DNA integrity, and fertilization ability. Biol Reprod. 2004;71(4):1167-73.

Chapter 13

Embryo Vitrification

Pankaj Talwar

INTRODUCTION

Human oocyte cryopreservation is performed either using conventional slow-rate freezing or vitrification.[1] With conventional freezing, cells are cooled to a very low temperatures slowly, thus minimizing intracellular ice crystal formation. At the same time low molarity cryoprotectants are used which reduce the unwanted influences of increased solute concentrations. On the other hand vitrification, a nonequilibrium approach to cryopreservation utilizes high concentrations of cryoprotectants that solidify without forming ice crystals as embryo/oocytes are dehydrated by short exposure to a high molarity cryoprotectant before plunging the samples directly into liquid nitrogen.

PRINCIPLES OF VITRIFICATION

Since freeze injury to embryos/oocytes is time dependent, the rationale is to prevent ice formation and injury by cooling at a rate fast enough to solidify the intracellular water before it can crystallize. At very low temperature water molecules form complex viscous material and does not freeze. When high concentration of sucrose is cooled slowly it can crystallize to form crystal sugar but when it is cooled rapidly it forms dense syrupy cotton candy.

Vitrification is accomplished by exposing the cell to high concentrations of cryoprotectant for a very short equilibration followed by ultra rapid cooling by plunging into liquid nitrogen. The high osmolarity of the vitrification medium rapidly dehydrates the cell and the submersion into liquid nitrogen quickly solidifies the cell before the remaining intracellular water has time to form damaging ice crystals.

PRINCIPLES OF WARMING

The vitrified embryos are sensitive to osmotic changes during warming. Stepwise dilution using varying concentrations of extracellular cryoprotectants and an osmotic buffer is commonly used to prevent excessive fluid movement across the cell membranes and lysis of the blastomers, as the permeating cryoprotectants are removed from the cell.

Two to four step dilutions with reducing concentrations of extracellular sucrose solutions has usually been used by various schools. Chen et al found that there were no differences in survival of vitrified human oocytes devitrified by three or four steps. Thus the four step dilution may not be necessary for human oocytes.[2]

Remember...
- Essential requirement of the vitrifying solutions and of this technique are the high osmolarity and the ability to vitrify (cool) and (warm) quickly enough to avoid ice crystal formation.
- Remember that vitrification solutions are very toxic at room temperature so we have to work fast in small volumes.
- The gradient of sucrose and the duration of warming in different solutions are important to prevent devitrification injuries.

UNIQUE VITRIFICATION DEVICES

Modern day vitrification works on the principle that higher the cooling/warming rates rate, the lower is the required cryoprotectant concentrations. Vitrification may be achieved, with relatively moderate volumes of cryoprotectants at room temperature.

A wide variety of cryodevices ate available to the embryologist. All have there advantages and drawbacks (Table 13.1).

Table 13.1
Vitrification devices

Vitrification device	Technique
• Open pulled straw (OPS) technique[3] • Glass micropipettes, GMP[4] • Super-finely pulled OPS, SOPS • Gel-loading tips • Sterile stripper tip • Volume of solution with media: (<1 μl)	• Loaded with a tiny amount of solution containing the sample and plunging it into the liquid nitrogen. • The achievable cooling and warming rates with these tools may be as high as 20,000°C/min.
• Cryoloop-A 20-μm nylon loop, 0.5 mm in diameter, mounted on a 20 mm steel tube, which is attached to the lid of the cryovial.[5]	• Thin solution film bridging the hole of the loop is formed and the oocytes/embryos are loaded onto this film. The film remains intact during immersion into liquid nitrogen. The solution volume is negligible, accordingly the cooling and warming rate may reach the estimated level of 7,00,000°C/min.[6] Storage is performed in cryovials.

Contd...

Contd...

Vitrification device	Technique
• Minimum drops size (MDS) • Volume of the sample loaded (<0.5 or even 0.1 µl)[7]	• Very small droplet containing the sample is placed onto a solid surface and immersed into the liquid nitrogen. Place small drops on precooling metal surface instead of liquid nitrogen for cooling. Originally, a metal block immersed into liquid nitrogen was used, but eventually a commercially available technique has also been produced (CMV, Cryologic, Australia).
• High security vitrification (HSV) kit • Volume of the sample loaded (<0.5 µl)	• This high security vitrification (HSV) kit makes it possible to place a micro droplet of cryoprotectant containing the embryos in the gutter of a capillary before inserting it in a mini-straw. It is heat sealed using a special welder which ensures a leak-proof seal.
• Cryotop The Cryotop consists of a 0.4 mm wide, 20 mm long, 0.1 mm thick flexible filmstrip attached to a rigid plastic handle. • Volume of the sample loaded (0.1 µl)	• To protect the filmstrip and the sample cryopreserved on it, a 30 mm long transparent plastic cap is also provided to cover this part during storage in liquid nitrogen. The device is sterilized, should be handled under aseptic conditions, and used only for one cycle of vitrification. • Cooling rates (23000°C/min). • Warming rate (42,000°C/min).

Contd...

Contd...

Vitrification device	Technique
• Cryotip A plastic straw container that can be sealed as a closed device to hold gametes or embryos during cryopreservation. Volume of solution with media: 1 μl	• Cooling rates 1200°C/min. • Warming rate 2400°C/min.
• Cryoleaf	• Oocytes or embryos are double protected from stress and contamination through an inner and outer cover system.
• Electron microscope grids	• Biological EM work is done on small copper discs called grids cast with a fine mesh. This mesh can vary a lot depending on the intended application, but is usually about 15 squares per millimeter (400 squares per inch). • On top of this grid, a thin layer of carbon is deposited by evaporating carbon graphite onto it. This carbon film on the grid holds the sample during the procedure. • Oocytes are placed on the electron microscope and directly plunged into liquid nitrogen (LN_2).

SUPERIORITY OF VARIOUS VITRIFICATION METHODS

Several studies compared superiority of vitrification techniques regarding oocytes or embryos survival and development. Kuwayama et al applied the cryotip method for human embryo vitrification. They found that the cryotip had the same efficiency as the cryotop, although the cooling rate of the cryotip is slightly lower than that of the cryotop.[8]

Using bovine oocytes, he found that more oocytes vitrified by the cryotop method cleaved and developed into blastocyst than those by conventional straws or OPS. With reference to the reports in the literature, for vitrification of human oocytes, the cryoleaf methods appear to have a higher survival rate than the grid method. The high security vitrification straws/cryotip methods have the advantage of being a closed system for embryo storage.

VITRIFICATION STEP BY STEP

Below we will describe the technique of Vitrification using vitrolife (Vitrification media) using cryoloop as the carrier. The cryoloop™ is a vitrification and storage device with greatly improved handling, making it very easy to load and store oocytes/embryos. The recommended maximum load of the cryoloop™ is 2-3 Oocytes or embryos.

The media is MOPS buffered so that the all steps can be performed outside the incubator and at room temperature. RapidVit™ Cleave contains three solutions for the vitrification of day 3 cleavage stage embryos. Timing with vitrification is critical.

> *Note:* For vitrification and warming, a relatively simple stereomicroscope equipped with zoom and capable of providing sharp, contrasted views is appropriate. There is no need to restrict background light if the sources are filtered for UV light. Use microscope lights only when required and at low intensity.

Protocol for Embryo Vitrification using Cryoloop and Vitrolife Vitrification Media (Figs 13.1 to 13.21)

Preparation of Styrofoam box with liquid nitrogen: A Styrofoam box, which is leak proof and has enough depth for storing the cryo-device after extraction from the cryo-container is used. Practically, it should be thick-walled foam box (approximately 20 cm long, 20 cm deep and 20 cm wide, with minimum 2 cm thick walls) with appropriate tightly fitting foam cover. The box should be placed on a suitable stable surface within easy reach of the embryologist. The box should be filled with the liquid nitrogen and lid placed tightly to retard its evaporation. All safety instructions related to work with liquid nitrogen should be strictly followed.

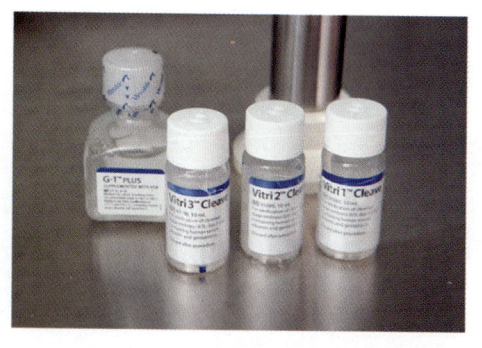

Fig. 13.1: The solutions consist of three MOPS buffered mediums containing gentamicin as an antibacterial agent.

- Vitri 1™ Cleave contains no cryoprotectants.
- Vitri 2™ Cleave contains ethylene glycol as a cryoprotectant.
- Vitri 3™ Cleave contains ethylene glycol, propanediol, ficoll and sucrose as cryoprotectants.

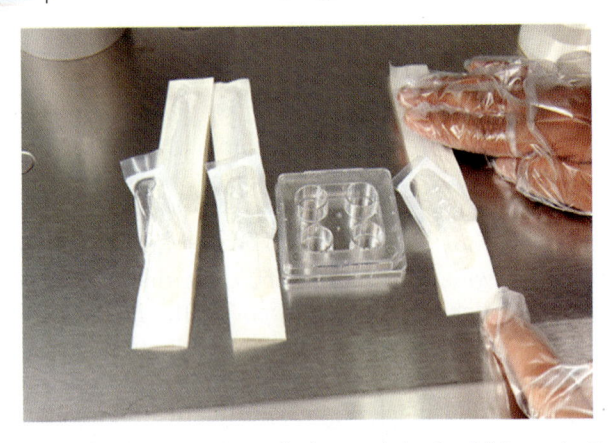

Fig. 13.2: Label the Nunc 4 well plate and the 3 ml falcon pipettes

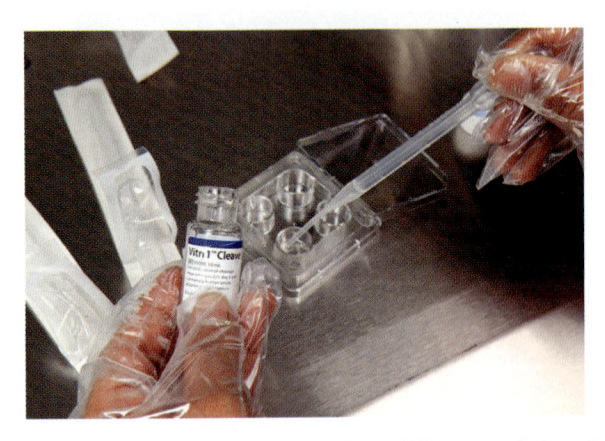

Fig. 13.3: Dispense 0.5 ml of each of the following solutions into separate wells of 4 well plate
- Well 1-Vitri 1™ Cleave, contact period with embryo, 5 minute
- Well 2-Vitri 2™ Cleave, contact period with embryo, 2 minute
- Well 3-Vitri 3™ Cleave, contact period with embryo, 30 seconds.

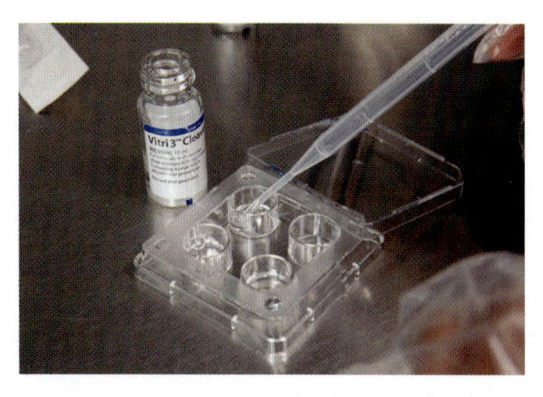

Fig. 13.4: Warm all the three media to 37°C over period of 30 minutes. If we keep the media plate for longer time at this temperature the vitrification media may evaporate and condense on the inner surface of the lid. Vitrification in such high osmolarity media may not produce desired results on cooling and warming

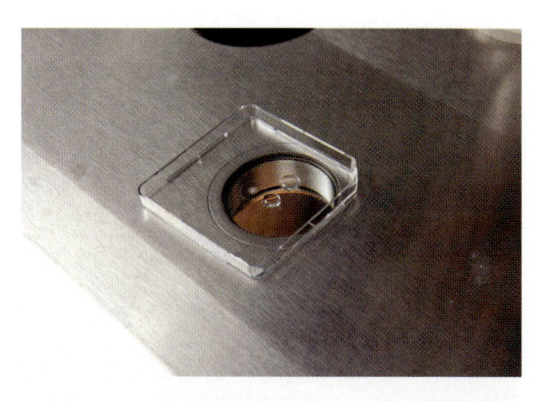

Fig. 13.5: Make two 20 μl droplet of Vitri 3™ Cleave on a lid of a culture dish. First drop is used for rinsing the embryos and equilibrating them for 10–15 seconds and the second drop is used for loading the embryos on the cryoloop. Total time permitted in Vitri™ is 30 seconds

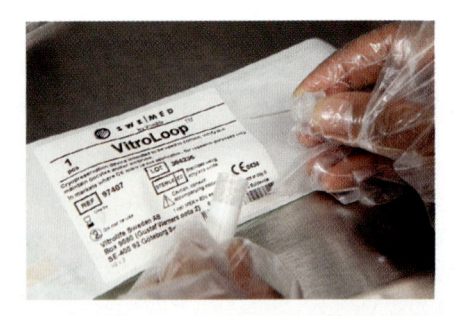

Fig. 13.6: VitroLoop™ is a cryopreservation device used to carry, vitrify and store oocytes and/or embryos.

VitroLoop™ consists of three parts:
1. A 20 μm nylon loop, 0.5 mm in diameter, mounted on a 20 mm steel tube, which is attached to the lid of the cryovial.
2. Cryovial lid is equipped with a magnetic plate for attachment of the magnetic wand for handling of the loop under liquid nitrogen.
3. A 1.8 ml cryovial is used for storage and protection of the loaded cryoloop

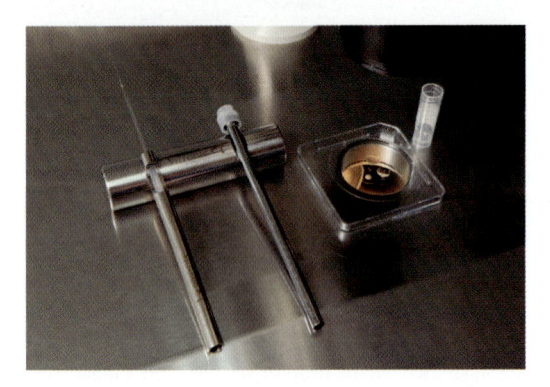

Fig. 13.7: Crystal wand with mounted magnetic cryovial screw cap with (loop). Wand allows us to load the embryos and handle the loop safely under liquid nitrogen. Also seen in the picture is swemed handle mounted with glass pipette

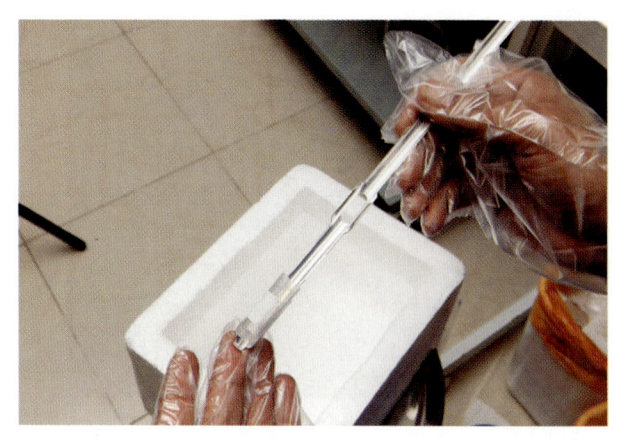

Fig. 13.8: Before starting the process of vitrification, attach the cryovial with aluminum cane, firmly

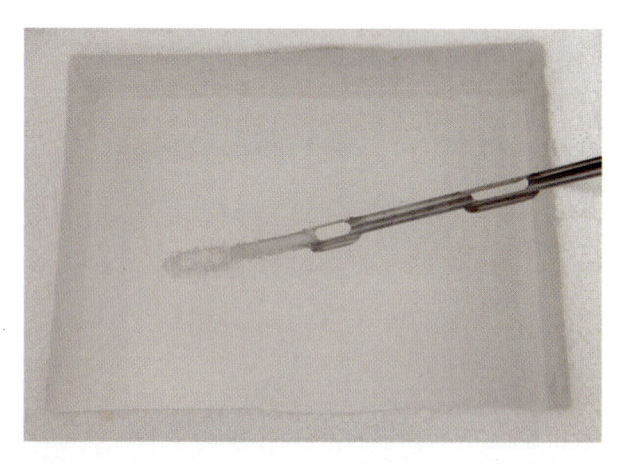

Fig. 13.9: Place the cryovial in liquid nitrogen, supported on an aluminum cryocane. This is done to fill the cryovial with LN_2 and cool the assembly to sub-zero temperatures

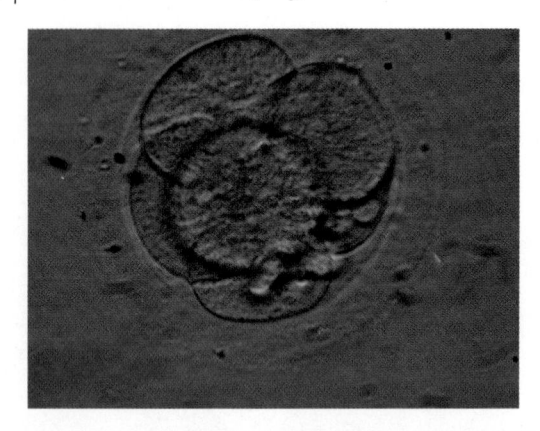

Fig. 13.10: Grade 1, 6-cell embryo with minimal fragments. Embryo is in Vitrolife G1 plus media and has been cultured for 50 hours in Vitrolife series of media. Blastomeres look healthy and zona pellucida is intact

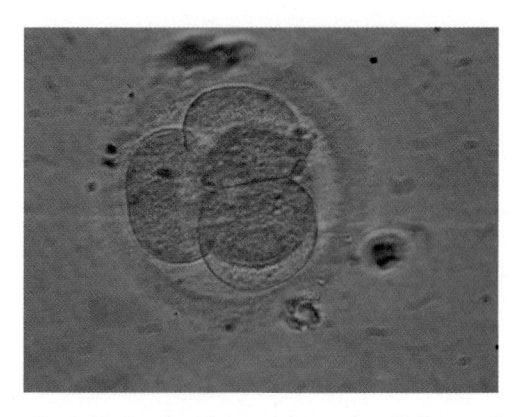

Fig. 13.11: Grade 1, 4-cell embryo embryo after 44 hour culture. The embryo is in G1 plus media. Regular blastomeres and zona pellucida are well appreciated. Blastomeres are translucent and there is no fragmentation

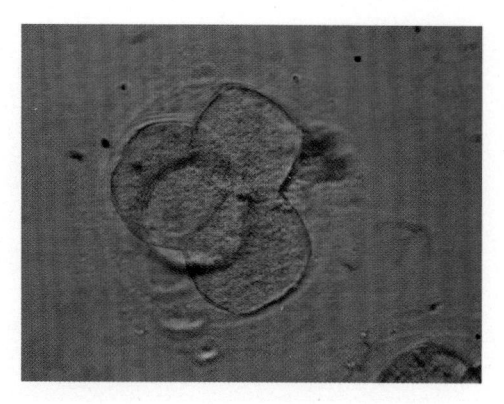

Fig. 13.12: A 4 cell embryo in vitri cleave 1 medium. Vitri 1™ Cleave does not contains any cryoprotectant. Embryos are equilibrated here for 5 minutes. Not much morphological change is appreciated here. This step is primarily carried out to equilibrate the embryos in vitrification media. This allows the embryos to adapt to change in buffer media from bicarbonate in G1 Plus media to MOPS in vitrification media

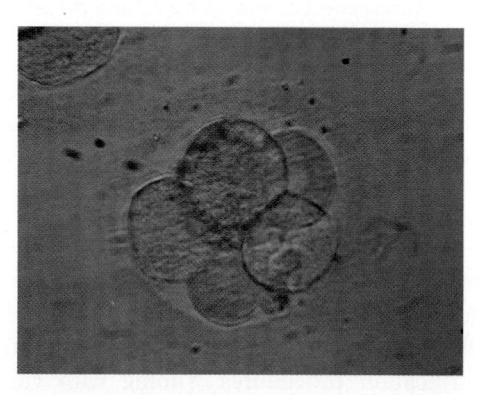

Fig. 13.13: A 6-cell, grade 1, embryo in Vitri 1™ Cleave. Contact period of the embryos with media is 5 minutes. This media contains no Cryoprotectants. No change in morphology of the embryos is appreciated

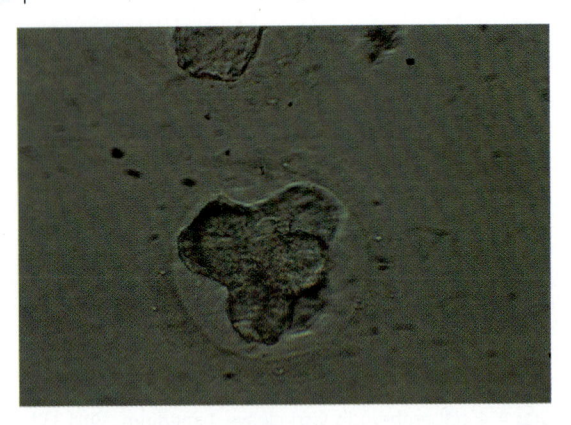

Fig. 13.14: A 6-cell grade I embryo now in Vitri 2™ Cleave containing ethylene glycol as a cryoprotectant. Contact period permitted is 2 minutes. We can appreciate sudden contraction of he blastomeres. Perivitelline space is contracted. Zona pellucida looks regular. Embryos are very fragile at this stage and require gentle handling. Use appropriate size pipettes to rinse the embryos. Before we move embryos from vitri cleave 1 to vitri cleave 2, rinse the pipette in virti cleave 2. Now spray some virti cleave 2 on the embryos' in vitri cleave 1. Such Spraying of the media will prevent embryos from sudden osmotic shock from being exposed to higher concentration of the cryoprotectant. Embryos are now aspirated and moved to vitri cleave 2

a. *Media for vitrification of cleavage stage embryos:* RapidVit™ Cleave contains three solutions for the vitrification of day 2/3 cleavage stage embryos. Vitrification should only be performed by staff trained in vitrification procedures. Timing with vitrification is critical please ensure that you follow the protocol precisely. We use cryoloop for vitrification procedure.
b. Label all the disposable lab-ware.

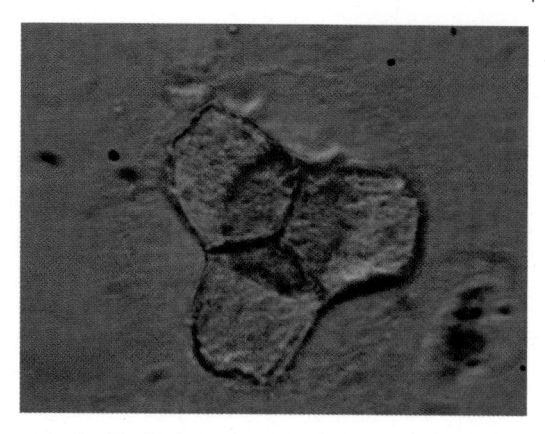

Fig. 13.15: A 4-cell embryos in vitri cleave 2 media after 1 min of exposure to ethylene glycol. Shrinking of the blastomeres is seen. Blastomeres membrane is crumpled as the cells are being dehydrated in Vitri 2™ Cleave containing ethylene glycol as cryoprotectant

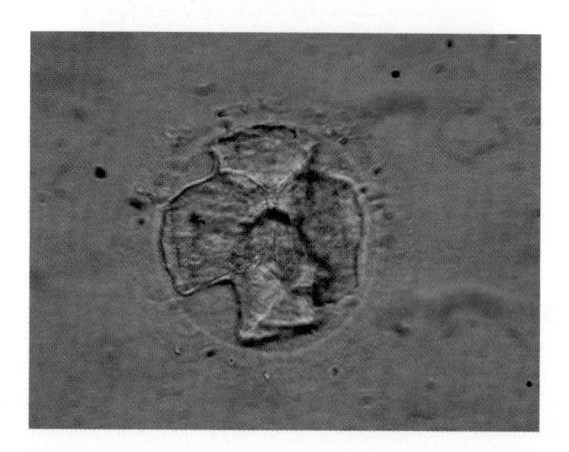

Fig. 13.16: A 6-cell, embryo in vitri cleaves 2 media containing ethylene glycol after 1 minute of contact. Embryos gradually expand as equilibration occurs over period of 2 minutes

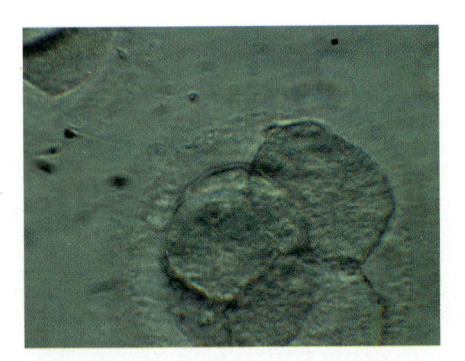

Fig. 13.17: A 4-cell grade , embryo in vitri cleave 2 media™ after contact period of 100 seconds we see that blastomeres are expanding and periviteline space is increasing. After 2 minutes in vitri cleave media™ the embryos are shifted to the Vitri 3™ Cleave containing ethylene glycol, propanediol, ficoll and sucrose as cryoprotectants

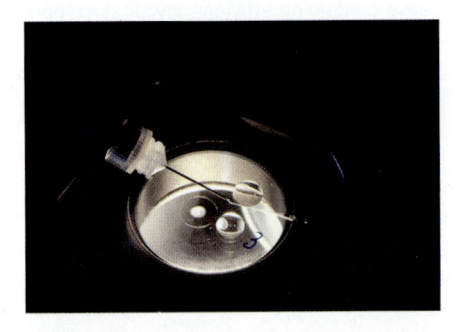

Fig. 13.18: Aspirate the embryos with a micropipette in minimal volume of vitri cleave 2 media. Now gently transfer the shrunken embryos to a first 20 microliter drop of vitro cleave media 3. Gently and quickly rinse the embryos and transfer them to second drop of vitro cleave media 2. Keeping embryos in vision, dip the nylon cryoloop in droplet of vitro cleaves media 2 so that a film is formed on the loop. Carefully aspirate the embryos and gently place them on the loop under microscope. All the work here is done under low magnification of stereo zoom microscope. Wide field of vision thus allows us to load the cryoloop easily

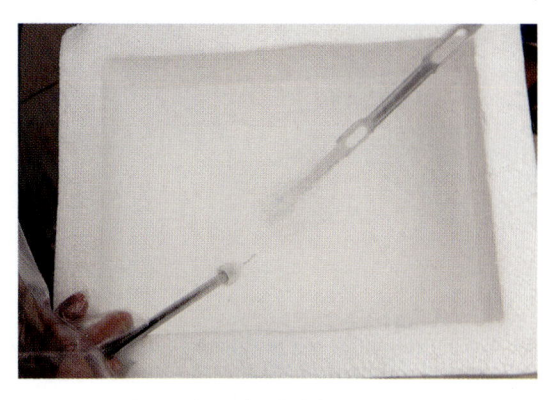

Fig. 13.19: Move the embryo-loaded loop into the liquid nitrogen immediately and keep it dipped for few seconds. This causes instant vitrification of the embryos. Now we place loop in the cryovial without touching the wall of the cryovial. If we accidently touch the nylon loop with the vial wall it may crack, as it is very fragile being at very low temperature. Such accidents may result in loss of embryos

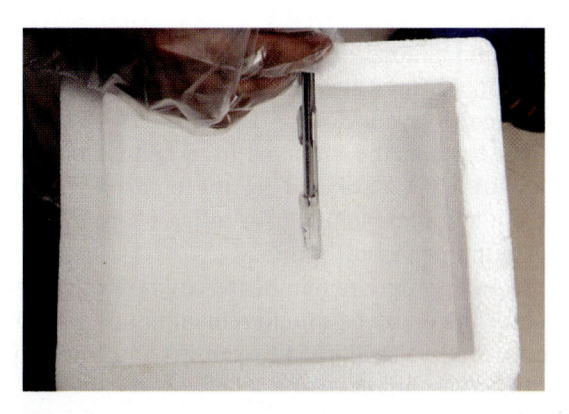

Fig. 13.20: Tighten the lid of the cryovial with the Crystal Wand Tab. The embryos are now vitrified and ready for storage. The cryoloop should not exposed to higher temperatures as it may lead to accidental warming and thus harm the embryos

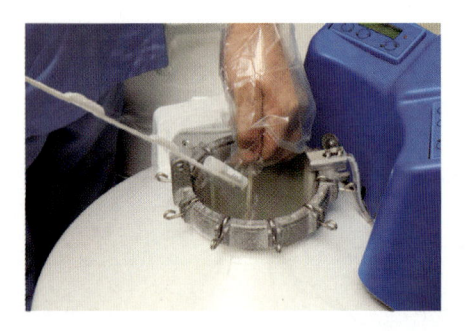

Fig. 13.21: Transfer the VitroLoop to the long-term storage tank. The loop must always be immersed in liquid nitrogen

c. Place 0.5-1 ml of each of the following solutions into separate wells and warm to 37°C:
   - Vitri 1™ Cleave : Well 1
   - Vitri 2™ Cleave : Well 2
   - Vitri 3™ Cleave : Well 3
d. All manipulations of the embryos are carried out at 37°C (on a heated stage).
e. Prepare the cryodevice for use.
f. Gently transfer the embryos from culture media into the Vitri 1™ Cleave and let the embryos remain in the equilibration solution for at least 5 min but for a maximum period of 10 min.
g. Move an appropriate number of embryos into Vitri 2™ Cleave. The embryos should remain in this solution for 2 min. Embryos will initially contract and latter expand in this cryosolution.
h. The embryos will tend to float to the surface due to sudden dehydration. Carefully aspirate and rinse them using an appropriate diameter pipette them and replace them at the bottom of the dish.

> *Note:* The embryos will tend to float to the surface due to sudden dehydration. Carefully aspirate and rinse them using an appropriate diameter pipette them and replace them to the bottom of the dish.

i. When 30 second remain, make a 20 µl droplet of Vitri 3™ Cleave on a nontoxic culture dish. Transfer the embryos in this droplet for maximum period of 30 seconds. Rinse them few times and meanwhile dip the loop in the vitrification media to create a fine film on it. Now load the embryos on the film on the cryoloop 2–3 at a time, under stereozoom microscopic vision.

Warming Steps (Figs 13.22 to 13.39)

Rapid Warm™ Cleave contains four solutions for the warming of vitrified day 2/3 cleavage stage embryos. The solutions consist of a MOPS buffered medium containing gentamicin as an antibacterial agent and human serum albumin.

a. Label the labware.
b. Place 0.5 ml of each of the following media into separate wells of a 4 well plate and warm to 37°C:
   - Warm 1™ Cleave
   - Warm 2™ Cleave
   - Warm 3™ Cleave
   - Warm 4™ Cleave
c. All manipulations of the embryos are carried out at 37°C (on a heated stage).
d. Carry the styrofoam box LN_2 and cryodevice close to the workstation.
e. Place the vitrified embryos quickly into Warm 1™ Cleave.
f. Allow the embryos to fall from the device and sink to the bottom. Leave for 10–30 sec.
g. Transfer the embryos into Warm 2™ Cleave and let the embryos remain in the solution for 1 min.

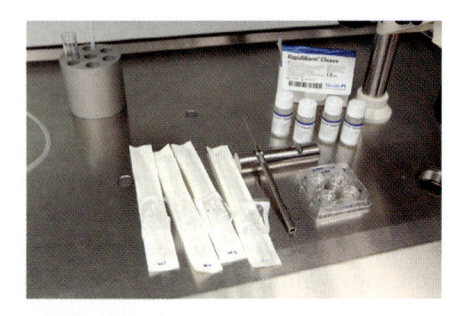

Fig. 13.22: The media and the disposable required for the rapid warming. 3 ml falcon pipettes and a 4 well nunc IVF plate should be labeled before the procedure. Appropriate size of the pipette should be selected to shift the embryos. RapidWarm™ Cleave contains four solutions for the warming of vitrified day 2/3 cleavage stage embryos. The solutions consist of a MOPS buffered medium containing gentamicin as an antibacterial agent and human serum albumin.

Warm 1™ Cleave contains sucrose as a cryoprotectant
Warm 2™ Cleave contains sucrose as a cryoprotectant
Warm 3™ Cleave contains sucrose as a cryoprotectant
Warm 4™ Cleave contains no cryoprotectant

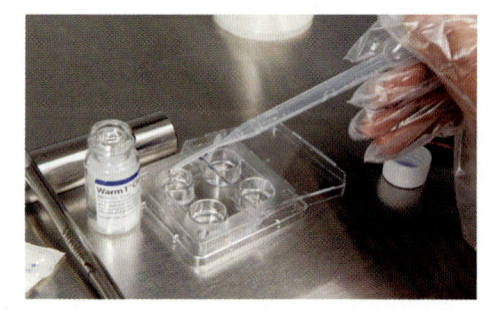

Fig. 13.23: Dispense 0.5 ml of all four warming media into separate wells of a labeled 4 well plate. Warm the media plate to 37°C.

All manipulations of the embryos are carried out at 37°C (on a heated stage)

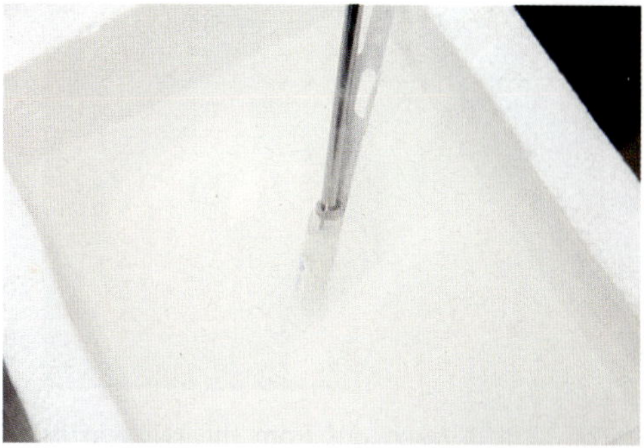

Embryo Vitrification | **349**

Fig. 13.24: Take out the embryo cryovial, fixed on the aluminum cane from the cryocan. Immediately place the vial in the Styrofoam box filled with LN_2. Fix the magnetic crystal wand to the cap of the cryovial and rotate the wand anticlockwise to unscrew the cryoloop, loop from the cryovial

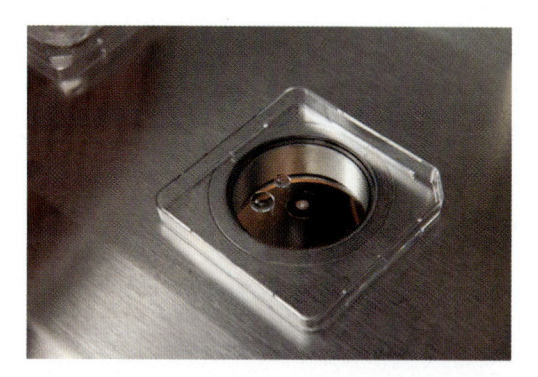

Fig. 13.25: Make 2 drops of Warm 1™ Cleave media on the lid of the IVF dish. This media contains sucrose as a cryoprotectant. The drops should be of approximately 20 microlitres size and should be maintained at 37°C. This droplet plate should be made immediately before warming the embryos otherwise the media may evaporate and cause change in osmolarity of the media

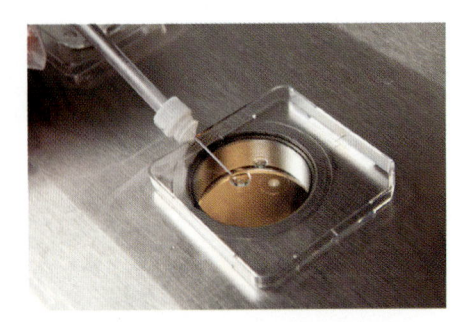

Fig. 13.26: The loop is taken out from the LN_2 and its nylon loop holding the embryos is touched to the first 20 microliters media droplet edge. Ensure that the stainless steel handle does not touch the media drop as this may lead to bubble formation in the droplet and loss of embryos. Vitrified embryos quickly fall into the Warm 1™ Cleave media. Allow the embryos to equilibrate for 10-20 sec. Aspirate the embryos from this droplet and wash them again second droplet. After a total of 30 sec. in warm cleave media 1 move the embryos to the warm 2 cleave media

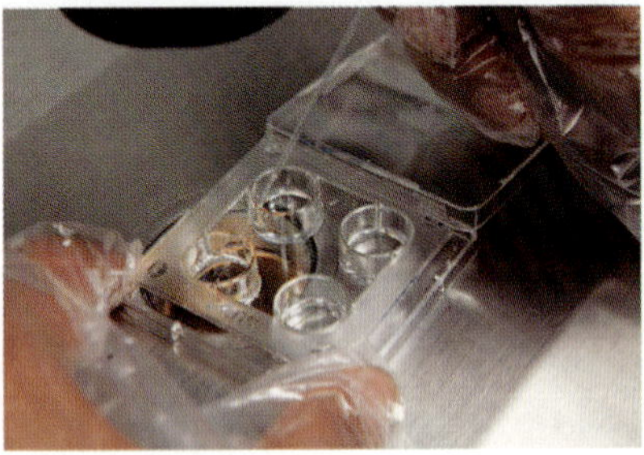

Fig. 13.27: Transfer the embryos into Warm 2™ Cleave and let the embryos remain in the warming solution for 1 minute. Embryos are still shrunken and difficult to visualize and they move towards the periphery of the media well. These are very fragile and should be handled very gently with appropriate sized pipette. We should work at low light and less magnification. This makes embryo aspiration and handling easier.

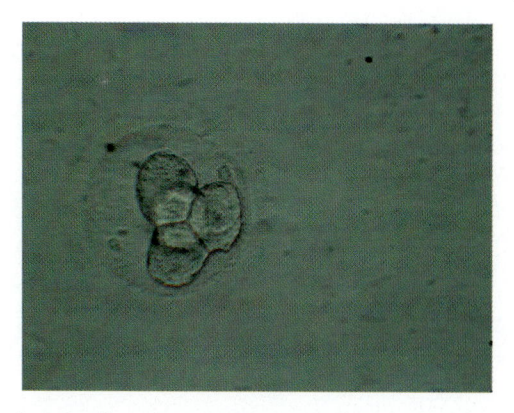

Fig. 13.28: A 4-cell, embryo in Warm 2™ Cleave solution containing sucrose as a cryoprotectant. Blastomeres are still contracted and there is wide perivitelline space observed. Cytoplasm looks granular and dark. This is a normal embryo and will have complete recovery, as it will be exposed to various concentrations of cryoprotectant solutions gradually

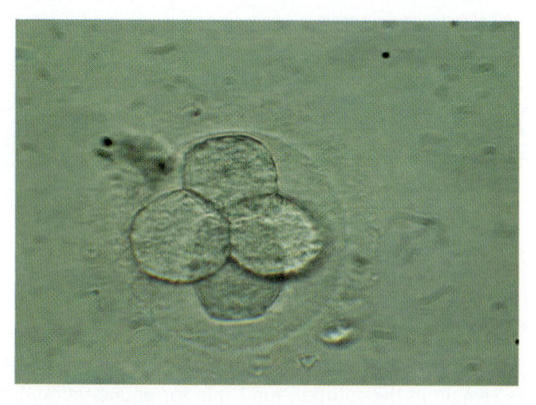

Fig. 13.29: A 4-cell, grade 1, embryo after 45 second contact with the warm 2 cleave solution containing sucrose. Blastomeres are expanding and PVS space is reducing. Blastomeres are equal in size and cell membrane looks healthy

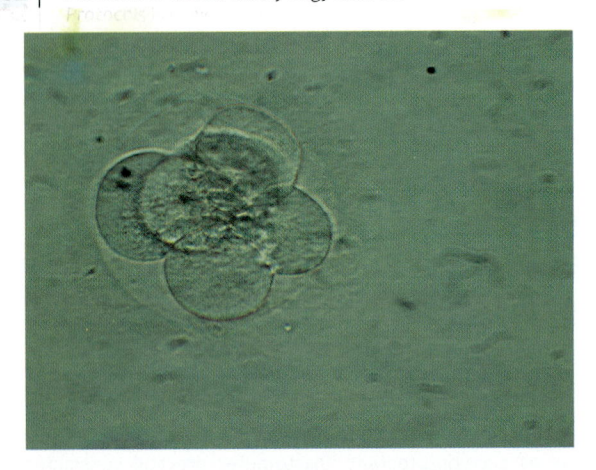

Fig. 13.30: A 6-cell grade 1, embryos after 45 second contact with the warm 2- cleave media solution containing sucrose

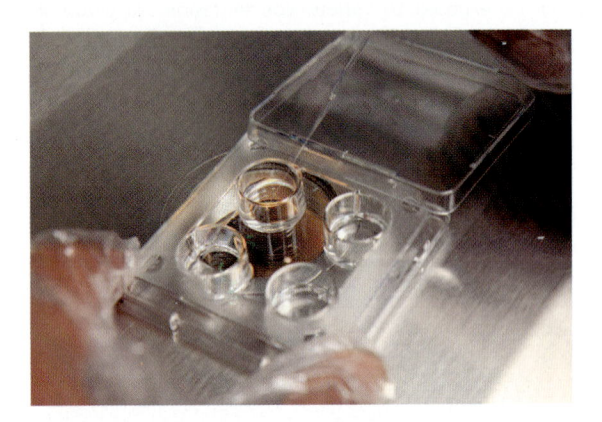

Fig. 13.31: Transfer the embryos into Warm 3™ Cleave and let the embryos remain in the solution for 2 min for equilibration. Embryos should be moved in minimal volume of the vitrification solutions. Always spray media from the higher well on the embryos in the lower well before aspirating them to avoid osmotic shock

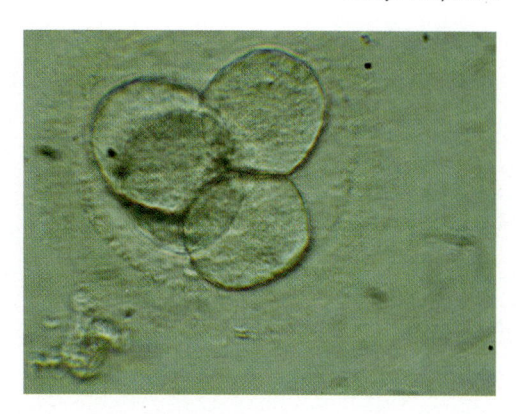

Fig. 13.32: A 4-cell embryo in warm 3 solution. Blastomeres can be seen expanding gradually. The wrinkling of the blastomere membranes will disappear with exposure to lower concentrations' of the cryoprotectants. Blastomeres are healthy and there is no evidence of cryodamage in terms of lysis of the cells

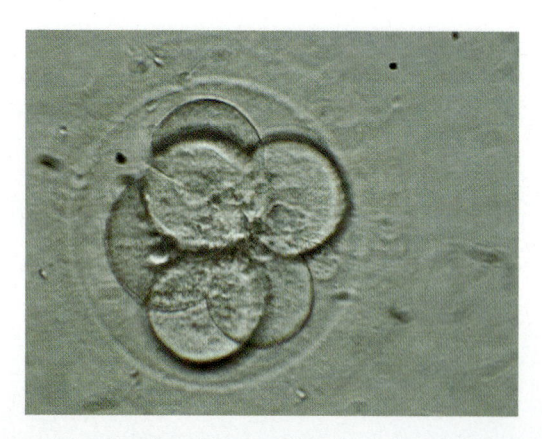

Fig. 13.33: A 6-cell embryo in warm 3 media. Embryo is recovering its original shape. Gradually the blastomeres become becoming more translucent and clear. The blastomeres are regular and compact. Zona pellucida is healthy and even with no cracks or irregularity

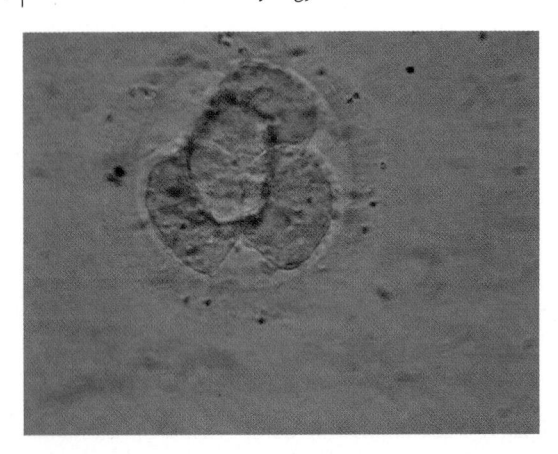

Fig. 13.34: Another 4-cell embryo after 1 minute exposure in warm 3 cleave media. Response of all embryos is not the same. Some may have delayed recovery

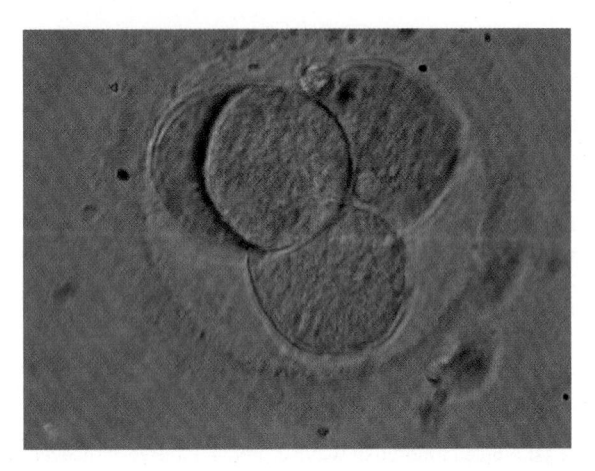

Fig. 13.35: A 4-cell, embryo in warm 3 media as seen with contrast imaging on inverted microscope. Blastomere edges are well seen. Their regularity and cytoplasmic contents are fully appreciated

Embryo Vitrification | **355**

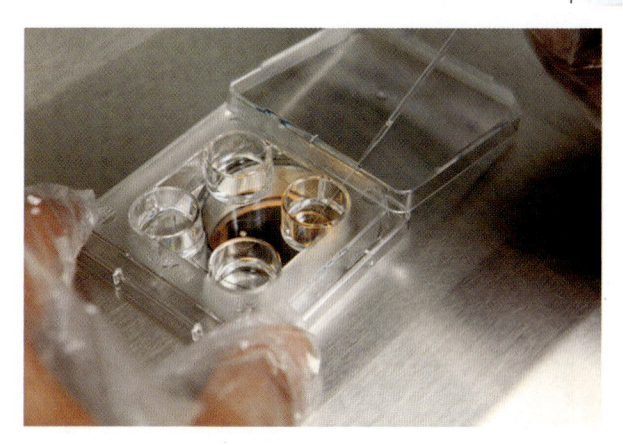

Fig. 13.36: Transfer the embryos into Warm 4™ Cleave and let the embryos remain in the solution for 5 minutes for equilibration

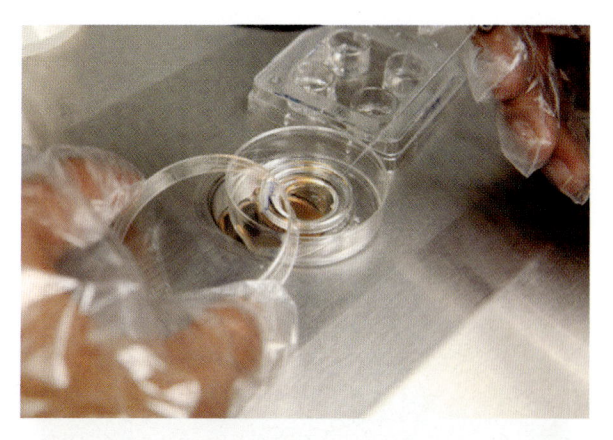

Fig. 13.37: Embryos being cultured in G2 plus media in a single well dish. Rinse the embryos in culture media several times and continue culture for 2 hours in CO_2 incubator before embryo transfer is carried out

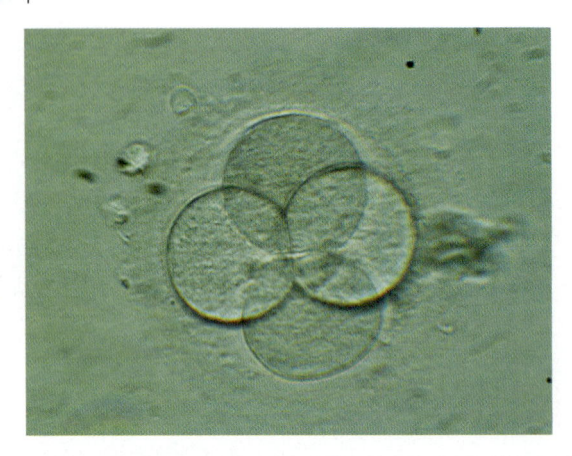

Fig. 13.38: A 4-cell, grade 1, fully recovered embryo after culture in G2 plus media. Blastomeres are regular and normal shape. Zona pellucida is intact and regular

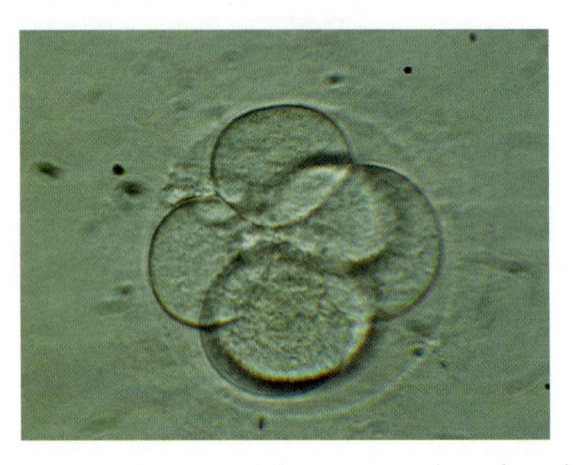

Fig. 13.39: A 6-cell, grade 1, fully recovered embryo after culture in G2 plus media. Blastomeres are regular and normal shape. Zona pellucida is intact and regular

h. Transfer the embryos into Warm 3™ Cleave and let the embryos remain in the solution for 2 mins.
i. Transfer the embryos into Warm 4™ Cleave and let the embryos remain in the solution for 5 min.
j. Rinse the embryos in culture media several times and continue culture according to laboratory practice.

> *Remember...*
> *Precautions during warming*
> - The container should be positioned close to the microscope to avoid delay in moving the cryocoop to the 4 well dish
> - The steroozoom microscope has to be focused at the center of the warming media dish under low magnification
> - The cryo-carrier for the oocytes/embryos should be soaked in the sucrose solution as quickly as possible, making sure the sample is never held in the air at room temperature
> - Dip only the nylon loop in the warming solution
> - Follow all movements of oocytes/embryos continuously, as they become transparent during this stage of warming and it is easy to lose them.

PREVENTING POTENTIAL CONTAMINATION FROM LIQUID NITROGEN

Recent vitrification methods using closed cryo devices have reduced the chances of contamination in the media, and to the conceptus. If using in open system we should use medical grade LN_2. However, a major concern regarding the potential risk to human oocytes or embryos from contaminated liquid nitrogen at the time of vitrification or storage remains.

The liquid nitrogen is filtered through a 0.2 µm pore-size filter and UV irradiated to make it medical grade LN_2. Many Minimum–volume vitrification techniques have been developed to avoid direct contact of the embryos with the liquid nitrogen. The method of solid surface vitrification (SSV) using metal surfaces for cooling does not involve loading of embryos into a closed system, like closed pulled straws (CPS) thus making the procedure simple and safe cryologic vitrification system uses pre-chilled vitrification blocks and fibreplugs to completely eliminate the chances of contamination. Kuwayama et al developed the Cryotip method using a heat-sealed pulled straw technique.[12]

Very recently, an aseptic vitrification approach based on the hemi-straw principles has also been developed. This high security vitrification kit (HSV kit) makes it possible to place a micro droplet (< 0.5 µl) of cryoprotecant containing the embryos in the gutter of a capillary before inserting it in a mini-straw.

CONCLUSION

Vitrification has the advantage of being simple, inexpensive, and rapid. This procedure leads to higher survival and developmental rates than those achievable with alternative slow freezing methods. Concerns regarding disease transmission are partially justified, but safer closed vitrification methods are now available to lessen this danger.

REFERENCES

1. Vajta G, Nagy PZ. Are programmable freezers still needed in the embryo laboratory? Review on vitrification. Reprod Biomed Online. 2006;12:779-96.
2. Chen SU, Lien YL, Chao KH, et al. Cryopreservation of mature human oocytes by vitrification with ethylene glycol in straws. Fertil Steril. 2000;74:804-8.
3. Vajta G, Holan P, Kuwayama M, Both PJ, et al. Open pulled straw (OPS) vitrification: a new way to reduce cryoinjuries of bouine ova and embryos. Mol Reprod Dev. 1998;51(1):53-8.

4. Kong IK, Lee SI, Cho SG, et al. Comparison of open pulled straw (OPS) glass micropipette (GMP) vitrification in mouse blastocysts.Theriogennology. 2000;53:1817-26
5. Lane M, Schoolcraft WB, Gardner DK, Vitrification of mouse and human blastocysts using a novel cryoloop container – less technique. Fertil Steril. 1999;72:l073-8.
6. Isachenko E, Isachenko V, Katkov II, et al. Vitrification of mammalian spermatozoa in the absence of cyroprotectants: from past partial difficulties to present success. Reprod difficulties to present success. Reprod BIOMed Online. 2003;6:191-200.
7. Arav A. Vitrification of oocytes and embryos. In: Layria A, Gandolfi F, End new trends in embryo transfer. Cambridge, UK; Portland press; 1992. pp. 255-64.
8. Kuwayama M, Vajta G, Kato O, et al. Highly efficient vitrification method for cryopreservation of human oocytes. Reprod BIOMED online. 2005;11:300-8.

Chapter 14

Endometrial Receptivity and Luteal Support

Surveen Ghumman Sindhu

Despite progress and research in the field of infertility the live birth rate with IVF has not gone beyond 30 percent. In 75 percent of the failed cases there is no cause for failure other than implantation forming a major obstacle to ART. The complexities of embryo apposition to invasion of the epithelium are only partly understood at the molecular level and still present a challenge to the infertility specialist.

Definition: Endometrial receptivity can be defined as the histological and molecular changes occurring in a temporal and spatial manner in the endometrium so as to facilitate embryonic implantation.

Under the influence of estrogen and progesterone, the endometrium undergoes these important changes so as to make it receptive to the implanting embryo and this period is known as the 'Window of receptivity' and lasts for approximately 4 days in women usually from day 20 to 24.[1] The key factor for implantation is the synchrony between embryo development and endometrial receptivity. The ability of the decidua to respond optimally to the invading trophoblasts is determined by endocrine and end-organ interactions that long precede ovulation. There are many causes of poor endometrial response (Table 14.1).

The implantation process, as described by Enders[2] consists of the three important phases:

Table 14.1

Causes of poor endometrial response

Poor hormonal environment	Suboptimal estrogens
	Suboptimal progesterones
	Out of phase development
	Excessive estrogen levels
	Hyperprolactinemia
	Hyperandrogenemia
Infections	Endometritis
	Tuberculosis
	Chlamydia
Anatomical	Uterine septum
	Leiomyomas submucous
	Multiple/large intramural
	Endometrial polyps
Foreign bodies	Lost intrauterine devices
Iatrogenic	Vigorous curettage
Adhesions	Intrauterine synechiae
Drugs	Clomiphene citrate
Endometrial	Squamous metaplasia
	Calcification/ossification

1. *Apposition:* The blastocyst at this phase ceases to move freely in the uterine cavity and comes in close proximity to the uterine epithelium.
2. *Adhesion:* Apposition leads to an interaction between the trophoectoderm and the endometrial epithelial cells, attaching the blastocysts to the uterine lining.
3. *Invasion:* It involves epithelial penetration and placentation. The trophoectoderm cells, taking advantage of the loss of polarity and tight junctions between the epithelial cells, that occurs during this period, invades into the endometrium.

Table 14.2 shows the number of factors effect implantation.

HISTOLOGICAL CHANGES

The most significant morphological change observed in this period is the development of pinopodes which are large cytoplasmic protrusions of the apical membranes of the secretory cells after they loose their microvilli. They develop 4 to 5 days after ovulation, i.e. day 18 of a 28-day cycle and are fully developed by day 20 after which they start regressing, largely disappearing by day

Table 14.2

Factors which affect implantation

1. General
   - Age
   - Hormonal control of endometrial preparation
   - Endometriosis
   - Hydrosalpinx
2. Uterine factors
   - Endometrial receptivity
   - Congenital uterine abnormalities
   - Fibroids/polyps
   - Endometritis
   - Poor uterine artery blood flow
3. Immunological function
   - Antiphospholipid syndrome
   - Lupus erythematosus
   - Rheumatoid Arthritis
   - Hashimoto's Thyroiditis
4. Embryological
   - Aneuploidy in embryos
   - Spindle damage

22.[3] They are thought to have a pinocytotic function and are involved in the apicobasal transport of fluids and macromolecules towards the stroma and are important markers of endometrial receptivity. The other important change seen at this time is the decrease in cell polarity and tight junctions between cells thus assisting in trophoblastic invasion.

BIOCHEMICAL AND MOLECULAR CHANGES

The various phases of implantation involve synchronized interplay of a variety of molecules. These molecules, expressed at the three stages of implantation are in accordance with the needs of that phase (Table 14.3). Biochemical markers of endometrial receptivity include mucins, integrins, trophinin, growth factors, cytokines,

Table 14.3
Molecules at three stages of implantation

1. Apposition—chemokines
   - Interleukin-8 (IL-8)
   - Monocyte chemo-attractant protein-1 (MCP-1)
   - Regulated on activation, T-cell expressed and secreted (RANTES)
2. Adhesion—cytokines
   - LIF
   - IL-1
   - HBGF
   - Integrins
   - HOXA10
3. Invasion—proteolytic enzymes
   - Serine proteases
   - Metalloproteases
   - Collagenases

calcitonin, HOXA-10, cyclo-oxygenase-2, fibronectin, insulin like growth factor binding protein-1 (IGFBP-1). The appropriate interaction between the preimplantation embryo and maternal endometrium is controlled by cytokines and growth factors and its receptors. While cytokines help in attachment and adhesions, the growth factors are involved in stromal invasion, vascular penetration and finally nidation. The cytokines may be adhesive or anti-adhesive molecules. It is the adhesive cytokines which help in implantation. Both the cytokines and growth factors may react through 'embryo-endometrial dialogue' by helpful or harmful responses. Mucins play a role in attachment. Mucin MAG's (mouse ascites Golgi) has been used as a marker for ER and 60 percent of unexplained infertility have an abnormal MAG expression.[4] The α-5, 3 integrins are emerging as important markers of endometrial receptivity and are absent in cases of unexplained infertility,[5] luteal phase defect, endometriosis and hydrosalpinx. Leukemia inhibiting factor and colony stimulating factor are decreased in women with unexplained infertility.[6] Newer molecules like glycodelin, uteroglobin, osteoprotegerin have shown an important role in endometrial receptivity.[7]

IMMUNOLOGICAL ASPECTS OF ENDOMETRIAL IMPLANTATION

It is postulated that the conceptus may be treated as foreign to the mother as it contains paternal antigen. According to responses either pregnancy is maintained or rejected. Large granular lymphocytes (LGL) comprise 70 to 80% of the endometrial leukocyte population and play a role in implantation and maintenance of pregnancy. Endometrium of women with unexplained infertility contain fewer CD56,

LGL and CD8 T cells as compared to fertile women suggesting that body immune system could regulate endometrial receptivity.

ENDOMETRIAL VASCULAR CHANGES

There are marked changes in the vascularity of the endometrium during the menstrual cycle. The lowest impedance to blood flow is during the secretory phase around implantation. This increase in vascularity leads to endometrial (epithelial and stromal) growth and efficient distribution as well as expression of molecular biomarkers required for preparation of the endometrium for implantation.

CURRENT STRATEGIES TO ASSESS ENDOMETRIAL RECEPTIVITY

Unfortunately there are no universally accepted markers of endometrial receptivity. Tests that assess receptivity can be grouped as in Table 14.4.

Endometrial Histology

1. *Endometrial histopathology:* This is done by endometrial biopsy taken during the late luteal phase. This has been the gold standard to assess endometrial maturity. There are certain limitations to this procedure, namely:
   a. It is performed in the late luteal phase and hence may give information only of the invasion phase.
   b. It is only representative of the endometrial changes within that cycle and cycle variations are well-known.
   c. Does not reflect the endometrium as a whole, regional variations being frequently encountered.

> **Table 14.4**
>
> **Methods of endometrial evaluation**
>
> *Tests to assess endometrial changes*
> 1. Endometrial histology
>   - Endometrial histopathology
>   - Study of pinopodes
> 2. Endometrial culture
> 3. Ultrasonography and Doppler, MRI
> 4. Hormonal evaluation
> 5. Hysteroscopy for anatomical and infectious cause
>
> *Markers of the embryo-endometrial dialogue*
>   - Biochemical markers—endometrial proteins
>   - Uteroglobin and glycodelin A

    d. Cannot be carried out in the cycle in which the patient is undergoing ART.

2. *Study of pinopodes:* Pinopodes are studied by electron microscopy only.

Endometrial Culture and Histopathology for Infections

Tuberculosis and chronic nonspecific endometritis has a high incidence in unexplained infertility, recurrent implantation failure and abortions. All cases with bacterial vaginosis have a high incidence of chronic nonspecific endometritis and should be screened. Chronic nonspecific endometritis is diagnosed by presence of plasma cells on histopathology. However, underdiagnosis because of nondetection of plasma cells is known and immunohistochemistry of syndecan 1 (a proteoglycan found on the surface of plasma cells) should be done for detection, specially in high-risk groups like those with recurrent implantation failure and abortions, unexplained infertility, abnormal uterine bleeding where no cause found and those with characteristic milieu of CE in which plasma cells not found on H and E stain.

A poor concordance is seen between endocervical, vaginal and endometrial cultures. Hence, an endometrial culture should be sent to confirm microorganism responsible for endometritis. Antimicrobial therapy should be initiated in chronic nonspecific endometritis only after organism is identified as besides chlamydia and gonococcus, other organisms like *E. coli, staphylococcus, streptococcus* and *U. urealyticum* have a high incidence.

Ultrasound and Color Doppler

Transvaginal sonography is a simple noninvasive modality used to assess endometrial receptivity. Using Doppler the impedance to blood flow of the uterine artery is expressed as the pulsatility index (PI) and is the lowest at the time of implantation.

a. *Endometrial thickness:* It is generally accepted that if the thickness is < 7 mm on ultrasound the implantation is poor. Similarly endometrial volume of < 2.5 ml on 3D ultrasonography is associated with a poor pregnancy rate.
b. *Echogenicity:* As thickness increases a distinct triple line or multilayered pattern is seen and is considered to be predictive of implantation. Further under the influence of progesterone the endometrium undergoes secretory changes and becomes more isoechoic and then hyperechoic. A nonmultilayered endometrium is associated with poor implantation.
c. *Endometrial vascularity:* Sub and intraendometrial vascularity is a prognostic factor for implantation if endometrium is more than 7 mm, irrespective of the morphological index. Uterine perfusion is maximum

during the mid-luteal phase. PI < 3 is associated with increased pregnancy rate. Absence of sub-endometrial blood flow on the day of LH surge is related to implantation failure.

Spiral artery perfusion is evaluated by color Doppler and the endometrium has been divided into four zones:
- *Zone* 1—only myometrial vessels surrounding endometrium are seen
- *Zone* 2—vessels penetrate through the hyperechogenic endometrial edge
- *Zone* 3—vessels reach the internal endometrial hyperechogenic zone
- *Zone* 4—vessels reach up to the endometrial cavity. A good vascularity in zone ¾th which relates to the surface of the endometrium suggests good endometrial receptivity.

Hormonal Levels

They are of not much use for assessment of endometrial receptivity.

Hysteroscopy

Hysteroscopy may detect anatomical lesions missed earlier and chronic nonspecific endometritis. Hysteroscopy may show evidence of endometritis in the form of focal or diffuse hyperemia, white spots, micropolyps and intrauterine adhesions.

Markers of the Embryo-endometrial Dialogue

Evaluation of the various biomarkers are mostly research tools. Kits for evaluation of integrins and mucins are now commercially available (see Table 14.3).

ENDOMETRIAL PREPARATION FOR FROZEN EMBRYO TRANSFER

Many regimes have been used for endometrial preparation in donor oocytes or frozen ET. Estradiol supplementation is started on day 1 with 2 mg/day and increased to 6 mg/day depending on endometrial response.[17] Beta-estradiol transdermal patches at steadily increasing dosage from 100 to 300 μg have been given for at least 12 days. This was increased by 100 μg after 7 days.

A recent Cochrane review showed no significant benefit for using GnRH agonists. No difference in pregnancy rate was demonstrated when no treatment was compared to aspirin, steroids, ovarian stimulation, or human chorionic gonadotropin (hCG) prior to embryo transfer. Starting progesterone on the day of oocyte pick-up (OPU) or the day after OPU produced a significantly higher pregnancy rate than when recipients started progesterone the day prior to OPU. So, there is insufficient evidence to recommend any one particular protocol for endometrial preparation over another with regard to pregnancy rates after embryo transfers.[8]

TREATMENT OF POOR UTERINE RECEPTIVITY

Treatment of poor uterine receptivity may be advocated in follicular or luteal phase (Table 14.5 and Flow chart 14.1).

Estrogens

Where endometrial response is suboptimal as often occurs with clomiphene induction, because of its antiestrogenic effect, treatment is given by supplementing estrogen from day 7 to 12 of cycle or till plasma estradiol is 400 to 700 pg/ml.

1. Ethinyl estradiol 0.05 mg/day.
2. Premarin 0.325 mg/day.
3. Estradiol valerate 2-8 mg.
4. Vaginal estradiol 0.1 mg twice a day.

Drugs to Improve the Endometrial Blood Flow

Aspirin: Low dose aspirin, 75 mg/day has shown favorable results.

Sildenafil: It is a type five specific phosphodiesterase inhibitor. When given in a dose of 25 mg four times a day intravaginally for 3 to 10 days, it has improved endometrial receptivity.[9] Uterine perfusion improved and pulsatility index decreased from 3 to 2.1 whereas there was no effect in placebo cases. This, however, is an observational study and is not supported by randomized control trials. It should be used with caution as it has side effects like headache, hypertension and occasional death.

Nitroglycerine: It is thought to be useful because of it vasodilating effect and is given in a dose of 800 mg sublingually 3 minutes before embryo transfer in IVF or as 5 mg daily patch on day of ET and then daily.

L-arginine: NO is formed from L-arginine and leads to increased vascularity and improves blood flow in the ovarian follicle. It is given in a dose of 16 gm/day.

Immunosuppression

Treatment regimes involving administration of IVIG (intravenous immunoglobulin) and LITT (leukocyte immunotherapy), are tried where paternal or donor leukocytes are injected into the mother in an attempt to alter the maternal immune response, making it favorable for implantation. Currently, there is no consensus of

Table 14.5
Improving uterine receptivity

1. Estrogens (Day 7-12)
    a. Ethinyl estradiol 0.05 mg/day
    b. Estradiol valerate 2-8 mg
    c. Vaginal estradiol 0.1 mg twice a day
    d. Premarin 0.325 mg/day
2. Increase blood flow
    a. Aspirin
    b. Sildenafil
    c. Nitroglycerine
    d. L-arginine
3. Immunotherapy
    a. Intravenous immunoglobulins
    b. Leukocyte immunotherapy
4. Reducing uterine contractility
    a. Ritodrine
    b. Piroxicam
5. Change of drugs which do not affect endometrial receptivity
    a. Letrozole
    b. Tamoxifen
    c. Gonadotropins
6. Luteal phase support
    a. Progestogens
    b. hCG
7. Surgical
    a. Hysteroscopic resection of endometrial synechia
    b. Drainage of hydrosalpinx
8. Treatment of endometritis

Endometrial Receptivity and Luteal Support | 373

Flow chart 14.1: Evaluation and management of poor uterine receptivity

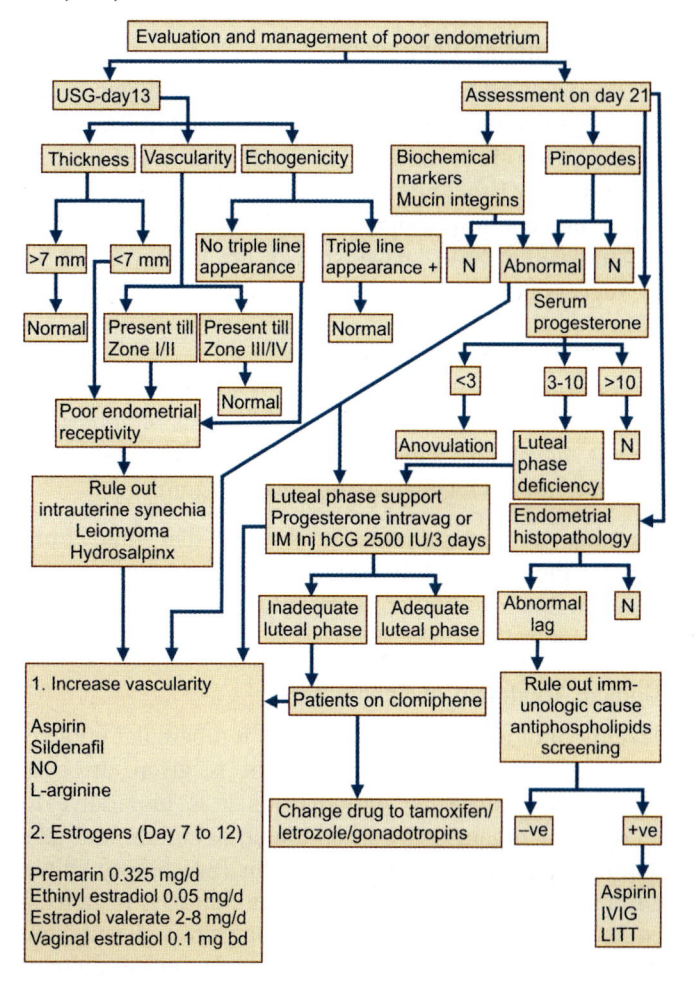

```
Evaluation and management of poor endometrium
├── USG-day13
│   ├── Thickness
│   │   ├── >7 mm → Normal
│   │   └── <7 mm → Poor endometrial receptivity
│   ├── Vascularity
│   │   ├── Present till Zone I/II → Poor endometrial receptivity
│   │   └── Present till Zone III/IV → Normal
│   └── Echogenicity
│       ├── No triple line appearance → Poor endometrial receptivity
│       └── Triple line appearance + → Normal
└── Assessment on day 21
    ├── Biochemical markers Mucin integrins
    │   ├── N
    │   └── Abnormal → Serum progesterone
    │       ├── <3 → Anovulation
    │       ├── 3–10 → Luteal phase deficiency → Endometrial histopathology
    │       │           ├── Abnormal lag → Rule out immunologic cause antiphospholipids screening
    │       │           │   ├── –ve
    │       │           │   └── +ve → Aspirin / IVIG / LITT
    │       │           └── N
    │       └── >10 → N
    └── Pinopodes
        ├── N
        └── Abnormal
```

Poor endometrial receptivity →
- Rule out intrauterine synechia, Leiomyoma, Hydrosalpinx
- Luteal phase support: Progesterone intravag or IM Inj hCG 2500 IU/3 days
  - Inadequate luteal phase → Patients on clomiphene → Change drug to tamoxifen/letrozole/gonadotropins
  - Adequate luteal phase

1. Increase vascularity

Aspirin
Sildenafil
NO
L-arginine

2. Estrogens (Day 7 to 12)

Premarin 0.325 mg/d
Ethinyl estradiol 0.05 mg/d
Estradiol valerate 2–8 mg/d
Vaginal estradiol 0.1 mg bd

opinion on either of these treatments and they are to be used in research setting only.

Reducing Uterine Contractility

1. *Ritodrine:* Administration of this drug has shown better pregnancy rate in randomized controlled trials.
2. *Piroxicam:* In a randomized controlled trial 10 mg of piroxicam 1 to 2 hours before embryo transfer showed 20 percent improvement in pregnancy rate. Recent studies, however, have shown no improvement in success rate.[10]

Surgical Treatment

Lysis of uterine synechia: In cases of adhesions following D and C or endometritis hysteroscopic lysis of adhesions should be done. Patients are treated with estrogens following this to regenerate the endometrium.

Drainage of hydrosalpinx: It is seen that fluid from hydrosalpinx impairs implantation. Hence, drainage of hydrosalpinx can be done by ultrasound guidance or laparoscopically.

Medical Treatment of Endometritis

Treatment of endometritis is a must. If tubercular etiology is present, antitubercular treatment is given. In case of chronic nonspecific endometritis it is imperative to identify the organism by an endometrial culture and give antimicrobial therapy accordingly. In case biopsy shows chronic nonspecific endometritis but culture is negative a course of metronidazole and azithromycin is given. Often these infections are difficult to eradicate and antibiotics may be needed for a longer period.

Luteal Phase Support

Normal formation and function of the corpus luteum and optimal endometrial preparation is a prerequisite for both nidation and normal progress of early pregnancy. This is dependent on normal follicular and ovulatory phase endocrine events. Luteal phase defect has remained a disorder of controversy since its description. Luteal phase defect is characterized by inadequate endometrial maturation due to a qualitative or quantitative disorder in corpus luteum function. Progesterone secreted by the corpus luteum is essential for the initiation and maintenance of normal gestation. Luteal support remains essential till about the seventh week of gestation, by which time the trophoblast acquires sufficient steroidogenic capacity to support the pregnancy. When pregnancy occurs chorionic gonadotropins are responsible for the prolongation of corpus luteum function.

Pathophysiologic mechanism: During folliculogenesis, there is a complex interplay between GnRH pulsatile patterns, FSH release and activity within the growing follicle, and peripheral steroid feedback. Disturbance in any of these factors leads to possible mechanisms for development of luteal phase defect (Flow chart 14.2). It was observed that there was a significantly low progesterone receptor content on endometrial glandular nucleus in luteal phase defect group. This resulted in a deficient endometrial response to progesterone stimulus. The result is a poorly prepared endometrium either due to inadequate progesterone receptor induction during the follicular phase or insufficient peripheral progesterone levels reaching the endometrium from the ovary leading to abnormal implantation or early pregnancy wastage.

Flow chart 14.2: Pathophysiology of luteal phase defect[11]

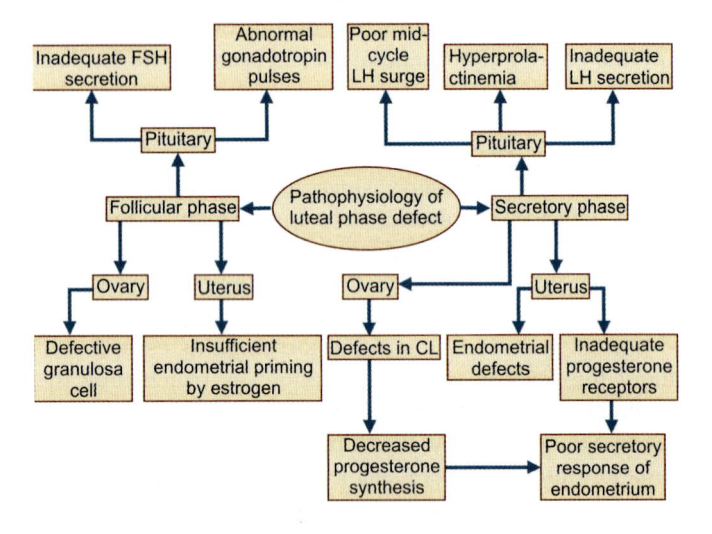

```
Inadequate FSH    Abnormal        Poor mid-      Hyperprola-   Inadequate
  secretion      gonadotropin     cycle         ctinemia      LH secretion
                    pulses        LH surge
       ↑             ↑               ↑              ↑              ↑
       └──Pituitary──┘               └──────Pituitary─────────────┘
              ↓                              ↓
        Follicular phase  ←  Pathophysiology  →  Secretory phase
              ↓                of luteal                ↓
                              phase defect
       ┌──────┴──────┐              ┌──────────┬──────────┐
     Ovary         Uterus          Ovary               Uterus
       ↓             ↓               ↓           ↓        ↓
   Defective    Insufficient      Defects    Endometrial  Inadequate
   granulosa    endometrial       in CL      defects      progesterone
     cell       priming by                                receptors
                estrogen             ↓                        ↓
                                Decreased              Poor secretory
                                progesterone    →      response of
                                synthesis              endometrium
```

Why Luteal Support is Needed in ART Cycles?

1. Supraphysiological estrogen levels seen in controlled ovarian hyperstimulation protocols may induce premature luteolysis.
2. Follicular phase downregulation may impair luteal phase luteinizing hormone release.
3. Some protocols may give only pure FSH thus leading to a relatively low LH value.
4. Ovarian aspiration may cause disruption of granulosa cells leading to aberrant steroidogenesis.
5. Controlled ovarian stimulation accelerates endometrial maturation hindering implantation.

The ability of the endometrium to respond to progesterone is an acquired property depending on the induction of adequate progesterone receptors by estradiol during the follicular phase of the cycle.

Hence, there is a concern in IVF/ICSI cycles of luteal phase defect. Hence, luteal phase is supported by progesterone, hCG, sometimes estradiol as a routine. Recently single dose of GnRH agonist has also been tried.

Risk Factors for Luteal Phase Inadequacy

It is mostly seen in:
1. Hyperprolactinemia.
2. Elevated circulating androgens.
3. Oligo-ovulation.
4. Extremes of reproductive age.
5. Treatment with ovulation inducing agents or ovarian suppressive agents.
6. Patients present with history of recurrent abortion.
7. Endometriosis.[11]
8. Following discontinuation of suppressive medical therapies.
9. Strenuous exercise.

Diagnosis is based on endometrial histopathology, basal body temperature, low luteal progesterone levels and transvaginal sonography. There are other tests like decidual prolactin, steroid receptor studies and endometrial biochemical markers which can be done (Table 14.6).

Treatment of Luteal Phase Defect

It is in the form of progesterone supplementation, hCG, and estradiol in recent years.

Progesterone Supplementation

Progesterone supplementation should commence after oocyte retrieval and continue till 12 weeks of gestation as the placenta takes over the role of progesterone production.

Table 14.6

Techniques for diagnosis of luteal phase defects

1. Basal body temperature charts—monophasic or rise of temprature for less than 11 days.
2. Luteal phase progesterone levels—less than 10 ng/ml.
3. Transvaginal ultrasonography and Doppler studies.
4. Endometrial biopsy and histopathology—lag of 2 days.
5. Serum prolactin measurement.
6. Decidual prolactin measurement.[12]
7. Steroid hormone receptor analysis.
8. Biochemical markers for endometrial receptivity.
9. Sonographic criteria for aberrant luteolysis
    i. Persistent perifollicular reaction
    ii. Rupture of follicle of <17 mm
    iii. Poorly formed or ill-defined dominant follicle
    iv. Luteinized unruptured follicle
    v. Lutein cyst formation
    vi. Absence of corpus luteum
    vii. Lack of endometrial echogenicity on 7th postovulation day.

Oral administration: Though progesterone is absorbed orally, more than 90 percent is metabolized during the first hepatic pass limiting its efficacy. Many micronized forms have become available to overcome this problem. Metabolites of orally administered progesterone may produce a hypnotic effect.

Intramuscular administration: It is the most reliable route to achieve desired concentration of progesterone. It is rapidly absorbed and peak level is reached in 8 hours. Serum progesterone levels remain sustained compared to other routes as it is administered in an oil vehicle. Allergic reactions may be seen. Intramuscular dose is 50 to 100 mg per day.

Vaginal administration: There is increased bioavailability and reduced variability when progesterone is given vaginally or rectally compared to oral route. This sustained level produces a more physiologic endometrial response. Micronized progesterone may exert a direct effect on the uterus by blocking the rejection of the embryo. It does not cause drowsiness or sleepiness but is inconvenient because of vaginal discharge. Patient is advised the use of progesterone vaginal suppositories after ovulation is confirmed. In a dose of 400 mg per day in 2 divided doses. This produces concentration similar to the luteal phase which is maximal within 1 to 8 hours and decrease over 24 hours. Vaginal gel also produces endometrial response as good or better than the intramuscular route and comparable to any other vaginal preparation. [13,14]

Dehydrogesterone: It is a retroprogesterone or stereoisomer of progesterone. It is closest to native progesterone. It was found that pregnancy and implantation rate was similar whether micronized progesterone or gel or dehydrogesterone was given in the luteal phase following IVF and ET. It is given in a dose of 20 to 30 mg/day.[15]

Human Chorionic Gonadotropin (hCG)

Administration of hCG stimulates the corpus luteum to produce progesterone. It is ineffective in the presence of inadequate number of LH receptors or a malfunctioning corpus luteum which is hypo-responsive to hCG. hCG is effective if there is a specific defect in postovulatory LH secretion or in trophoblastic hCG production.

In order to achieve complete luteinisation of the preovulatory follicle, 10,000 IU of hCG should be administered at the time of ovulation followed by a dose of 2500 IU every 3 to 4 days. The long half-life of hCG renders pregnancy testing invalid for 7 days after the last hCG injection.

As hCG was associated with a higher risk of OHSS, it should be avoided (Cochrane Review 2011).[16]

Estradiol Supplementation in Luteal Phase

Supplementation in the luteal phase with estradiol in doses of 2 mg, 4 mg and 6 mg/day is being used. In initial studies conducted significantly higher implantation rate and PR were recorded in those who received low dose E2 supplementation compared with no substitution (PR 23.1 vs 32.8%). The best implantation and pregnancy results were found significantly in the group with high dose E2 supplementation (PR 51.3%).[17] However, more recent studies showed no difference in terms of pregnancy and implantation.[18]

Single-dose GnRH Agonist in the Luteal Phase

The exact mechanism is still not known. It was suggested that GnRH-a can help in the maintenance of the corpus luteum, acting directly on the endometrium via local receptors, a direct effect on the embryos or by some combination of these possibilities. A single dose of GnRH agonist (0.5 mg leuprolide acetate) was administered subcutaneously on day 6 after ICSI. A metanalysis showed that the luteal-phase single-dose GnRH-a administration can increase implantation rate in all cycles and CPR per transfer and ongoing pregnancy rate in cycles with GnRH antagonist ovarian stimulation protocol.[19] GnRH agonist addition during the luteal phase significantly increases the probability of live birth rates.[20]

A recent Cochrane review (2011) favored progesterone for luteal phase support, favoring synthetic progesterone over micronized progesterone. Estrogen or hCG did not seem to improve outcomes. There was no evidence favoring a specific route or duration of administration of progesterone There were significant results showing a benefit from addition of GnRH agonist to progesterone for the outcomes of live birth, clinical pregnancy and ongoing pregnancy.[16]

Poor endometrial receptivity and luteal phase deficiency is an important cause of IVF failure. Considerable research is ongoing in this area to unravel the mystery of implantation. The ART success rate will improve if we can selectively modulate implantation.

REFERENCES

1. Psychosos A. Endocrine control of egg implantation. In: Greep RO, Astwood EG, Geiger SR (Eds). Handbook of Physiology. American Physiological Society, Washington DC, USA, 1973; 187-225.
2. Enders AC. Contributions of comparative studies to understanding mechanisms of implantation. In: Glasser SR, Mulholland J, Psychosis A (Eds). Endocrinology of Embryo-Endometrium Interactions. Plenum Press: New York and London 1994.pp.11-16.
3. Nikas G. Pinopodes as markers of endometrial receptivity in clinical practice. Hum Reprod 1999;14 (suppl 2):3-16.
4. Fienberg RF, Kilman HJ. MAG (mouse ascites Golgi) mucin in the endometrium: a potential marker of endometrial receptivity to implantation. In: Diamond MP, Osteen KG (Eds): Endometrium and Endometriosis. Blackwell Science, Malden, MA, USA, 1997.pp.131-9.
5. Lessey BA, Castlebaum AJ, Sawin SJ, et al. Integrins as markers of uterine receptivity in women with primary unexplained infertility. Fertil Steril 1995;63:533-42.
6. Hambartsoumann E. Endometrial leukemia inhibitory factor (LIF) as a possible cause of unexplained infertility and multiple failures of implantation. Am J Reprod Immunol 1998;39:137-43.

7. Alok A, Karande AA. The role of glycodelin as an immune-modulating agent at the feto-maternal interface. J Reprod Immunol. 2009;83(1-2):124-7.
8. Glujovsky D, Pesce R, Fiszbajn G, Sueldo C, Hart RJ, Ciapponi A. Endometrial preparation for women undergoing embryo transfer with frozen embryos or embryos derived from donor oocytes. Cochrane Database Syst Rev. 2010;(1):CD006359.
9. Sher G, Fisch JD. Effect of vaginal sildenafil on the outcome of *in vitro* fertilization (IVF) after multiple IVF failures attributed to poor endometrial development. Fertil Steril 2002;78(5):1073-6.
10. Dal Prato L, Borini A. Effect of piroxicam administration before embryo transfer on IVF outcome: a randomized controlled trial. Reprod Biomed Online 2009;19(4):604-9.
11. Cunha-Filho JS, Gross JL, Bastos de Souza CA, Lemos NA, Giugliani C, Freitas F, Passos EP. Physiopathological aspects of corpus luteum defect in infertile patients with mild/minimal endometriosis. J Assist Reprod Genet 2003;20(3):117-21.
12. Garzia E, Borgato S, Cozzi V, Doi P, Bulfamante G, Persani L, et al. Lack of expression of endometrial prolactin in early implantation failure: A pilot study. Hum Reprod 2004;19(8):1911-6.
13. Polyzos NP, Messini CI, Papanikolaou EG, Mauri D, Tzioras S, Badawy A, Messinis IE. Vaginal progesterone gel for luteal phase support in IVF/ICSI cycles: a meta-analysis. Fertil Steril. 2010 ;94(6):2083-7.
14. Yanushpolsky E, Hurwitz S, Greenberg L, Racowsky C, Hornstein M. Crinone vaginal gel is equally effective and better tolerated than intramuscular progesterone for luteal phase support in *in vitro* fertilization-embryo transfer cycles: a prospective randomized study. Fertil Steril. 2010;94(7):2596-9.
15. Ganesh A, Chakravorty N, Mukherjee R, Goswami S, Chaudhury K, Chakravarty B. Comparison of oral dydrogestrone with progesterone gel and micronized progesterone for luteal support in 1,373 women undergoing *in vitro* fertilization: a randomized clinical study. Fertil Steril. 2011;95(6):1961-5

16. van der Linden M, Buckingham K, Farquhar C, Kremer JA, Metwally M. Luteal phase support for assisted reproduction cycles. Cochrane Database Syst Rev. 2011;10:CD009154.
17. Lukaszuk K, Liss J, Lukaszuk M, Maj B. Optimization of estradiol supplementation during the luteal phase improves the pregnancy rate in women undergoing *in vitro* fertilization-embryo transfer cycles. Fertil Steril. 2005;83(5):1372-6.
18. Tonguc E, Var T, Ozyer S, Citil A, Dogan M. Estradiol supplementation during the luteal phase of *in vitro* fertilization cycles: a prospective randomised study. Eur J Obstet Gynecol Reprod Biol. 2011;154(2):172-6.
19. Oliveira JB, Baruffi R, Petersen CG, Mauri AL, Cavagna M, Franco JG Jr. Administration of single-dose GnRH agonist in the luteal phase in ICSI cycles: a meta-analysis. Reprod Biol Endocrinol. 2010 8;8:107.
20. Kyrou D, Kolibianakis EM, Fatemi HM, Tarlatzi TB, Devroey P, Tarlatzis BC. Increased live birth rates with GnRH agonist addition for luteal support in ICSI/IVF cycles: a systematic review and meta-analysis. Hum Reprod Update. 2011;17(6):734-40.

Chapter 15

Ovarian Hyperstimulation Syndrome

Surveen Ghumman Sindhu

Ovarian hyperstimulation syndrome (OHSS) is one of the known complications of controlled ovarian stimulation. It is a syndrome with a wide spectrum of clinical and laboratory symptoms and sign, due to a fluid shift from the intravascular to the third space because of increased intravascular permeability, manifesting as ascites, pleural effusion, hemoconcentration, oliguria, electrolyte imbalance and hypercoagulability. It is accompanied by ovarian enlargement.

INCIDENCE

OHSS is classified as mild, moderate and severe with the incidence ranging from 3 to 23% of inductions.[1] The incidence varies with the ovarian stimulation protocols and the risk profile of the population being treated. Incidence of mild moderate or severe OHSS is 8 to 23%, 0.005 to 7% and 0.008 to 2% respectively. It occurred in 0.008 to 23% of hMG/hCG cycles and 0.6 to 14% in GnRH –a/hMG/hCG cycle.

CLASSIFICATION

It presents after hCG administration or rise of hCG due to an early pregnancy. It can be 'Early onset', within 3 to 7 days of hCG administration, or 'late onset' 12 to 17 days after hCG because of early pregnancy.

1. *Golan's classification:* Golan proposed an acceptable classification with greater practical advantages (Table 15.1). It incorporates clinical signs, symptoms,

Table 15.1
Golan's classification of OHSS[2]

Grade	Mild	Moderate	Severe
1.	Abdominal discomfort/distention		
2.	Features of grade 1 along with nausea, vomiting and/or diarrhea. Ovaries enlarged 5–12 cm		
3.		Features of mild OHSS and USG evidence of Ascites	
4.			Feature of moderate OHSS plus clinical evidence of ascites and/or hydrothorax with/or difficulty in breathing
5.			All of the above plus change in blood volume, increased blood viscosity due to hemoconcentration, coagulation disturbances and diminished renal perfusion and function

ultrasonographic findings and laboratory findings to yield three stages and five grades of OHSS severity.[2]

2. *Navot's classification (Table 15.2):* This classification further defined the severest degree of OHSS as given by Golan into severe and critical life threatening stage based on a multitude of clinical and biochemical findings.[3] In this classification generalized edema and

Table 15.2

Clinical Signs and laboratory criteria of ovarian hyperstimulation syndrome[3]

	Mild to moderate	Severe	Critical
Ovarian enlargement	5–12 cm	>12 cm	Variable
Abdominal distension	Moderate	Severe	Tense
Clinical ascitis	None	Yes	Tense
Hydrothorax	None	Possible	Yes
Pericardial effusion	None	Infrequent	Infrequent
Decreased renal function	None	Infrequent	Frequent
Renal failure	None	None	Possible
Thromboembolism	None	None	Possible
ARDS	None	None	Possible
Hemoconcentration (Hematocrit)	<45%	45–55%	>55%
WBC count	<15,000	15,000–25,000	>25,000
Liver enzymes	Normal	Elevated	Elevated
Creatinine (ng/ml)	<1.0	1.0–1.5	>1.6
Creatinine clearance (ml/min)	>100	50–100	<50

liver dysfunction are considered additional signs of severe OHSS while adult respiratory distress syndrome, a tense ascitis, severe hemoconcentration (>55%) and profound leukocytosis (>25,000) are signs of the severest life threatening form and need aggressive medical and surgical intervention.

PATHOPHYSIOLOGY OF OHSS

The complicated pathophysiology of OHSS has still yet not been completely elucidated.

Two major events are, however recognized.
1. *Neovascularization:* Neovascularization leads to increased vascularity
2. *Increased vascular permeability of mesothelial surfaces:* The increased capillary permeability of the ovarian vessels and other mesothelial surfaces leads to acute fluid shift to the third space (Flow chart 15.1). This is triggered by release of vasoactive substances secreted by the ovary under the influence of hCG. These are prorenin and active renins, interleukins, nitric oxide, and vascular endothelial growth factor.

CLINICAL FEATURES

The clinical features associated with OHSS are due to the shift of fluid into the third space because of vascular permeability (Tables 15.1 and 15.2). The patient may have clinical features like
- Lower abdominal pain and distension.
- Symptoms of nausea, vomiting and diarrhea.
- Progressive lethargy

Ovarian Hyperstimulation Syndrome

Flow chart 15.1: Pathophysiology of OHSS

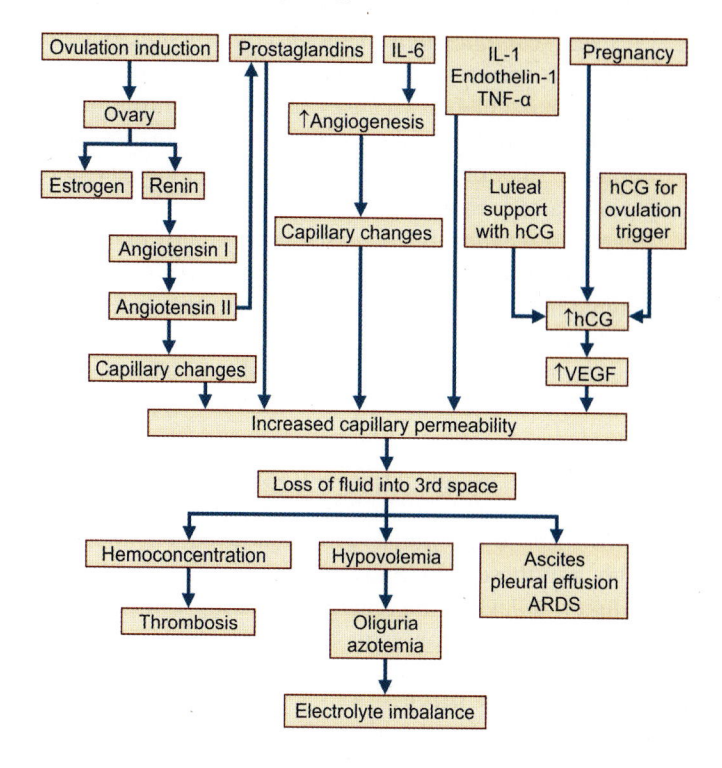

- History of decreased urine output.
- Increased pulse rate, shortness of breath, fluid collection at the base of lungs.
- Significant fluid electrolyte imbalance.
- Dehydration in severe cases.
- Hypercoagulability of blood causing thrombosis.

FATAL COMPLICATIONS

1. *Vascular complications:* Venous compression due to enlarged ovaries and ascites, immobility and a state of hypercoagulability causes deep vein thrombosis. Cerebrovascular complications subsequent to thromboembolic phenomenon may lead to hemiplegia and carotid artery embolism.
2. *Liver dysfunction:* The increased permeability in hepatic vasculature leads to edema, damage to hepatic cells and altered hepatic function. These changes may persist for 60 days.
3. *Respiratory complications:* Ascites, pleural effusion and ARDS are due to fluid shift into the third space.
4. *Renal complications:* Prerenal failure occurs due to hypovolemia secondary to fluid transudate.
5. *Gastrointestinal complications:* Gastrointestinal symptoms may be the initial symptoms a patient presents with, and these help to diagnose the syndrome early.
6. *Adnexal torsion:* The enlarged ovaries can undergo torsion leading to an acute abdomen.

MANAGEMENT OF OHSS

The most effective treatment of OHSS is precise prediction and active prevention. This can be done effectively with the combined use of ultrasonography and serum estradiol levels.

Prevention

1. *Identify patients who are at high-risk:* This is the first step in prevention (Table 15.3). Monitoring of induction of ovulation is done to identify high-risk cases. A number of factors are related to increased risk of OHSS

Table 15.3
Risk factors for OHSS

Predicting factors	High-risk	Low-risk
Age	Young (<35 years)	Older (>36 years)
Cause of anovulation	Polycystic ovarian disease	Hypogonadotropic hypogonadism
Build	Asthenic habitus	Heavy build
Number of follicles	Multiple follicles (>35)	Fewer follicles (<20)
Ultrasonography of ovary	Necklace sign present	Absent
Outcome of IVF cycle	Pregnancy	No pregnancy
Luteal supplementation	hCG luteal supplementation	Progesterone/no supplementation
Ovulation induction protocol	GnRH agonist protocol	GnRH antagonist protocol
History of OHSS	Present	Absent

a. *Size and number of follicles:* Women with a large number of follicles (>15), decreased fraction of large follicles and a high proportion of small and intermediate size follicles, are more prone to OHSS.
b. *Serum estradiol:* At serum estradiol levels of 4000 pg/ml or above hCG is withheld though studies have even quoted values above 3500 pg/ml.
c. *Age:* Young patients are more prone to develop OHSS
d. *Built:* Thin patients are at higher risk of OHSS
e. *PCOS:* At the start of the cycle PCOS patients have a large number of small follicles which are all likely to respond to the dose of gonadotropins once the FSH threshold is reached. This would lead to hyperstimulation.

f. *OHSS in previous cycle:* A history of OHSS in previous cycle, increases risk of recurrence in next cycle.
g. *Protocol of ovarian stimulation:* GnRH agonist protocol has higher risk of OHSS compared with an antagonist protocol.
h. *Pregnancy:* Patient who conceived, and more so with multiple pregnancy, were more prone to OHSS.
i. *Trigger for inducing follicular rupture:* If hCG was used as a trigger for follicular rupture there were higher chances of OHSS.
j. *Luteal support:* With hCG as a luteal support, the chances of development of OHSS were higher.
k. *Basal antimullerian hormone (AMH):* The basal serum AMH level predicted OHSS with a sensitivity of 90.5% and specificity of 81.3%.[4]

2. *Withholding hCG:* The criterion for withholding hCG varies in different centers. It is mostly based on more than one parameter like are number and size of follicles, estradiol levels, slope of rise of estradiol, history of OHSS in previous cycle and presence of PCOS.

   a. *Level of estradiol:* hCG is withheld when estradiol levels are more than 3000 pg/ml. Incidence of severe OHSS was 1% if serum estradiol levels are 3000 to 3999 pg/ml and it increases to 5.97% if the levels are more than 4000 pg/ml. Hence, many prefer to take a cut off value of 4000 pg/ml. However, many cases of OHSS can occur in normal estradiol levels and often, high estradiol levels may lead to no overstimulation.[5]

   Slope of rise of the plasma estradiol level: If values are more than doubling during 2 to 3 days (steep slope) then it should be regarded as a serious warning sign, and hCG should be withheld in that cycle.

   b. *Number of follicles on ultrasonography:* When there is an increase in fraction of the small and intermediate size follicles there was greater chance of OHSS developing. Presence of 15 to 20 follicles which are mainly immature (9 mm) should be taken as a cut off. The final decision must see multiple parameters.

3. *Delaying hCG (Coasting):* Withholding gonadotropins causes decreased FSH which causes downregulation of LH receptors reducing number of granulosa cell available for luteinization and a concomitant decrease in vasoactive substances causing OHSS. When estradiol levels are high hCG is delayed, while GnRH agonist is continued witholding HMG till E2 falls below 3000 pg/ml. At this level hCG is given. Longer period of coasting beyond 5 days, is associated with lower pregnancy rates.[6] A recent Cochrane review has stated that coasting has no beneficial role in preventing OHSS.[7]

4. *Decreasing dose of hCG:* Lower dosage may avoid hyperstimulation by exerting shorter periods of stimulation. 5,000 IU of hCG is given instead of 10,000 IU as an ovulation trigger.

5. *The use of GnRH agonist as a trigger:* Since period of stimulation is lesser with GnRH agonist surge, there is no hyperstimulation. The pregnancy rates are similar after an agonist or hCG trigger.[8] A recent Cochrane review (2011) recommends it in patients at high-risk of OHSS.[9]

6. *Luteal phase support:* Progesterone, intravaginally or intramuscularly, is given for luteal support instead of hCG when patients are at high-risk of OHSS.

7. *Follicle aspiration:* Follicle aspiration was found to decrease the incidence of OHSS.[10] Hence if women are showing signs of being at risk of hyperstimulation follicles should be aspirated.
8. *Post oocyte retrieval Albumin or Hydroxyethyl starch administration:* Albumin helps by increasing serum oncotic pressure and reversing the leakage of fluid into the third space. Albumin has a half life of 10 to 15 days, and needs timely administration at oocyte recovery, in a dose of 50 to 100 gm. The disadvantage is its oncotic action lasts for less than 36 hours, following which it moves into the interstitial compartment drawing fluid out of the intravascular space. A recent Cochrane review (2011) states there is limited benefit from intravenous albumin but better results with hydroxyethyl starch in preventing OHSS.[11]
9. *Cryopreservation of embryo and subsequent replacement:* OHSS decreases by the tenth day if no pregnancy occurs, but continues for a longer time with viable pregnancy. Cryopreservation of embryos helps decrease chances of OHSS due to pregnancy. However, a recent Cochrane review did not support this.[12]
10. *Steroids:* Methyl Prednisolone has been tried in cases of OHSS.[13] However, most studies have not shown a protective effect.
11. *Step up low dose regime of gonadotropins:* Low dose of gonadotropins are given in cases at high-risk for hyperstimulation like PCOS and gradually stepped up.
12. *Metformin:* Addition of metformin to ovulation induction regimen in polycystic ovarian disease results in decreased incidence of OHSS (Cochrane review 2009)[14]
13. *Dopamine agonists:* The dopamine receptor 2 agonists cabergoline and bromocriptine inactivate VEGF

receptor-2 and prevent increased vascular permeability. It is given in a dose of 0.5 mg/d administered from the day of human chorionic gonadotropin for 8 days.[15] Bromocriptine also decreased incidence of OHSS.[16]

Investigation and Monitoring of an OHSS Patient

1. *General condition:* General condition is monitored by regular charting of vital signs, weight charts, abdominal girth measurement and a strict fluid balance record.
2. *Biochemical tests:* A complete biochemical assessment includes hematocrit, electrolytes, liver function tests, kidney function tests and coagulation profile. Blood gases and acid base balance is required if there is a respiratory or renal compromise. Serum β hCG is done to rule out pregnancy. Serum and urinary osmolarity and urinary electrolytes may be needed in more severe forms of the disease. The frequency of these tests is guided by the severity of the disease.
3. *Ultrasonographic examination:* Ultrasound gives important information on ovarian size, amount of ascites, presence of hydrothorax or pericardial effusion, and detection of pregnancy, whether single or multiple.
4. *Chest X-ray:* A chest X-ray can rule out pleural effusion.
5. *Serum ß hCG:* It is done to confirm pregnancy making the women at a high-risk for developing severe disease.
6. *Invasive hemodynamic monitoring:* When OHSS becomes critical monitoring of pulmonary artery pressure and central venous pressure may be required.

Treatment

The condition usually resolves within 10 to 14 days. Treatment is based on severity of the disease.

Mild OHSS

In mild cases the treatment is usually conservative and is done at outpatient level with close follow-up. Reassessment is required if increase in weight is more than 2 kg or worsening of symptoms occurs.

Grade I: Woman is reassured and advised to have plenty of fluids and avoid exertion. She is counseled on warning signs like dyspnea, decreased urinary output, abdominal pain or distension and any other alarming symptom.

Grade II: Patient should be advised minimum physical activity and plenty of fluids. Serum electrolytes, hematocrit and ultrasonography should be done. Analgesics and antiemetics may be used if required. Intake output monitoring must be recorded.

Indication of hospitalization

Hospitalization should be considered in higher grades of the disease or if condition worsens and patient is not responding to treatment.

I. In cases of grade II or III admission is required, if there is:
   1. Intolerable nausea and vomiting
   2. Hypotension
   3. Signs of pleural effusion
   4. Ascitis
   5. Hematocrit >48%
   6. Potassium level >5.0 mg/L
   7. Serum creatinine >1.2 mg
II. All cases of grade IV and V should be hospitalized

Severe OHSS

Aim of Therapy after admission
1. Correction of circulatory volume electrolyte imbalance

2. Maintenance of renal function
3. Prevention of thrombosis

1. *Maintenance of intravascular volume and electrolyte imbalance:* The aim must be to restore normal intravascular volume and preserve adequate renal function. Colloid expander may be used for this purpose but, they have the disadvantage that after a short while they redistribute into the extravascular space worsening the ascitis. Low salt albumin is the expander of choice and is given in a dose of 50 to 100 gm every 2 to12 hours. It reverses hematocrit changes, improves renal function and is safe from viral contamination. Other options tried are mannitol, dextran and fresh frozen plasma. Dextran can cause ARDS. Only if there is hyponatremia, normal saline with or without glucose is the crystalloid used for replacement. Upto 1.5 to 3 liters may be needed. Other electrolyte imbalances like hyperkalemia are corrected.
2. *Prevention of thrombosis:* Low dose heparin should be given, as prophylaxis, in cases where there is an altered coagulation profile.
3. *Diuretics:* These drugs are usually not used but can be given after hemodilution is achieved if oliguria is persisting or in cases of pulmonary edema.
4. *Dopamine:* Dopamine may help to avoid fluid and salt retention by improving the renal blood flow in oliguric patient.
5. *Management of ascitis:* Paracentesis under ultrasound guidance is done where there is severe discomfort, compromise of venous return leading to a decreased cardiac output and hypotension, renal compromise, respiratory distress or hemoconcentration unresponsive to medical therapy. Repeat aspiration may be required

6. *Paracentesis of hydrothorax:* This should be done if dyspnea is present because of severe pleural effusion.

Critical OHSS

Critical OHSS causes multisystem failure and requires multidisciplinary intensive care.

1. *Renal failure:* Dopamine central venous pressure line and hemodialysis may be required in severe cases.
2. *Pulmonary compromise:* Arterial blood gas monitoring, thoracocentesis or assisted ventilation is required if they do not respond to basic treatment.
3. *Thromboembolic events:* Patients with thromboembolic episodes require therapeutic anticoagulation with heparin.
4. *Termination of pregnancy:* If critical condition does not improve one may consider termination of pregnancy.
5. *Laparotomy:* Laparotomy is required if the cysts undergo torsion, hemorrhage or rupture. Laparoscopic unwinding can be done in cases of torsion.

OHSS is an iatrogenic complication of controlled ovarian stimulation and may sometimes lead to life threatening complications. Prevention is the best way to manage OHSS. Proper monitoring is essential and a balance between a conservative and aggressive approach is ideal to prevent unnecessary cycle cancellation.

REFERENCES

1. Schenker IG, Weinsyein D. Ovarian overstimulation syndrome: a current survey. Fertil Steril. 1978;30:255-68.
2. Golan A, Ron-El-R, Herman A, et al. Ovarian hyperstimulation syndrome: an update review Obstet Gynecol Survey. 1989;44:430-40.

3. Navot D, Bergh PA, Lanfer N. Ovarian hyperstimulation syndrome in novel reproductive technologies; Prevention and treatment. Fertil Steril. 1992;58:249-61.
4. Lee TH, Liu CH, Huang CC, Wu YL, Shih YT, Ho HN, Yang YS, Lee MS. Serum anti-mullerian hormone and estradiol levels as predictors of ovarian hyperstimulation syndrome in assisted reproduction technology cycles. Hum Reprod. 2008;23:160-7.
5. Levy T, Orvieto R, Homberg R, Dekel A, Peleg D, Ben-Rafael Z. Severe hyperstimulation syndrome despite low plasma estrogen levels in hypogonadotropic hypogonadal patient. Hum Reprod. 1996;11:1177-9.
6. Cheema P, Gelbaya TA, Horne G, Fitzgerald CT, Pease EH, Brison DR, Lieberman BA. The optimal length of 'coasting protocol' in women at risk of ovarian hyperstimulation syndrome undergoing in vitro fertilization. Hum Fertil (Camb). 2006;9(3):175-80.
7. D'Angelo A, Brown J, Amso NN. Coasting (withholding gonadotrophins) for preventing ovarian hyperstimulation syndrome. Cochrane Database Syst Rev. 2011 Jun 15;(6):CD002811.
8. Shapiro BS, Daneshmand ST, Garner FC, Aguirre M, Ross R. Comparison of human chorionic gonadotropin and gonadotropin-releasing hormone agonist for final oocyte maturation in oocyte donor cycles. Fertil Steril. 2007;88(1):237-9.
9. Youssef MA, Van der Veen F, Al-Inany HG, Griesinger G, Mochtar MH, Aboulfoutouh I, Khattab SM, van Wely M Gonadotropin-releasing hormone agonist versus hCG for oocyte triggering in antagonist assisted reproductive technology cycles. Cochrane Database Syst Rev. 2011 Jan 19;(1):CD008046.
10. Zhu WJ, Li XM, Chen XM, Zhang L. Follicular aspiration during the selection phase prevents severe ovarian hyperstimulation in patients with polycystic ovary syndrome who are undergoing in vitro fertilization. Eur J Obstet Gynecol Reprod Biol. 2005;122(1):79-84.

11. Youssef MA, Al-Inany HG, Evers JL, Aboulghar M. Intravenous fluids for the prevention of severe ovarian hyperstimulation syndrome. Cochrane Database Syst Rev. 2011 Feb 16;(2):CD001302.
12. D'Angelo A, Amso N. Embryo freezing for preventing ovarian hyperstimulation syndrome. Cochrane Database Syst Rev. 2007 Jul 18;(3):CD002806.
13. Laines T, et al. Administration of methyl prednisolone to prevent severe ovarian hyperstimulation syndrome in patients undergoing *in vitro* fertilization. Fertil Steril. 2002;78:529-34.
14. Tso LO, Costello MF, Albuquerque LE, Andriolo RB, Freitas V. Metformin treatment before and during IVF or ICSI in women with polycystic ovary syndrome. Cochrane Database Syst Rev. 2009 Apr 15;(2):CD006105.
15. Youssef MA, van Wely M, Hassan MA, Al-Inany HG, Mochtar M, Khattab S, van der Veen F. Can dopamine agonists reduce the incidence and severity of OHSS in IVF/ICSI treatment cycles? A systematic review and meta-analysis. Hum Reprod Update. 2010;16(5):459-66.
16. Sherwal V, Malik S, Bhatia V. Effect of bromocriptine on the severity of ovarian hyperstimulation syndromeand outcome in high responders undergoing assisted reproduction. J Hum Reprod Sci. 2010; 3(2):85-90.

Chapter 16

Multifetal Pregnancy Reduction

Preeti Chauhan

The last century witnessed an explosion of science and technology and one of the greatest advancements has been that of assisted reproduction. Assisted reproductive technology (ART) has revolutionized infertility management over the last couple of decades. While it has been a boon to millions of childless couples, it also brought with it numerous difficulties and one of its major problems has been multiple or high order pregnancies as a result of the transfer of many embryos. According to the Center for Disease Control, 30% pregnancies that result from ART are multiple as opposed to 2% that occur spontaneously.[1] In the United States, this has increased the incidence of high order pregnancy (triplets and beyond) to over 44% over the period between 1980 and 1996.[2] The National ART Registry of India (NARI) also reports a steady increase in multiple pregnancies resulting from IVF cycles each year.[3] Such pregnancies bring with them their own attendant risks both for the mothers and for the children. This is further compounded by the fact that women are bearing these children at advanced ages as compared to women of the past where child birth was at a younger age. There is a higher risk of total pregnancy loss, preterm labor, pre-eclampsia, gestational diabetes and difficult labor. For the babies, there is increased fetal wastage; small for dates babies, and decreased survival during the first year of life. Most children require a long stay in neonatal intensive care unit. This is a major emotional and financial burden for the couple who have already spent a fortune in achieving the pregnancy and for poor resource countries like India who are already reeling under the burden of their overpopulation. To address these problems, multifetal pregnancy reduction (MFPR) was developed with the aim to improve the poor prognosis of pregnancies with three or more fetuses. Utilization of the procedure has increased dramatically as IVF has become commonplace, but the average starting number has decreased with the transfer of fewer embryos.

The first report of fetal reduction came in 1978 when it was carried out in a twin pregnancy with a genetic defect.[4] Technically, this was a selective reduction where the affected twin was targeted, but this formed the basis for attempting selective fetal abortion in normal fetuses in multiple gestation in an effort to increase the chances of survival of the remaining fetuses (principle of proportionality, i.e. "therapy to achieve the most good for the least harm").[5] Thus, Dumez and Oury in 1986,[6] described their experience of 15 women with starting number of embryos from 3 to 6 reduced to 1 or 2 by suction evacuation under ultrasonographic visualization. The success of this small series in reducing the risk of severe prematurity led the other investigators to explore it further. The first American report by Evans and coworkers in 1988[7] was followed by report from Berkowitz and coworkers (1988)[8] and later by Wapner and coworkers (1990).[9] The technique gradually evolved in the last century as we grouped to find the ideal method that would eliminate the risks completely. Success rates from fetal reduction improved as a function of increasing experience, better ultrasound and lower starting numbers. The largest database of the procedure and its variations appeared in 2000 reporting improved results due to increasing experience and 12% losses from 1995 to 2000.[10]

Several terms have been used to describe this procedure of reducing the number of fetuses in a multiple pregnancy. A consensus has been reached to use the term 'selective termination' for a procedure performed due to an abnormality in one fetus and 'MFPR' when the indication is solely fetal number without an apparent fetal defect.[11]

METHODS

Several methods of MFPR have been described over the years which are based on different combinations of three components: (i) the use of embryotoxic agent; (ii) the timing of procedure; and (iii) the route of approach. However, it is difficult to determine which one is a better option because prospective randomized studies or simultaneous comparisons among these variable methods are difficult to perform.[12] Depending upon the preferred route three different methods have been used: (i) transcervical aspiration; (ii) transabdominal reduction; and (iii) transvaginal fetal reduction.

Transcervical Aspiration

Transcervical aspiration was described by Domez et al.[13] It is performed early in pregnancy till 7–8 weeks gestation. Vagina is cleaned with povidone iodine solution and a suction cannula number 8 is introduced through the cervix after gentle cervical dilatation. The whole procedure is performed under transabdominal ultrasound guidance. The most easily accessible sac—usually the lowest sac is targeted. A 50 ml syringe is attached to the suction catheter and the contents of the sac are aspirated by building up manual suction through the syringe. This method is, however, no longer used since it was thought to be associated with an increased incidence of bleeding and fetal loss due to infection caused by introduction of bacteria from the cervix or due to cervical incompetence brought about by cervical dilatation.[14]

Transabdominal Reduction

As suggested by the name itself, in this procedure, the abdominal route is used for fetal reduction. The procedure is performed in an outpatient setting usually between 9 and 14 weeks of pregnancy and preferably between 11th and 12th postmenstrual week of gestation. This timing is ideal because the nuchal translucency can be measured and an early anatomic survey can be performed. Before starting the procedure, a detailed ultrasound examination is carried out to verify the number of viable fetuses, their crown rump length or fetal maturity and accessibility as well as their chorionicity and dizygotic or monozygotic nature. A broad-spectrum antibiotic is administered prior to the procedure. The maternal abdomen is cleaned and draped. A sterile cover is placed on the ultrasound transducer and sterile ultrasound gel is placed on the maternal abdomen. A 22-gauge needle is introduced under direct ultrasound guidance into the cardiac or pericardiac area of the most easily accessible fetus and an embryotoxic agent like potassium chloride (KCl) 2–3 mEq is injected into it and kept in place for 1 minute after the asystole to see that there is no resumption of the cardiac activity. The same procedure is repeated for other fetuses undergoing termination. Care should be taken so that the lowermost fetus near the cervix is not disturbed unless it is the selected fetus.

With the technique of color flow mapping or color Doppler, fetal demise can be confirmed immediately following the procedure and this greatly reduces the chances of a repeat procedure being required by the patient. The most important advantage of using color is easy identification of cardiac motion and its disappearance after injection KCl.[15]

A repeat scan is done 2 hours after the procedure to confirm asystole in the reduced fetuses and then again, it is done one week later. Patient can go home 4–6 hours after the procedure.

A variation of the procedure is to use 0.9% NaCl instead of KCl. Cardiac asystole in this case is due to combination of the injected solution as well as mechanical damage caused to the thorax by needle penetration.[16]

In certain cases of MFPR, where difficulty is encountered in reaching the thorax due to the fetal position as well as the location of membranes and placenta, an alternative approach may be the insertion of the needle to the fetal cranium and injection of KCl.[17]

Many centers prefer to use the transabdominal route as it allows selective fetal reduction to be performed, but it is technically more challenging and has a longer learning curve than transvaginal approach. It is also difficult to perform in obese patients, in presence of uterine fibroids and abdominal scarring.

Transvaginal Fetal Reduction

Transvaginal fetal reduction uses the vaginal route to access the fetuses. The optimum time to perform this procedure is around 7–9 weeks. Again a mapping ultrasound is done before the procedure is started. A dose of broad-spectrum antibiotic is administered intravenously and short general anesthesia is used for the procedure. Patient is placed in lithotomy position and vagina is cleaned with povidone iodine solution. The uterus is scanned, and the configuration and the position of each gestational sac relative to the uterine cavity and to each other is identified. An oocyte retrieval needle (18-gauge, 30 cm) is introduced through the puncture guide on the vaginal probe and is advanced through the lateral or posterior vaginal fornix and the uterine wall aligned with the biopsy needle guideline on the screen into the most easily accessible sac. The needle tip is introduced into the fetal thorax and 1–2 mEq of KCl is injected. This results in immediate asystole and needle is kept in position for 1 minute to confirm cessation of cardiac activity. The same procedure is repeated for other embryos to be reduced.

As described in transabdominal approach, 0.9% NaCl has also been used for injection.

Another reported method using the transvaginal approach has been the aspiration of embryonic contents. The initial procedure is exactly the same as above. Once the needle is positioned in the fetal echo, the fetal contents are aspirated using an aspirator or creating suction pressure with a 20–50 ml syringe. This procedure may be performed earlier in gestation than the injection of potassium chloride, from approximately 7 weeks gestation. Researchers found this method to have a significantly lower rate of total pregnancy loss with an overall loss rate of 6.7% prior to 24 weeks gestation. In a subset of 39 women with higher order gestational pregnancies ($\geq$4), significant improvement was seen with the reduction of initial quadruple (or higher) pregnancies with a loss rate of 2.6%.[18] Another support for the use of embryonic aspiration is the potential risk of toxicity from the potassium chloride on the remaining fetuses. The fetus may be pushed away from the needle during the injection procedure causing the potassium chloride to diffuse into the amniotic sac and perhaps to other sacs causing harm to other fetuses.[19]

A disadvantage of embryo aspiration can be that amniotic fluid aspiration may make it difficult to visualize embryonic heart activity throughout the procedure and may also favor trophoblastic detachment.[20]

In order to reduce the morbidity of the procedure, different techniques have been used by different workers[21] (Table 16.1). Iberico et al.[21] reported an early transvaginal intracardiac embryo puncture until asystole is verified without the injection of any substances as an effective and safe technique. The authors have reported a small series using transvaginal needling of the fetus till asystole was noted. The procedure was performed at 8.5 weeks gestation with no pregnancy loss and 55.5% delivering between 35 and 37 weeks of gestation.[22] In yet another recent report, KCl has been injected into the cranium rather than the thorax.[23] In the absence of a meta-analysis on the ideal method for MFPR, an elaborately designed study was carried out to understand which method gives best results.[12] The patients were divided into early and late KCl and non-KCl groups. It was found that least morbidity was present in the early non-KCl group.

The advantages of transvaginal reduction are higher resolution, better visualization, shorter needle path and the ability to direct the needle more precisely, thereby reducing the risk of injury to adjacent gestational sacs or pelvic organs.

Reproductive physicians are more comfortable with transvaginal MFPR because the procedure is similar to ovum aspiration under transvaginal ultrasonographic guidance. Thus, transvaginal MFPR requires fewer technical considerations than transabdominal MFPR.[12]

Some of the disadvantages of using transvaginal route may be the possibility of spontaneous fetal reduction at this

Table 16.1

Gestational age at procedure and miscarriage rate of the different techniques—a literature review[21]

Reference	Technique	No of patients	Gestational age (weeks)	Miscarriage rate (%)
Shalev et al. (1989)	Abd + KCl	10	10–13	40.0
Evans et al. (1994)	Abd + KCl	846	11.3	16.2
Sebire et al. (1997)	Abd + KCl	127	7–13	12.6
Antsaklis et al. (1999)	Abd + KCl	158	9–11	10.6
Dechaud et al. (1998)	Abd	2145	—	16.7
Salat-Baroux et al. (1988)	C + As	42	7–12	12.0
Bollen et al. (1993)	C + As	14	8–9	21.4
Dechaud et al. (1998)	C	363	—	24.8
Evans et al. (1994)	V and C	238	9.3	13.1
Shalev et al. (1989)	V + KCl	10	8–11	10.0
Mansour et al. (1999)	V + KCl	30	7.2	30.0
Yovel et al. (1992)	V + NaCl	16	8–10	10.0
Itskovitz-Eldor et al. (1992)	V + As	19	7–8	5.3
Coffler et al. (1999)	V + As	90	7.5	6.7
Timor-Tritsch et al. (1993)	V	148	8–10	12.0
Dechaud et al. (1998)	V	248	—	10.9
Mansour et al. (1999)	V + As	45	7.2	8.8
Present study	V + Pu	149	7.8	7.3

(Abbreviations: Abd—transabdominal technique; As—aspiration; C—transcervical technique; KCl—potassium chloride; NaCl—sodium chloride; Pu—intracardiac embryo puncture; V—transvaginal technique)

stage of gestation, the inability to perform first trimester fetal screening to identify a structural or chromosomal abnormality and the possibility of increasing infections.

When considering which fetuses to reduce, some physicians recommend selecting the fetuses according to the accessibility of the gestational sacs, while others prefer selecting based on the size of sac or smallest crown to rump length (CRL) or on basis of chromosomal analysis by chorionic villus sampling.[24] One study describes the preference for fetuses with fundal implantations on separate sides of the uterus to prevent competition and low implantation, thereby increasing the chance of positive pregnancy outcomes.[25]

Optimal timing of embryo reduction remains controversial. There have been studies that suggest that fetal reduction should be delayed until the late first trimester based on the expectation of a natural reduction of fetus and detection of structural and chromosomal anomalies,[26,27] but the proponents of early reduction argue that early reduction is easier to perform and is more acceptable to the patients from a psychological point of view, also there is a lesser burden of reduced fetuses left in the body.[18]

There are also concerns whether embryotoxic agents should be used or not. Potassium chloride is widely used for embryo reduction, but the safety and efficacy of this agent are debatable. Cases of anencephaly[28] and limb amputation[29] have been reported, and total pregnancy loss may result if the KCl solution accidentally reaches the amniotic fluid of remaining fetuses.[30] It has been suggested that the development of an inflammatory response to the resorbing dead fetoplacental tissue with subsequent release of cytokines and stimulation of prostaglandins is a cause of pregnancy loss, preterm delivery and other complications following MFPR.[31-33] The use of KCl for embryo reduction may cause or aggravate the inflammatory process and induce premature rupture of membranes and preterm birth. Several reports have demonstrated that preterm premature rupture of membranes is associated with matrix degrading enzymes such as plasminogen activators (PAs) and matrix metalloproteinases (MMPs).[34-36] Moreover, in animal studies, investigators found that KCl can induce a release of tissue plasminogen activator in the hypothalamo-neurohypophysial system[37] and an upregulation in MMP-9 activity in the retina, which promote retinal damage.[38] Although no study has been conducted on the roles of KCl in relation to matrix degrading enzyme activity in the intrauterine system, Jung et al.[12] hypothesize that KCl can cause preterm premature rupture of membranes by inducing matrix degrading enzymes in the uterus after MFPR. KCl has also been reported as a possible risk factor for periventricular leukomalacia in premature newborns.[33]

There is some debate about the number of fetuses to be reduced. Although everyone agrees to the benefits achieved by reducing quadruplets and higher order pregnancies, there is some controversy over reducing triplets to twins or singletons and even whether twins should be reduced to singleton pregnancy. A collaborative study by Evans et al. in 1996[39] reaffirmed that gestational age at delivery is inversely related to either the initial number of fetuses or the final number of fetuses remaining after reduction. The typical duration of pregnancy in case of twins is 36 weeks, in triplets 33 weeks, in quadruplets 29 weeks and in quintuplets 24 weeks.[40] The 2001 collaborative data demonstrated that the outcome of triplets reduced to twins and quadruplets reduced to twins now perform essentially as if they started as twins.[41] Yaron et al.[42] compared triplets reduced to twins data to unreduced triplets with two large cohorts of twins. The data show substantial improvement of reduced twins as compared to triplets. In their study, the observed pregnancy loss was 25% for nonreduced triplets and 6.2% for triplets reduced to twins. The severe prematurity rate was 25% in nonreduced triplets and 4.9% in triplets reduced to twins, and the birth weight for nonreduced triplets was 1636 +/- 645, while it was 2381 +/- 602 for triplets reduced to twins. Antsaklis et al.[43] showed a reduction of losses from 15.41 to 4.76% for twins and diminishment of low birth weight from 28 to 11%. Blickstein[44] has reported that triplets do worse than reduced twins in every perinatal category in his large database.

Yet, due to the relatively high chance of successful outcome with careful management and cesarean delivery, some physicians do not recommend reducing triplet pregnancies.[45]

Reduction to a single fetus is controversial and it has been noticed that this type of reduction is usually requested by elderly couples, whose reasons are probably of a psychological and or financial nature.[21,46] Almost all the authors agree that nonselective reduction to a single fetus is not justified, though one might consider exceptions for medical reasons like bicornuate uterus, prior premature delivery of less than 30 weeks or monoamniotic twins in triplets.[47] Because studies have shown that even twin pregnancy poses higher risks to both the mother and fetus than a singleton pregnancy, some physicians recommend fetal reduction to a singleton fetus.[48] This is a debate which is going to intensify in the coming times as more and more elderly women conceive. An ever increasing situation involves the inclusion of a monoamniotic pair of twins in a higher order multiple pregnancy.[49] Provided the "singleton" seems healthy, the best outcomes are achieved by reduction of then monoamniotic twins. Obviously if the singleton is not healthy, then keeping the twins is the next choice.[50]

Even though it seems that the inherent tendency for early delivery of a high order pregnancy is not completely eliminated by reducing the total number of fetuses in that pregnancy; nonetheless the rate of very dangerous early prematurity is significantly reduced.

COMPLICATIONS OF PREGNANCY REDUCTION

The procedure of MFPR is recommended to reduce the burden of pregnancy loss and complications, but it is a paradox that the procedure itself may lead to similar situations. One of the major complications after reduction is miscarriage or loss of all remaining fetuses. A collaborative report by Evans et al. in 1996 estimated that following MFPR, the overall pregnancy loss rate before 24 weeks is 11.7% and the early premature delivery rate between 25 and 28 weeks is 4.5%. The reported pregnancy loss rate was 7.6% when the initial number of embryos was three and increased to 15.3% with quadruplets and higher order multiple gestation. In the study by Coffer et al., the rate of pregnancy loss after transvaginal aspiration for triplets was 6.7% before 24 weeks and that for higher order multiple pregnancies was just 2.6%. Most of the pregnancy losses occur 4–10 weeks after the procedure. The most common causes for pregnancy loss are chorioamnionitis, premature rupture of membranes, uterine contractions and bleeding.

Occasionally, severe bleeding may occur while carrying out the procedure[51] due to which an incomplete procedure may have to be prematurely abandoned leading to the birth of a physically handicapped child.

Another complication that is often overlooked is its psychological impact on the patient. The studies that have been done suggest that patients experience feelings of grief and bereavement after the reduction. The birth of healthy children helps reduce the traumatic impact of fetal reduction but parents often feel guilty as they contemplate the babies they have, and think about the one, or ones, they reduced.[52]

ETHICAL ISSUES

According to Evans et al. 1988, MFPR is ethically controversial for several reasons: the procedure is a direct termination of a fetus, which is more objectionable than an abortion; some may see it as a precedent to euthanasia and, because the safety and efficacy of the procedure, has gradually improved, there is the increased risk that it may be employed casually.

The committee on Ethics of the American College of Obstetrics and Gynecology (ACOG) in its 2007[53] opinion on MFPR states that there is a complex interrelationship between the intention to reduce the morbidity of a smaller number of surviving fetuses and the intentional sacrifice of others that demands an ethical as well as a medical assessment of the relative benefits and risks of MFPR. It recognized that "counseling should be an ongoing process, beginning before treatment decisions are made and continuing throughout the patients care". The committee implies that before starting infertility treatment, the patient should clearly understand not only that multiple pregnancy can result but also the various risks of multiple pregnancy including the possibility of a recommendation for selective reduction. At the time of counseling for MFPR, the patient must be given clear information regarding procedural risks, adverse outcomes and complications.

To conclude, the association of an increased rate of multifetal pregnancies with infertility treatment deserves serious attention. Some multifetal pregnancies will inevitably occur despite the best of intentions, knowledge, skill and equipment, but it is essential that those providing infertility treatment exercise a high degree of diligence to minimize the problem (ACOG).

MFPR has been described as a medical solution to an iatrogenic problem.[54] Our ultimate goal should be to reduce the occurrence of multiple pregnancies. With single embryo transfer becoming the norm in many countries, MFPR will soon become rare. However, selective fetal reduction may still need to be carried out for monozygotic twins and other such situations. It is also possible that women may want only one child and ask for a reduction of a twin to a singleton.

REFERENCES

1. CDC 1997 ART success rates. National Summary and Fertility Clinic Reports, 1999.
2. Latest birth statistics for the nation released. News Release, 1998.
3. National ART Registry of India (NARI), 2004-2006.
4. Aberg A, Mitelman F, Cantz M, et al. Cardiac puncture of fetus with Hurler's disease avoiding abortion of unaffected co-twin. Lancet. 1978;2:990-1.
5. Strauss A, Paek BW, Genzel-Boroviczeny O, et al. Multifetal gestation–maternal and perinatal outcome in 112 pregnancies. Fetal Diagn Ther. 2002;17:209-17.
6. Gwyer B, MacDorman M, Marrtin J, et al. Annual summary of vital statistics–1998. Pediatrics. 1998;102:1333-49.
7. Evans MI, Fletcher JC, Zador IE, et al. Selective first trimester termination in octuplet and quadruplet pregnancies: clinical and ethical issues. Obstet Gynecol. 1988;71:289-96.
8. Berkowitz RL, Lynch L, Chitkara U, et al. Selective reduction of multiple pregnancies in the first trimester. N Engl J Med. 1988;318:1043-7.
9. Wapner RJ, Davis GH, Johnson A. Selective reduction of multifetal pregnancies. Lancet. 1990;335:90-3.

10. Evans MI, Berkowitz RI, Waapner RJ, et al. Improvement in outcomes of multifetal pregnancy reduction with increased experience. Am J Obstet Gynecol. 2001;184(2):97-110.
11. Multifetal pregnancy reduction and selective fetal termination. ACOG committee opinion: Committee on Ethics Number 94-April 1991. Int J Gynaecol Obstet. 1992;38:140-2.
12. Lee JR, Ku SY, Jee BC, et al. Pregnancy outcomes of different methods for multifetal pregnancy reduction: a comparative study. J Korean Med Sci. 2008;23(1):111-6.
13. Dumez Y, Oury JF. Method for first trimester selective abortion in multiple pregnancy. Contrib Gynecol Obstet. 1986;15:50-3.
14. Dommergues M, Nisand I, Mandelbrot L, et al. Embryo reduction in multifetal pregnancies after infertility therapy: obstetrical risks and perinatal benefits are related to operative strategy. Fertil Steril. 1991;55:805-11.
15. Desai SK, Allahbadia GN, Dalal AK. Selective reduction of multifetal pregnancies in the first trimester using colour Doppler ultrasonography. Hum Reprod. 1993;8(4):642-4.
16. Yovel I, Yaron Y, Amit A, et al. Embryo reduction in multifetal pregnancies using saline injection: comparison between the transvaginal and transabdominal approach. Hum Reprod. 1992;7:1173-5.
17. Lembet A, Selam B, Bodur H, et al. Intracranial injection with KCl: an alternative method in selected cases of multifetal pregnancy reduction. Fetal Diagn Ther. 2009;26(3):134-6.
18. Coffler MS, Kol S, Drugan A, et al. Early transvaginal embryo aspiration: a safer method for selective reduction in high order multiple gestations. Hum Reprod. 1999;14:1875-8.
19. Mansour RT, Aboulghar MA, Serour GI, et al. Multifetal pregnancy reduction: modification of the technique and analysis of the outcome. Fertil Steril. 1999;71(2):380-4.
20. Vauthier-Brouzes D, Lefebvre G. Selective reduction in multifetal pregnancies: technical and psychological aspects. Fertil Steril. 1992;57:1012-6.
21. Iberico G, Navarro J, Blasco L, et al. Embryo reduction of multifetal pregnancies following assisted reproduction: a modification of the transvaginal ultrasound-guided technique. Hum Reprod. 2000;15(10):2228-33.

22. Malik S, Sharma R Pregnancy outcome following transvaginal needling of fetal heart under USG guidance, retrospective analysis of 18 cases. International Journal Obstet Gynecol (India). 2008;12(6).
23. Lembet A, Selam B, Bodur H, et al. Intracranial injection with KCl: an alternative method in selected cases of multifetal pregnancy reduction. Fetal Diagn Ther. 2009;26(3):134-6.
24. Brambati B, Tului L, Baldi M, et al. Genetic analysis prior to selective termination in multiple pregnancy: technical aspects and clinical outcome. Hum Reprod. 1995;10:818-25.
25. Evans MI, Fletcher JC, Zador IE, et al. Selective first trimester termination in octuplet and quadruplet pregnancies: clinical and ethical issues. Obstet Gynecol. 1988;71:289-96.
26. Lipitz S, Shulman A, Achiron R, et al. A comparative study of multifetal pregnancy reduction from triplets to twins in the first versus early second trimesters after detailed fetal screening. Ultrasound Obstet Gynecol. 2001;18(1):35-8.
27. Dickey RP, Taylor SN, Lu PY, et al. Spontaneous reduction of multiple pregnancy: incidence and effect on outcome. Am J Obstet Gynecol. 2002;186(1):77-83.
28. Boulot P, Pelliccia G, Molenat F. Pronostic obstetrical des grossesses multiples. Contracept. Fertil Sex (Paris). 1992;20:315-30.
29. Roze RJ, Tschupp MJ, Arvis PH, et al. Selective interruption of pregnancy and embryonic malformations of the limbs. J Gynecol Obstet Bioreprod (Paris). 1989;18:673-7.
30. Tabash KM. Transabdominal multifetal pregnancy reduction-report of 40 cases. Obstet Gynecol. 1990;75:739-41.
31. Sebire NJ, Sherod C, Abbas A, et al. Preterm delivery and growth restriction in multifetal pregnancies reduced to twins. Hum Reprod. 1997;12(1):173-5.
32. Silver RK, Helfand BT, Russell TL, et al. Multifetal reduction increases the risk of preterm delivery and fetal growth restriction in twins: a case-control study. Fertil Steril. 1997;67(1):30-3.
33. Geva E, Lerner-Geva L, Stavorovsky Z, et al. Multifetal pregnancy reduction: a possible risk factor for periventricular leukomalacia in premature newborns. Fertil Steril. 1998;69(5): 845-50.

34. Liu YX, Hu ZY, Liu K, et al. Localization and distribution of tissue type and urokinase type plasminogen activators and their inhibitors type 1 and 2 in human and rhesus monkey fetal membranes. Placenta.1998;19:171-80.
35. Maymon E, Romero R, Pacora P, et al. Evidence for the participation of interstitial collagenase (matrix metalloproteinase 1) in preterm premature rupture of membranes. Am J Obstet Gynecol. 2000;183(4):914-20.
36. Athayde N, Edwin SS, Romero R, et al. A role for matrix metalloproteinase-9 in spontaneous rupture of the fetal membranes. Am J Obstet Gynecol. 1998;179(5):1248-53.
37. Miyata S, Nakatani Y, Hayashi N, et al. Matrix-degrading enzymes tissue plasminogen activator and matrix metalloprotease-3 in the hypothalamo-neurohypophysial system. Brain Res. 2005;1058:1-9.
38. Mali RS, Cheng M, Chintala SK. Intravitreous injection of a membrane depolarization agent causes retinal degeneration via matrix metalloproteinase-9. Invest Ophthalmol Vis Sci. 2005;46(6):2125-32.
39. Evans MI, Dommergues M, Wapner R, et al. International collaborative experience of 1789 patients having multifetal pregnancy reduction: a plateauing of risks and outcome. J Soc Gynecol Invest. 1996;3:23-6.
40. Taden I, Roje D, Banovic I, et al. Fetal reduction in multifetal pregnancy-Ethical Dilemmas. Yonsei Med J. 2002;43(2):252-8.
41. Evans MI, Berkowitz R, Wapner R, et al. Multifetal pregnancy reduction: improved outcomes with increased experience. Am J Obstet Gynecol. 2001;184:97-103.
42. Yaron Y, Bryant PK, Dave N, et al. Multifetal pregnancy reductions of triplets to twins: comparison with nonreduced triplets and twins. Am J Obstet Gynecol. 1999;180:1268-71.
43. Antsaklis A, Souka AP, Daskalakis G, et al. Embryo reduction versus expectant management for twin pregnancies. J Matern Fetal Neonatal Med. 2004;16:219-22.
44. Blickstein I. How and why are triplets disadvantaged compared to twins. Best Pract Res Clin Obstet Gynecol. 2004;18:631-44.

45. Lipitz S, Reichman B, Paret G, et al. The improving outcome of triplet pregnancies. Am J Obstet Gynecol. 1989;161:1279-84.
46. Evans MI, Hume RF, Polak S, et al. The geriatric gravida: multifetal pregnancy reduction, donor eggs and infertility treatments. Am J Obstet Gynecol. 1997;177:875-8.
47. Lipitz S, Reichman B, Uval J, et al. A prospective comparison of the outcome of triplet pregnancies managed conservatively or by multifetal reduction to twins. Am J Obstet Gynecol. 1994;170:874-9.
48. Kiely JL, Kleinman JC, Kiely M. Triplets and higher-order multiple births. Am J Dis in Child. 1992;146:862-8.
49. Yakin K, Kahraman S, Comert S. Three blastocyst stage embryo transfer resulting in a quintuplet pregnancy. Hum Reprod. 2001;16(4):782-4.
50. Evans M, Britt D. Multifetal pregnancy reduction. Glob Libr Women's Med. (ISSN: 1756-2228) 2009; DOI 10.3843/GLOWM.10214.
51. Malik S, Kumar N. Live birth after selective multifetal pregnancy reduction–a case report. Poster, ASRM 1998.
52. McKinney M, Downey J, Timor-Tritsch I. The psychological effects of multifetal pregnancy reduction. Fertil Steril. 1995;64(1):51-61.
53. Multifetal pregnancy reduction. ACOG Committee opinion No 369. American College of Obstetricians and Gynecologists. Obstet Gynecol. 2007;109:1511-5.
54. Maymon R, Herman A, Shulman A, et al. First trimester embryo reduction: a medical solution to an iatrogenic problem. Hum Reprod. 1995;10(3):668-73.

Chapter 17

Ultrasound Assessment of Endometrial Receptivity and Oocyte and Embryo Quality

Ashok Khurana

The endometrium is a uniquely specialized organ which undergoes cyclical changes that are critical in menstruation, embryo implantation and pregnancy. Fertilization triggers embryonic development and ovulation sparks off endometrial differentiation. The latter is consequential to corpus luteum progesterone production. These two synchronous processes coordinate about 1 week after their occurrence to optimize the implantation of the blastocyst into an optimally receptive endometrium.[1]

PHYSIOLOGICAL AND BIOCHEMICAL BASIS OF IMPLANTATION

Implantation is a phenomenon that involves a cascade of events between the embryo and maternal endometrium.[2] In a menstrual cycle, there is a brief and specific time period in which the maternal-embryonic interaction is optimal and culminates with adhesion and invasion of the blastocyst into the progesterone-induced secretory endometrium. This period is referred to as the "nidation window" or "implantation window." The implantation window is characterized by changes in endometrial epithelial morphology marked by the appearance of membrane projections called pinopodes. Pinopodes are progesterone-dependent organelles that look like apical cellular protrusions appearing between days 20 and 21 of a 28-day natural menstrual cycle.

Implantation in humans is a complex process that involves embryo apposition and attachment to the maternal endometrial epithelium, traversing adjacent cells of the epithelial lining, and invasion into the endometrial stroma.[3] Implantation of the blastocyst in endometrium requires establishment of a coordinated molecular dialog between the embryo and the endometrium. Biological molecules that bring about preparation of a receptive endometrium arise from the hypothalamic-pituitary-gonadal axis. These molecules modulate gene expression that drives the endometrium through sequential changes in each menstrual cycle. During each cycle, a series of synchronized, architectural, morphological, cytochemical and molecular changes ultimately lead to the preparation of a receptive endometrium during the putative "receptive period" or "implantation window." It is during this critical period that a well-orchestrated dialog is established between an implanting blastocyst and a receptive endometrium. If, for any reason, this dialog is not established or is perturbed, the embryo is aborted. In the absence of implantation, a second set of changes commences that ultimately leads to menstruation. These processes involve a variety of molecules, which are not unique in themselves, but play unique roles in the process of implantation. The molecular dialog that occurs between the implanting conceptus and the endometrium involves cell-cell and cell-extracellular matrix interactions, mediated by lectins, integrins, matrix degrading enzymes and their inhibitors, prostaglandins, and a variety of growth factors, cytokines, and angiogenic peptides, their receptors and modulatory proteins.[3] It is likely that each of these, when appropriately expressed or inhibited, contributes to endometrial receptivity or nonreceptivity to an implanting conceptus.

Currently, a scientific understanding of a receptive versus a nonreceptive endometrium is incomplete. Consequently, there is no single definitive investigative marker for the adequacy of an endometrium for implantation. Receptivity is being evaluated by a large variety of parameters with varying sensitivity and specificity. These include serum biochemical markers which reflect molecules that are induced or are present in a receptive endometrium; assessments using tissue samples for conventional microscopy, histochemistry and scanning electron microscopy, and, of late, newer ultrasound imaging techniques. This chapter evaluates the assessment of endometrial receptivity using ultrasound imaging.

LESSONS FROM IVF AND OVUM DONATION CYCLES

Until recently it was believed that implantation is consequent to good embryo quality. This is certainly true. What has been realized additionally, though, is that the quality of the endometrium is equally significant.[4]

Uterine receptivity is diminished in *in vitro* fertilization (IVF) cycles because of high estradiol (E2) levels,[5] and altered estradiol/progesterone ratios.[6] These high levels result from the use of ovulation inducing agents, which are used to recruit more oocytes. Histological studies,[7] electron microscopy[8] and biochemistry of endometrial fluid[9] confirm this finding. E2 levels of greater than 3000 pg/ml on the day of hCG administration, regardless of the number of oocytes and serum progesterone level are detrimental to uterine receptivity without affecting embryo quality.[10] Pregnancy and implantation rate in recipients of embryos derived from high responders (greater than 15 follicles) are similar to normal responders.

Ovum donation is a program in which patients receive oocytes donated by young women. As a consequence, ovum recipients are not stimulated with gonadotropins, and the endometrial factor is better that in IVF patients.[11,12] Implantation can be improved by optimizing the time of embryo transfer (ET) taking into consideration the individualized period of apparition, development and regression of pinopodes detected by scanning electronic microscopy.[13] The objective is to achieve a better individual synchronization between embryo and endometrium at the moment of ET in order to enhance implantation rate. Precocious luteal transformation and endometrial advancement observed in IVF cycles has a deleterious effect on implantation.[14]

Since endometrial evaluation for morphology, pinopodes, beta integrins and various biochemical factors involves an invasive procedure; however minor, there has been an earnest endeavor to find ultrasound markers of appropriate and impaired endometrial receptivity in order to enhance pregnancy and take-home baby rate. The noninvasive nature of ultrasound places it in a unique position to take on the challenge of assessing methods that enhance reproductive outcomes in assisted reproductive technology (ART) patients. Along with methods that enhance embryo quality, ultrasound evaluation of uterine receptivity constitutes an important step towards meeting the challenge of statistically better results in this new millennium.[15]

GRAY SCALE, POWER DOPPLER AND 3D ULTRASOUND

Currently available ultrasound techniques of evaluation for endometrial receptivity include gray-scale sonography using high frequency transvaginal scans, conventional color Doppler studies, power Doppler, three-dimensional (3D) and real time three-dimensional (4D) studies and tomographic ultrasound imaging.

The parameters that have been studied over the past two decades, more so, the last four years, include endometrial thickness, endometrial volume, endometrial ultrasound morphology, subendometrial peristalsis, endometrial and subendometrial vascularization, myometrial echogenicity, myometrial power Doppler, spectral analysis of uterine artery flow velocity waveforms and perifollicular vascularization.

Endometrial thickness below 6 to 8 mm (Fig. 17.1) is rarely associated with conception.[16-19] Increase in endometrial thickness above this level, however, does not enhance implantation rates, and there is no difference in

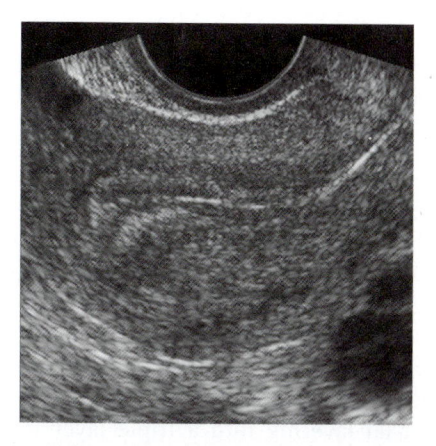

Fig. 17.1: Proliferative phase endometrium which has achieved a thickness of only 7 mm at the time of follicular maturation. Endometrial thickness is measured in the region of maximum anteroposterior extent in the subfundal area and should include the anterior and posterior layer. Such an endometrial thickness is almost never receptive to implantation

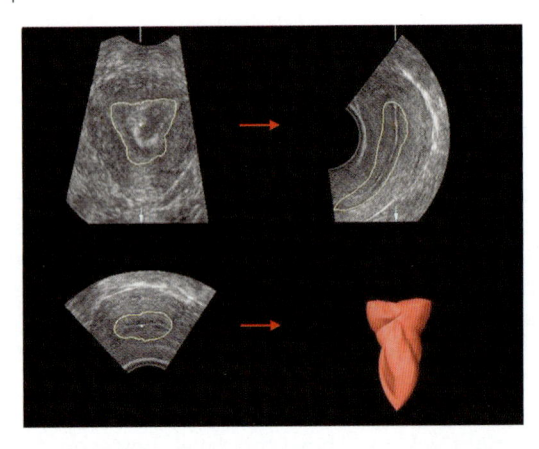

Fig. 17.2: 3D volume measurement of the endometrium. Using branded software called VOCAL, outline of the endometrium is traced through an acquired volume. The machine automatically calculates endometrial volume and displays it as shown in the bottom right hand picture. The other three frames show an orthogonal multiplanar display of the endometrium. The minimum volume associated with implantation is 1.59 ml

the mean endometrial thickness in patients who become pregnant and those who do not become pregnant in ART cycles.[20] The minimum endometrial volume (Fig. 17.2) associated with pregnancy is 1.59 ml as calculated by three-dimensional ultrasound.[18] This is calculated using a manual or semi-automated planimetry and automated software called virtual organ computer aided analysis (VOCAL).

Endometrial layering into a triple layer is associated with good implantation rates (Fig. 17.3). Conversely, a homogeneous or a heterogeneous (Fig. 17.4) endometrium in the proliferative and midcycle phases is associated with poor outcomes.[16,18] Premature echogenic transformation of the endometrium (Fig. 17.5), a consequence of progesterone action, if observed on the day of hCG administration

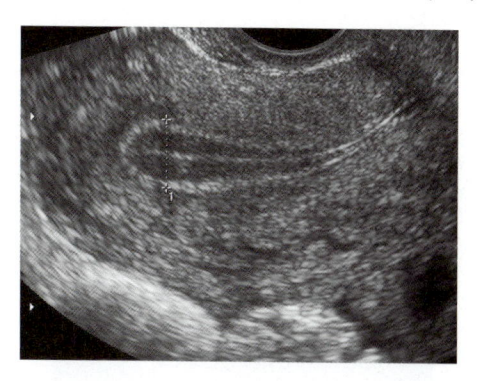

Ultrasound Assessment of Endometrial Receptivity | **425**

Fig. 17.3: Triple layered endometrium 10–11 mm thick. Note the hypoechoic anterior and posterior layer between the echogenic lines of triple layer. This shows no speckling and such an endometrium is highly conducive to implantation during the nidation window

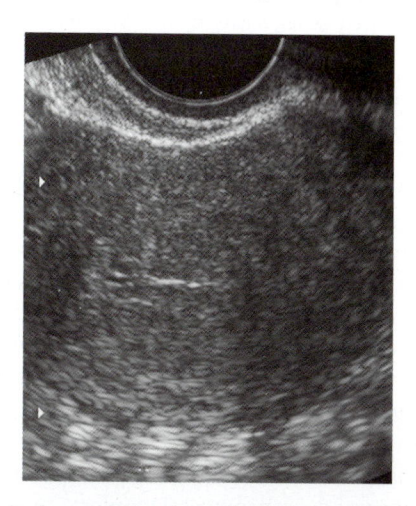

Fig. 17.4: A homogeneously echogenic endometrium or a heterogeneous echogenicity of the endometrium in a proliferative phase of the cycle reflects a disordered hormonal milieu or an endometritis, and is associated with a poor reproductive outcome consequent through failure of implantation

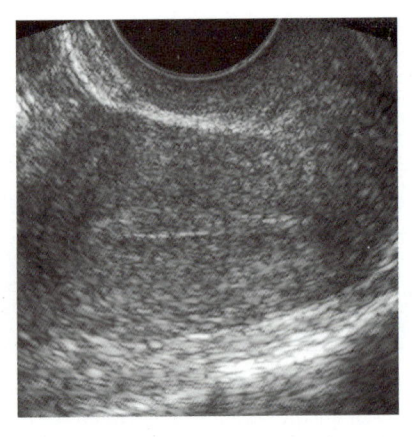

Fig. 17.5: Increased progesterone subsequent to an LH surge results in intracellular changes in the endometrium. On ultrasound, this is seen as increased echogenicity of the endometrium. Premature echogenic transformation of the endometrium is associated with poor implantation rate. It is termed premature if it is observed on the day of hCG administration or the day of ovum pick-up

or on the day of ovum pick-up is associated with poor implantation rates.[14]

Less than three peristaltic contractions of the subendometrial myometrium over a 2 minutes interval on the day of hCG administration are associated with poor implantation rates.[17] An inhomogeneous, poorly vascular myometrium is usually associated with poor implantation although the statistical significance of this preliminary observation needs further proof.[17]

By far the best correlation with implantation rates are being observed with power Doppler[17] and 3D power Doppler studies (Fig. 17.6).[21-23] Ultrasound delineation and quantification of endometrial and subendometrial angiogenesis is emerging as a reliable and reproducible

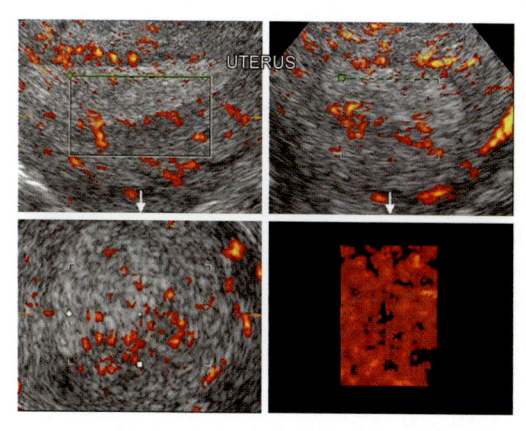

Fig. 17.6: Proliferation of spiral arteries and their subsequent growth into the endometrium is reflected as morphologic and quantitative increase in endometrial vascularity when imaged by power Doppler. This is seen in the late proliferative and periovulatory phases. The deeper the vascularization into endometrium, better the endometrial receptivity. 3D multiplanar studies with appropriate rendering afford an accurate delineation and quantification of angiogenesis in the endometrium. The illustration shows endometrial neovascularization in the longitudinal, axial and coronal planes along with the morphological rendering of endometrial vessels

indicator of endometrial receptivity.[24,25] Basic static 3D and VOCAL, and 3D shell imaging have been used to assess and quantify endometrial and subendometrial vascularization.[21-23] The vascularization index (VI), flow index (FI) and vascularization flow index (VFI) of endometrial and subendometrial vessels increases during the proliferative phase, peaks 3 days prior to ovulation and decreases to a nadir 5 days post-ovulation.[23] VI is the ratio of color voxels to the total number of voxels inside the volume of interest and reflects the number of vessels in the volume being studied.

FI is the ratio of the sum of color intensities to the number of color voxels inside the volume being interrogated. It reflects the amount of blood flow. VFI is the ratio of the sum of color intensities to the total number of voxels inside the volume of interest. This reflects vessel presence and blood flow. Endometrial and subendometrial VI/FI/VFI is significantly lower in stimulated cycles than in natural cycles.[22] Smoking is associated with significantly lower VI and VFI. Patients who become pregnant have a significantly lower resistive index (RI) of subendometrial vessels: 0.53 compared to 0.64 +/- 0.04 in pregnant and nonpregnant patients respectively.[21] Nondetectable subendometrial artery flow (Fig. 17.7) is not associated with a lower implantation rate.[18]

Uterine artery flow velocity waveforms show a remarkably good correlation with endometrial receptivity and

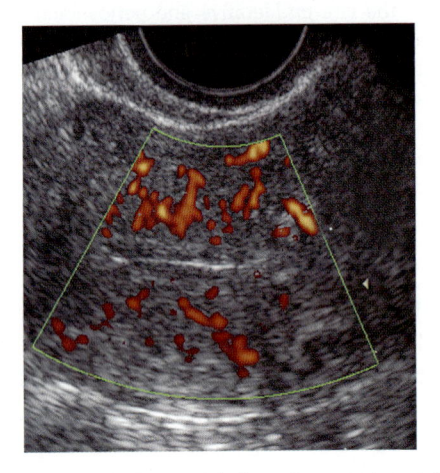

Fig. 17.7: When subendometrial flow is not detectable in the proliferative phase, this does not imply a lower implantation rate. Intraendometrial vascularization can proceed rapidly even after hCG administration. This endometrium shows absent intraendometrial and subendometrial flow

implantation rates. These should be recorded and measured from the segments of artery near the cornual aspect of the uterus. This downstream location compared to upstream location of the same artery near the cervix is a logically better reflector of cyclical uterine neovascularization. The assessment of uterine artery flow is easily accomplished and is also easily reproducible. Pregnant patients show considerably lower RI and pulsatility index (PI) values compared with the nonpregnant group, 5 to 6 days after ET.[20] The chance for pregnancy is almost zero if the PI is more than 3.019 (Fig. 17.8) on the day of hCG administration.

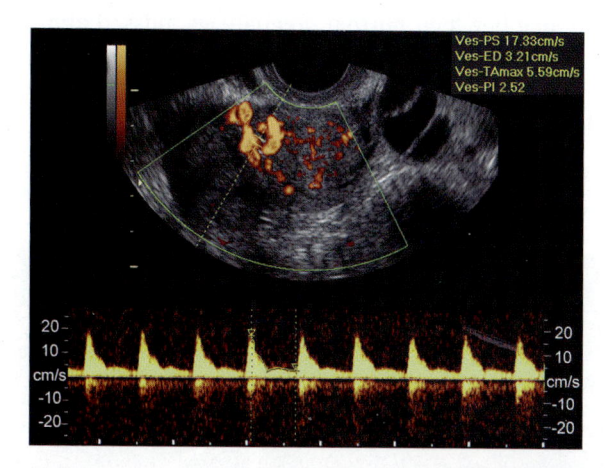

Fig. 17.8: In the late proliferative phase of cycle and particularly by the time of LH trigger, extensive myometrial and endometrial vascularization result in a lowered impedance flow through the uterine arteries. The quantification of flow should be done in the cornual areas of the uterus and signals should be obtained from the terminal portions of the uterine artery after it has given off the tubal branch and turned medially. This lowered impedance persists for 5–6 days after embryo transfer. A PI of greater than 3.019 is almost never associated with successful implantation

Inner zone vascularization (Figs 17.9A and B) of the endometrium observed on the day of hCG administration or on the day of ET is associated with higher pregnancy rates. This can be assessed subjectively by direct observation, but may be more objectively evaluated by quantification. Quantification can be done using the power Doppler area technique, which measures the vascularized area in any one endometrial plane or with VOCAL which involves a 3D acquisition followed by semi-automated planimetry. Pre-retrieval hCG does not enhance endometrial PI although more embryos are generated.[26] Interestingly, impedance in the uterine and spiral arteries does not show any significant difference between normal pregnancies, missed abortions and anembryonic pregnancies.[27]

OOCYTE AND EMBRYO QUALITY

Ovarian antral follicle number, ovarian volume (Fig. 17.10), and ovarian stromal blood flow 3D quantification (Fig. 17.11)

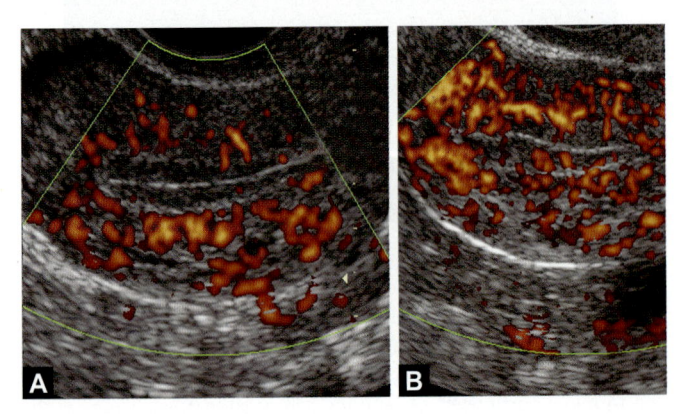

Figs 17.9A and B: (A) Vascularization into the mid-zone of the endometrium; (B) Extensive endometrial vascularization upto the cavity

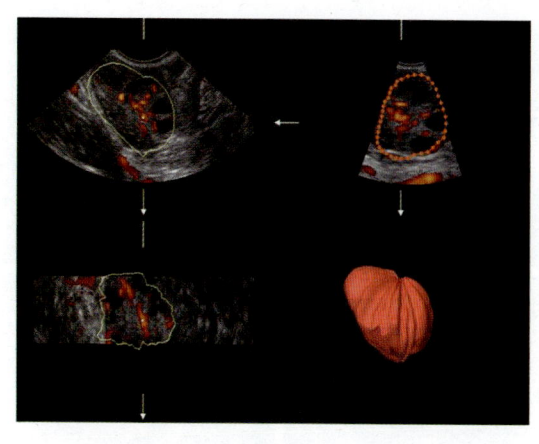

Ultrasound Assessment of Endometrial Receptivity | **431**

Fig. 17.10: Ovarian volume using 3D acquisition techniques and 3D quantification software is more accurate than 2D methods. However, volumes correlate well with embryo quality and fertilization rate, but not with endometrial receptivity

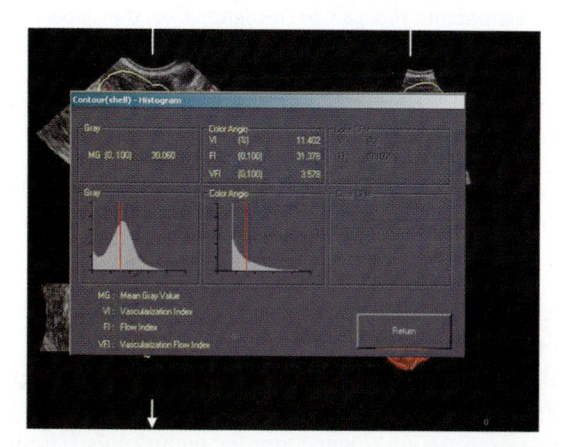

Fig. 17.11: Grey scale and power Doppler acquisition of ovarian morphological data, and stromal blood flow can be quantified using 3D software. Stromal blood flow correlates well with oocyte yield and embryo quality, but not with implantation rate

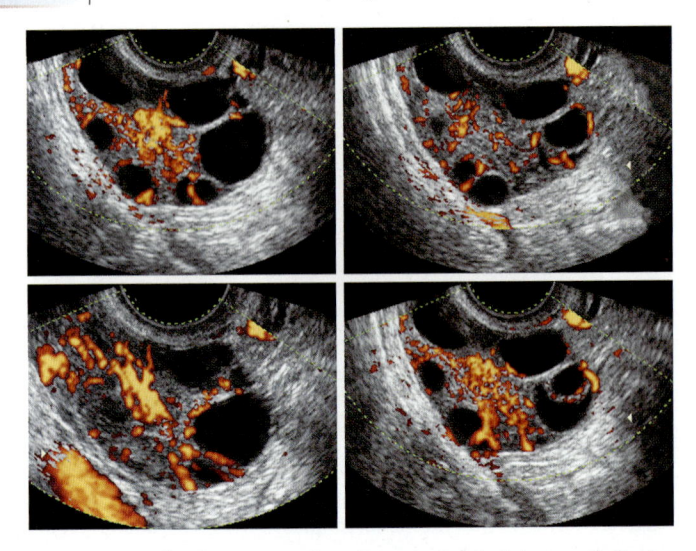

Fig. 17.12: Follicular maturation is accompanied by perifollicular neovascularization. This can be recognized by the appearance of occasional perifollicular vascular signals when the follicle reaches 12–14 mm in size, which then progress to 50–100% of perifollicular vascularization as the cycle progresses. This phenomenon correlates well with parameters of oocyte quality, such as the level of follicular fluid E2, pH, follicular fluid pO_2 and absence of oocyte aneuploidy. This neoangiogenesis, however, does not correlate well with endometrial receptivity

and perifollicular vascularization (Fig. 17.12) correlate well with embryo quality and fertilization rates.[22-24]

Vascularization of maturing follicles has been graded on the percentage of follicular circumference seen to be vascularized using power Doppler techniques (Grade 1 < 25%, Grade 2 < 50%, Grade 3 < 75% and Grade 4 > 75%). Mean follicular diameter, oocyte retrieval rate, number of mature oocytes recovered and fertilization rates are all higher, and triploidy rates significantly lower from follicles with more than 50% vascularity. PI values of perifollicular flow do not correlate with pregnancy outcome. However, the peak systolic velocity (PSV) is an excellent parameter to assess the chances of obtaining mature oocytes and high grade pre-implantation embryos. The chances of producing a Grade I or II embryo is 75% if the PSV is more than 10 cm/second. Interestingly, during the ovulatory process, there are prominent changes in the regional blood flow of the follicle with a marked increase in flow to the base of the follicle and a concomitant decrease of blood flow to the apex. These changes may be essential for the release of a mature oocyte.

The antral follicle count[28-32] done on any day between cycle days 2 to 5, yields a count of less than 4 to 5 in poor responders. The count correlates well with number of follicles later in the cycle, E2 levels on the day of hCG administration, number of oocytes, fertilization rates and pregnancy rates. This can be done by 2D manual methods or a 3D computer assisted model[28,33] (Figs 17.13 to 17.16). Smaller ovarian diameter and ovarian volumes also correlate fairly well with poor response to ovarian stimulation and poor pregnancy rates. In patients with lower antral follicle counts, the ovarian response to gonadotropins can be modified by using an increased dose at the commencement of the cycle and by instituting medication that enhances ovarian flow.[28]

Patients with a PSV of more than 10 cm/second in ovarian stromal arteries after pituitary suppression yield significantly higher mature oocytes and achieve a higher clinical pregnancy rate.

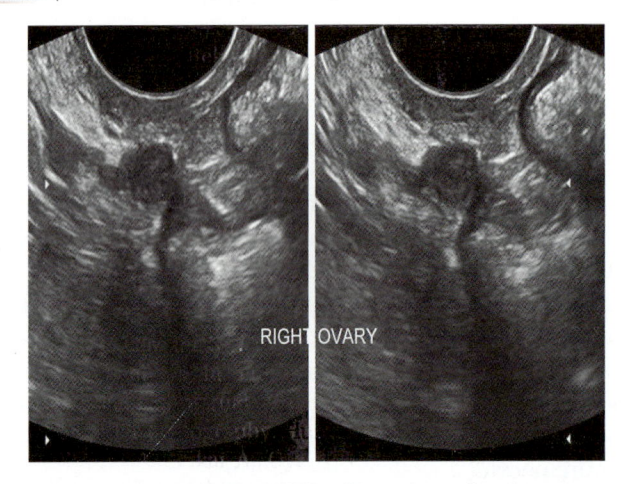

Fig. 17.13: Transvaginal sonogram of an ovary showing no antral follicles. This is a reliable marker for a poor response to gonadotropin stimulation

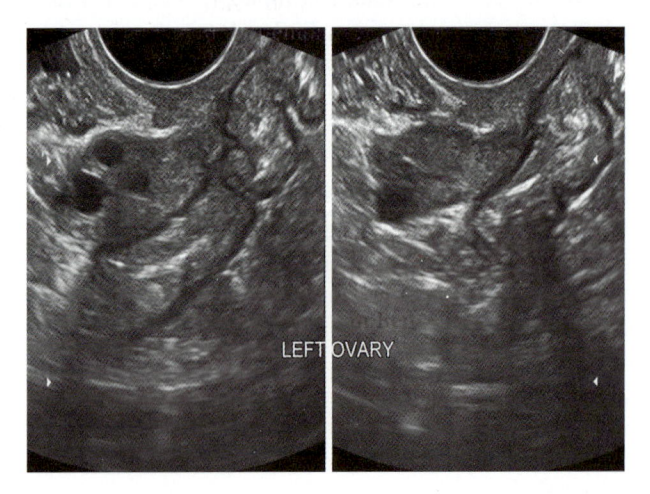

Fig. 17.14: Transvaginal sonogram of an ovary showing four antral follicles. Five or less antral follicles are a marker of poor responders

Ultrasound Assessment of Endometrial Receptivity | **435**

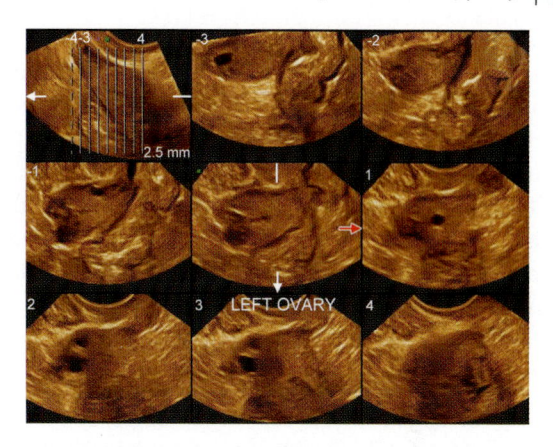

Fig. 17.15: Accurate and reproducible antral follicle counts can be obtained by 3D tomographic ultrasound imaging studies. In this technique, the ultrasound beam is programmed to fan across the entire region of interest and all tissue information in the volume of interest is digitally stored and processed by 3D hardware and software. It can then be visualized in an infinite number of planes

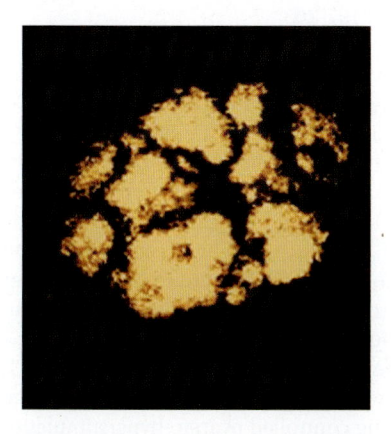

Fig. 17.16: 3D inversion mode rendering of a day 5 ovary. This mode facilitates an easier and more accurate antral follicle count

Threshold endometrial thickness, endometrial morphology, subendometrial and endometrial perfusion and uterine artery flow velocity waveforms have emerged as a reliable method of assessing the receptive and the impaired endometrium. Further improvements in image resolution and flow sensitivity, and availability of sophisticated software are likely to enhance endometrial receptivity evaluation and the application of this information to enhance reproductive outcomes.

REFERENCES

1. Nikas G. Endometrial receptivity: changes in cell-surface morphology. Semin Reprod Med. 2000;18(3):229-35.
2. Cavagna M, Mantese JC. Biomarkers of endometrial receptivity—a review. Placenta. 2003;24(Suppl. B):S39-47.
3. Giudice LC. Potential biochemical markers of uterine receptivity. Hum Reprod. 1999;14(Suppl. 2):3-16.
4. Tabibzadeh S, Shea W, Lessey BA, et al. From endometrial receptivity to infertility. Semin Reprod Endocrinol. 1999;17(3):197-203.
5. McLean-Morris J, Van Wagenen G. Interception: the use of the preovulatory estrogens to prevent implantation. Am J Obstet Gynecol. 1973;115:101-6.
6. Gidley-Baird AA, O'Neil C, Sinosich MJ, et al. Failure of implantation in human *in vitro* fertilization and embryo transfer patients: the effects of altered progesterone/estrogen ratios in human and mice. Fertil Steril. 1986;45:69-75.
7. Garcia JE, Acosta AA, Hsiu JG, et al. Advanced endometrial maturation after ovulation induction with human menopausal gonadotropin/human chorionic gonadotropin for *in vitro* fertilization. Fertil Steril. 1984;41:31-7.
8. Kolb BA, Najmabadi S, Paulson RJ. Ultrastructural characteristics of the luteal phase endometrium in donors undergoing controlled ovarian hyperstimulation. Fertil Steril. 1997;67:625-30.

9. Simon C, Mercader A, Frances A, et al. Hormonal regulation of serum and endometrial IL-1a, IL-1b and IL-1ra: IL-1 endometrial microenvironment of the human embryo at the apposition phase under physiological and supraphysiological steroid level conditions. J Reprod Immunol. 1996;31:165-84.
10. Simon C, Cano F, Valbuena D, et al. Clinical evidence for a detrimental effect on uterine receptivity of high serum oestradiol concentrations in high and normal responder patients. Hum Reprod. 1995;10:2432-7.
11. Hadi FH, Chantler E, Anderson E, et al. Ovulation induction and endometrial steroid receptors. Hum Reprod. 1994;9:2405-10.
12. Devroey P, Bourgain C, Macklon NS, et al. Reproductive biology and IVF: ovarian stimulation and endometrial receptivity. Trends Endocrinol Metab. 2004;15(2):84-90.
13. Bourgain C. Endometrial biopsy in the evaluation of endometrial receptivity. J Gynecol Obstet Biol Reprod (Paris). 2004;33(1 pt 2):S13-7.
14. Bourgain C, Devroey P. The endometrium in stimulated cycles for IVF. Hum Reprod Update. 2003;9(6):515-22.
15. Fanchin R. Assessing uterine receptivity in 2001: ultrasonographic glances at the new millennium. Ann N Y Acad Sci. 2001;943:185-202.
16. Pierson RA. Imaging the endometrium: are there predictors of uterine receptivity? J Obstet Gynaecol Can. 2003;25(5):360-8.
17. Baruffi RL, Contart P, Mauri AL, et al. A uterine ultrasonographic scoring system as a method for the prognosis of embryo implantation. J Assist Reprod Genet. 2002;19(3):99-102.
18. Schild RL, Knobloch C, Dorn C, et al. Endometrial receptivity in an *in vitro* fertilization program as assessed by spiral artery blood flow, endometrial thickness, endometrial volume, and uterine artery blood flow. Fertil Steril. 2001;75(2):361-6.
19. Ardaens Y, Gougeon A, Lefebvre C, et al. Contribution of ovarian and uterine color Doppler in medically assisted reproduction techniques (ART). Gynecol Obstet Fertil. 2002;30(9):663-72.

20. Chien LW, Lee WS, Au HK, et al. Assessment of changes in utero-ovarian arterial impedance during the peri-implantation period by Doppler sonography in women undergoing assisted reproduction. Ultrasound Obstet Gynecol. 2004;23(5):496-500.
21. Kupesic S, Bekavac I, Bjelos D, et al. Assessment of endometrial receptivity by transvaginal color Doppler and three-dimensional power Doppler ultrasonography in patients undergoing *in vitro* fertilization procedures. J Ultrasound Med. 2001;20(2):125-34.
22. Ng EHY, Chan CCW, Tang OS, et al. Comparison of endometrial and subendometrial blood flow measured by three-dimensional power Doppler ultrasound between stimulated and natural cycles in the same patients. Hum Reprod. 2004;19(10):2385-90.
23. Raine-Fenning NJ, Campbell BK, Kendall NR, et al. Quantifying the changes in endometrial vascularity throughout the normal menstrual cycle with three-dimensional power Doppler angiography. Hum Reprod. 2004;19(2):330-8.
24. Yokota A, Nakai A, Oya A, et al. Changes in uterine and ovarian arterial impedance during the periovulatory period in conception and nonconception cycles. J Obstet Gynaecol Res. 2000;26(6):435-40.
25. Kupesic S. Three-dimensional ultrasonographic uterine vascularization and embryo implantation. J Gynecol Obstet Biol Reprod (Paris). 2004;33(1 Pt 2):S18-20.
26. Buckett WM, Chian RC, Tan SL. Human chorionic gonadotropin for *in vitro* oocytes maturation: does it improve the endometrium or implantation? J Reprod Med. 2004;49(2):93-8.
27. Carbillon L, Perrot N, Uzan M, et al. Doppler ultrasonography and implantation: a critical review. Fetal Diagn Ther. 2001;16(6):327-32.
28. Kupesic S, Kurjak A. Predictors of IVF outcome by three-dimensional ultrasound. Hum Reprod. 2002;17(4):950-5.
29. Hendriks DJ, Mol BW, Bancsi LF, et al. Antral follicle count in the prediction of poor ovarian response and pregnancy after *in vitro* fertilization: a meta-analysis and comparison

with basal follicle-stimulating hormone level. Fertil Steril. 2005;83(2):291-301.
30. Scheffer GJ, Broekmans FJ, Dorland M, et al. Antral follicle counts by transvaginal ultrasonography are related to age in women with proven natural fertility. Fertil Steril. 1999;72(5):845-51.
31. Frattarelli JL, Lauria-Costab DF, Miller BT, et al. Basal antral follicle number and mean ovarian diameter predict cycle cancellation and ovarian responsiveness in assisted reproductive technology cycles. Fertil Steril. 2000;74(3):512-7.
32. Bancsi LF, Broekmans FJ, Looman CW, et al. Impact of repeated antral follicle counts on the prediction of poor ovarian response in women undergoing *in vitro* fertilization. Fertil Steril. 2004;81(1):35-41.
33. Scheffer GJ, Broekmans FJ, Bancsi LF, et al. Quantitative transvaginal two- and three-dimensional sonography of the ovaries: reproducibility of antral follicle counts. Ultrasound Obstet Gynecol. 2002;20(3):270-5.

Chapter 18

Ethical and Legal Aspects in ART

Shashi Prateek, Surveen Ghumman Sindhu

The birth of children and their socialization as members of a given society has been and continues to be an underlying concern in all societies globally. The rules regulating reproduction and the social norms associated with it may vary within different regions, and within the same region over time. Assisted reproduction raises complex ethical, legal and social dilemmas criticism of assisted reproduction arises in the context of a broad spectrum of cultural, religious and social attitudes in societies towards technical intervention in human reproduction. Although the necessity for some form of regulation in reproductive medicine is obvious, there has been an ongoing debate in society regarding the best approach to regulate assisted reproduction. The development of clinical practice guidelines may be a more effective approach to regulate assisted reproduction. However, these clinical guidelines must be formalized by means of legislation.

The ready availability of donor sperm and the ease of artificial insemination have long enabled couples with refractory male infertility to achieve successful pregnancy. Controversial issues in reproductive medicine concern the restriction of assisted repro-duction techniques including IUI based on age, marital status or sexual orientation, the impact of multiple births on health and healthcare resources, the donation of gametes, the cryopreservation of gametes and rights of the child born through donor insemination.

In most cases, progression from an ethical debate to legislation may not occur because of insufficient social concerns or cultural and religious beliefs of the society regarding legitimacy of these clinical solutions. Donor insemination is one such area. Donor sperms have been used in the treatment of male infertility for more than one hundred years. It has taken a century for us to subject it to legislative control.

Social Impact of Donor Insemination

The biological link builds a complex structure of human relationships which has considerable psychological and social significance. Donor insemination erodes this biological link which forms the foundation on which family relationships are built. It seems that nature versus nuture, genetic versus environmental and biological versus sociological interpretations of personal identity are resurfacing once again. We have to accept that donor insemination has implication still not accepted by the society. This is a fact, well-proven by the secrecy associated with donor insemination, desire for donor anonymity, and public uncertainty, leading to need for legislation. Reproduction involves factors much more complex than a biological event.

Assessment of Prospective Parents

Before going in for donor insemination the prospective parents must be evaluated as potential parents within their family structure. Aspects, such as commitment to bringing up a child, their ages, and medical histories, chances of multiple pregnancy and impact on other members of the family have to be considered. Assessment of whether parents can cope up with a child's queries, when growing up, is important. Attitudes of other family members, and its implication on the child, must be taken into account. Support structure should be emphasized if an unmarried female is being inseminated.

Counseling and Psychological Consultation

The decision to proceed with donor insemination is a complex one, and patients and their partners may benefit from psychological counseling to aid the decision. Counseling could be on:

- Information
- Implications
- Support
- Therapeutic.

All relevant information must be given to the patient before a treatment is given. No one is obliged to accept counseling but it is generally recognized as being beneficial, and couples should be encouraged to take it. Thus, before starting treatment, information should be given to the patient on the limitations and results of the proposed treatment, possible side effects, the techniques involved, comparison with other available treatments, the cost of the treatment, the rights of the child born through ART, and the need for the clinic to keep a register of the outcome of a treatment.

All ART Clinics must be registered with an appropriate authority.

Age of Recipient

In India as marriages often take place at a younger age the lower age limit needs to be defined.

No women younger than 21 years should have an ART procedure as per Indian Council of Medical Research (ICMR) recommendations.[1]

Choosing Donor Characteristics

The couple should be encouraged to list the characteristics which they desire in a prospective donor including race, ethnic group, height, body build, complexion, eye, and hair color. Consideration should be given to blood group and Rh type, specially in Rh negative women.

Consent

Suitable time for reflection by patient, after receiving information, should be allowed to elapse before consent is obtained.[2] No treatment should be given without the written consent of the couple to all the possible stages of that treatment. A standard consent form, recommended by the accreditation authority, should be used by all ART clinics. The consent would also state that the child born would be the legal heir of the couple in case of donor gamete. Specific consent must be obtained from couples who have their gametes frozen, in regard to what should be done with them if they die. He/she must consent to have no direct or indirect contact with the recipient, and to not disclosing his personal identity to the recipient. He/she must give up any legal right on the child and vice versa. No ART procedure is done in India without consent of the husband.[1]

Commercial Restriction

The ART clinic must not be a party to any commercial element in donor programs or in gestational surrogacy.

HIV Positive Status

As per the ASRM guidelines for sperm donation the following was recommended.[3]

HIV positive women: An HIV-positive woman shall not be refused ART but appropriately counseled about the possibility of the mother-to-child transmission of the AIDS virus.

HIV positive husband: An HIV negative woman should not be refused artificial insemination with donor sperms even if the husband is sero-positive for HIV.

HIV positive donor: The current FDA guidelines do not entirely preclude the use of semen from HIV positive donor/husband. However, in the opinion of ASRM, HIV positive donors should not be used, even if recipient wishes so, because the risk of viral transmission cannot be eliminated completely.

Testing for HIV in couple: Even with donor insemination the HIV status of both partners must be done to address potential medicolegal issues that could arise if the recipient seroconvert during or after treatment.

Storage and Handling of Gametes

Controlled access to areas where gametes are stored is only allowed to named individuals. The 'highest possible standards' in the storage and handling of gametes and embryos in respect to their security, and in regard to their recording and identification, should be followed. Gamete source and subsequent fate should be traceable at all times. Transfer of gametes must be undertaken with care. No woman should be treated with gametes or with embryos derived from more than one man during any one-treatment cycle.

Confidentiality: Any information about clients and donors must be kept confidential. No information about the treatment of couples provided under a treatment agreement may be disclosed to anyone other than the accreditation authority or persons covered by the license, except

- With the consent of the person to whom the information relates
- Medical emergency concerning the patient
- A court order.

It is the person's right to decide what information will be passed on and to whom.

Record Management

The nearly universal practice of physicians using donor gamete has been to keep confidential the identity of both donors and recipients. Records, including those pertaining to donor suitability, quality assurance, collection, processing, storage, medical and laboratory data, must be retained for at least ten years after insemination. This allows for donors and recipients to be tracked in the event of a medical problem in the donor or donor's family being discovered To maintain appropriate, detailed record of all donor eggs, sperm or embryos used, the manner of their use (e.g. the technique in which they are used) and the individual/couple/surrogate mother on whom they were used is important. If the ART clinic/center is wound up before 10 years, the records must be transferred to a central repository maintained by ICMR.[1]

All records must be maintained for at least 10 years by the ART clinic as per ICMR recommendations.[1]

The data of every accredited ART clinic must be accessible to an appropriate authority of the ICMR for collation at the national level. Any publication or report resulting out of analysis of such data by the ICMR will have the concerned members of the staff of the ART clinic as co-authors.

Rights of a Single Woman to ART

There is no legal bar on an unmarried woman going for artificial donor insemination (AID) provided other criteria mentioned are fulfilled. However, it is universally recommended that AID should be performed only on married women.

A child born to a single woman through AID is deemed to be legitimate and will have all the legal rights on the woman.[1]

Right of Homosexuals and Lesbians

According to the guidelines of American Society of Reproductive Medicine, IUI can be offered to lesbian and homosexual couples. However, in India there still is a need for clear guidelines because of lack of acceptability.[3]

LEGAL ISSUES OF ART IN MARRIAGE

Adultery in Case of ART

With consent of husband: ART in a married woman, with the consent of the husband, does not amount to adultery on part of the wife or the donor, as there is no sexual intercourse involved.[1]

Without consent of husband: AID without the husband's consent can be ground for divorce or judicial separation.

Consummation of Marriage in Case of AIH

Conception of the wife through artificial insemination with husband's sperm (AIH) does not necessarily amount to consummation of marriage, and a decree of nullity may still be granted in favor of the wife, on the ground of impotence of the husband, or his willful refusal to consummate the marriage.[1]

RIGHTS OF A CHILD BORN BY DONOR GAMETE

Legitimacy

A child born through AID shall be presumed to be the legitimate child of the couple, married or unmarried or a single parent. Therefore, this child shall have a right to parental support and inheritance.[1]

Right to Information

Children born through the use of donor gametes shall have a right to available medical or genetic information about the genetic parents, that may be relevant to the child's health, but no right, whatsoever, to know the identity (such as name, address, parentage, etc.) of their genetic parent(s). A child thus born will, however, be provided all other information about the donor when the child becomes an adult. While the couple will not be obliged to provide the above "other" information to the child on their own, no deliberate attempt should be made by the couple or others concerned to hide this information from the child, as and when asked for by the child.[1]

Divorce

In case of a divorce during the gestation period, if the offspring is of a donor program – be it sperm or ova – the law of the land, as pertaining to a normal conception, would apply.[1]

SEMEN BANKS

Who can Set it?
- ART clinic or suitable independent organization.[1]
- If set up by an ART clinic, it must operate as a separate identity.

Accreditation: Accreditation committee consisting of scientists, technologists and sociologists would regulate semen banks.

Advertisement: Can advertise for semen donors and legally give them financial compensation.

Confidentiality: The bank must ensure confidentiality in regard to the identity of the semen donor.

Who can be a Donor?
Use of sperm donated by a relative or a known friend of either the wife or the husband is not permitted, as per ICMR recommendations.

ASRM guidelines state that no owner, operator, lab director or employee of a facility providing AID can donate sperms. Neither can treating physician, or person performing the actual insemination, be a sperm donor.[3]

Directed donations (nonanonymous or known): They are not allowed in India but ASRM guidelines allow it provided it is acceptable to all parties. Directed donors have to undergo the same screening tests as anonymous donors. Use of semen which is not quarantined for 6 months can be justified in sexually intimate couples according to the ASRM guidelines.

Age of Donors

ICMR requires age of donor to be between 21 and 45 years.[1]

Male donors should be between 18 and 55 years in UK.[2] An upper limit of age has been defined, as there is progressive increase in prevalence of aneuploid sperm in older men.

ASRM guidelines on sperm donation recommend the upper age limit to be 40 years, with the lower limit being the legal age.[3]

Requirements for a Sperm Donor

Medical history: Hypertension, diabetes, psychiatric disorders, sexually transmitted diseases like herpes, chronic hepatitis and venereal warts or any other major illness, should be ruled out.

Personal history: ASRM has recommended that all men with personal history which makes them high risk for aquiring HIV like homosexuals, multiple sexual partners and IV drug users should be excluded.[3]

Genetic evaluation: Identifiable and common genetic disorders, such as thalassemia, should be ruled out. Chromosomal analysis is not a must.

Screening for infections: The individual must be free of HIV and hepatitis B and C infections. ASRM also recommends screening for CMV, HTLV 1 and 2, urethral swabs for *Neisseria gonorrhoea*.

Retesting: Semen should only be released after a quarantine period of 6 months to recheck donor for seroconversion. Retesting at 6 monthly intervals should be done as long as donor is active.

Semen analysis: An analysis must be carried out on the semen of the individual, preferably using a semen analyzer, and the semen must be found to be normal according to WHO method manual for semen analysis, if intended to be used for ART.

Blood group and Rh status: The blood group and the Rh status of the individual must be determined and placed on record.

General information: Other relevant information in respect of the donor, such as height, weight, age, educational qualifications, profession, color of the skin and the eyes, record of major diseases including any psychiatric disorder, and the family background in respect of history of any familial disorder, must be recorded in an appropriate proforma.

DNA Fingerprinting

If DNA fingerprinting technology is available, the ART clinic may offer to the couple, a DNA fingerprint of the donor without revealing his identity, against appropriate payment towards the cost of the DNA fingerprint. An ART clinic will then have DNA fingerprinting done of the couple and keep the DNA fingerprints on its records.

Donor Rights

1. Information on method of gamete collection, HIV screening and quarantine is provided to donor.
2. Anonymity of donor is protected and only non-identifying information is released. Donor has the right to decide what information is to be passed.
3. Donor has no right on the child and no responsibility towards the child.

4. Donor can specify limit of live children by donation.[2]
5. Storage of sperms can be for 5 years or longer if required for personal use.
6. Donor can specify for whom the sperms are to be used.
7. Donor has no right to know identity of recipient.

Donor Anonymity

It will be the responsibility of the ART clinic to obtain sperm from appropriate banks; neither the clinic nor the couple have a right to know the donor identity and address, but both the clinic and the couple, however, will have the right to have the fullest possible information from the semen bank on the donor such as height, weight, skin color, educational qualification, profession, family background, freedom from any know diseases or carrier status (such as hepatitis B or AIDS), ethnic origin and the DNA fingerprint (if possible), before accepting the donor semen. The information about the donor (including a copy of the donor's DNA fingerprint if available, but excluding the individual's personal identity) should be released by the ART clinic after appropriate identification, only to the offspring and only if asked by him/her after he/she reaches the age of 18 years, or as and when specified and required for legal purposes, and never to the parents (excepting when directed by a court of law).[1]

It will be the responsibility of the semen bank and the clinic to ensure that the couple does not come to know the identity of the donor.

Is Anonymity of the Donor Justified?

It is difficult for the child to accept refusal to access information about genetic parents when a record of such information exists. The child will grow into an adult and these donor conceived adults may become their best advocates for pressing for greater openness about donors. A situation where legislation is introduced which reduces secrecy about donor insemination, while maintaining donor anonymity, creates unfair fueling of the child's curiosity and demands resolution.

The other aspect being a hesitancy in donating sperms if identity is known on the part of the donor due to underlying fear of social criticism, interference with his own family life and potential for responsibility towards the child in unforeseen circumstances. This may reduce number of donors available.

Records

- Semen banks must keep record of all semen received, stored and supplied with details of use of each donor and pregnancy resulting from donor recorded for 10 years after which they are transferred to department of health research, Government of India.[1]
- On request for semen by ART clinic, the bank will provide the clinic with a list of donors (without name and address but with a code number) giving all relevant details.

Who can Use the Semen?

It could be used exclusively on the donors wife or any other woman designated by the donor. If not specified may be used for anyone.

Cryopreservation

Facilities for cryopeservation with accepted standards, must be provided.

Semen samples must be cryopreserved for at least six months before first use, at which time the semen donor must be tested for HIV and hepatitis B and C.[1-4]

Charges of Semen Banking

A semen bank may store a semen preparation for exclusive use on the donor's wife or on any other woman designated by the donor for use at a later date as in cases of malignancy.

An appropriate charge may be levied by the bank for the storage. In the case of non-payment of the charges when the donor is alive, the bank would have the right to destroy the semen sample or give it to a bonafide organization to be used only for research purposes.

Consanguinity and Limiting Donor

The risk of potential unknown consanguinity is not absent in gamete donation because donors may have their own children. This raises the responsibility of fertility clinics to limit the number of donor attempts for donor safety. Couples should be counseled about the rare possibility of unknown consanguinity.[5] This is a problem in small communities, in which a very limited supply of donors is available. It is far less likely where there are large commercial sperm banks. It has been suggested by ASRM in its guidelines for sperm donation, that in a population of 800,000, limiting a single donor to no more than 25 pregnancies would avoid inadvertent consanguineous conception.[3] UK allows only 10 pregnancies to one donor.[2]

The ART clinic can use a sample from the semen bank only once on a single recipient. ICMR has recommended that a single donor cannot donate more than 75 times and no more than 10 pregnancies must come from a single donor to avoid consanguinity.[1]

Problem: However, the problem lies in the fact that only 20% to 30% of the pregnancies produced through commercial donations are ever reported to the sperm banks in India.

Payment of Donors

A bank may advertise suitably for donors, who may be appropriately compensated financially, for their time and expenses, but the fee should be such that monetary incentive is not the primary motivation for sperm donation.[3] It is seen that majority of men, who donate sperm, are young single students, who are motivated predominantly by payment. If such payments are withdrawn, there is a possibility that the availability of donor sperm may decline. In the UK, the Human Fertilisation and Embryology Authority has suggested that minimal payment can be given.[2] This issue has been widely debated. In USA, men have always been paid to provide gametes. It has been suggested that donors should be paid incon-venience allowances similar to payment made to health volunteers who take part in drug and treatment trials. However, the question still remains unanswered–

In a country where sale of organs is illegal should gametes be allowed to be sold?

Death of Donor

In case of death of a donor, the semen becomes the property of the legal heir, or the nominee of the donor. All other conditions that apply to the donor would now apply to the legal heir, excepting that he cannot use it for having a woman of his choice inseminated by it.

If after the death of the donor, there are no claimants, the bank would have the right to destroy the semen sample or give it to a bonafide organization to be used only for research purposes.

Collection of Sperm from a Dying Person

Collection of gametes from a dying person will only be permitted if the spouse wishes to have a child.

Posthumous AIH through a Sperm Bank

A child born to a woman artificially inseminated with the stored sperms of her deceased husband is considered to be a legitimate child.[1]

OOCYTE DONATION

Indian Council of Medical Research has put down certain guidelines for oocyte donation.[1]

- No woman can donate more than six times with a minimum interval of 3 months
- Oocytes from a single donor can be shared between only 2 recipients provided each has at least 7 oocytes
- All excess oocytes must be preserved by the ART clinic for the same recipient or used for research by a bonafide organization
- Sale of any gametes or transfer to another country is completely prohibited in India.

How Long should Gametes be Stored?

Gametes should not be stored for more than 5 years.[1] Longer periods may be allowed in other circumstances like for personal use after treatment for malignancy.

After a period of five years or if commissioning parents die the embryo is destroyed or used for research. If one partner dies the embryo can be used by the other partner provided a consent has been taken.

SURROGACY

Surrogacy has been encompassed by a number of legal problems. Indian Council of Medical Research came out with the following guidelines in 2010 to decrease problems associated with surrogacy:[1]

- Surrogacy would not be allowed if the women can carry the pregnancy naturally
- A surrogacy agreement must be signed between the parties
- The identity of the surrogate is kept confidential
- All medical and insurance related expenses of surrogate must be borne by the couple seeking surrogacy
- Surrogate mother may receive monitory compensation
- A surrogate has to relinquish all rights on the child
- No woman less than 21 years and more than 35 can act as a surrogate
- No woman can act as a surrogate for more than 5 successful births in her life including her own children
- A surrogate should be screened for all medical diseases
- A surrogate mother is registered in her own name in the hospital with the address of the couple for whom she is a surrogate
- No surrogate shall undergo embryo transfer more than three times for the same couple
- The birth certificate shall bear the names of the parents who commissioned the surrogacy
- The couple is legally bound to accept responsibility of the child irrespective of any abnormality in the child
- Surrogate mother cannot act as an oocyte donor
- Consent of the spouse is required if the surrogate is married
- A relative or known person can act as a surrogate provided they are of the same generation

- For a foreign couple a legal guardian is appointed who will look after the child till the couple take the child. The foreign couple will have to produce a letter from their country stating that surrogacy is recognized and that the child will be permitted entry into the country as a biological child of the couple. The child will not be considered an Indian citizen even if donor gametes have been used.
- A couple cannot have the services of more than one surrogate at a time
- A couple cannot have simultaneous embryo transfer in the surrogate and the female partner.

The law needs to move along with medical advancements, and be suitably amended, so that it does not give rise to dilemma or unwarranted harsh situation. Burning debates still exist as to whether the donor has a right, independent of his existing or future family affiliations, to donate his gametes. There are many issues which are unsettled, some of which may have no answers. Yet it is important for guidelines to come into practice for ethical practice of reproductive technologies. Subfertility guidelines, besides assisting healthcare professionals, and patients, in the decision-making process regarding appropriate, safe and cost-effective care, may also serve as a means of external control of ethical, legal and social issues in reproductive medicine.

REFERENCES

1. Indian Council of Medical Research. The Assisted Reproductive Technology (regulation). Bill 2010—Draft. New Delhi, Ministry of Health and Family Welfare, India 2010.
2. Code of Practice. Human Fertilization and Embryology Authority, Clements House, 14-18 Gresham Street, London EC2V 7JE, 1991.

3. ASRM Practice Guideline: 2006 Guidelines for gamete and embryo Fertil Steril 2006;86:S38-50.
4. Guilhem D: New reproductive technologies, ethics and legislation in Brazil: A delayed debate. Bioethics 2001;15(3): 218-30.
5. Doyle P. The UK Human Fertilisation and Embryology Authority. How it has contributed to the evaluation of assisted reproduction technology. Int J Technol Assess Health care 1999;15(1):3-10.

INDEX

Page numbers followed by *f* refer to figure and *t* refer to table

A

Abnormal
  spermatozoa 57
  sperms 57*f*
Accessory sex gland epididymal dysfunction 42*t*
Acid phosphatase 42*t*
Acrosome detection 62
Adnexal torsion 390
Adultery in case of ART 447
Advantages of
  GnRH
    agonists 91
    antagonists over GnRH agonist in ART 97
  long protocol 88
  recombinant FSH 78
  short protocol 89
Agglutination 48
Aggregation 48
Air bubble technique during embryo transfer 110
American College of Obstetrics and Gynecology 413
Amino acid turnover pace 105
Amorphous heads 57
Analgesia 128
Andrologist 8
Anesthesia 128
Aniline blue 41*t*
Anti-Müllerian hormone 26
Antisperm antibody 46, 53, 63
  tests 42*t*
Antivibration microscope table 14

Antral follicle count 26, 26*t*
Artificial donor insemination 447
Aspirated follicular fluid 141*f*
Aspiration of follicle 143
Aspirin 371
Assessment of
  BMI and weight and lifestyle changes 22
  fertilization 240, 241
  nutritional status and role of supplements 23
  post-thaw fertility 313
  sperm DNA damage 65
Assisted reproductive technology 401, 422
Azoospermia 49, 50

B

Basal
  anti-Müllerian hormone 392
  follicle stimulating hormone levels 24, 25*t*
Basic infrastructure 1
Basis of centrifugation 221
Bed rest after embryo transfer 111
Binocular microscope 12
Biochemical measurement of sperm function 62
Blastocyst 163
  embryos 162*f*
  grading 254*t*
  scoring 161
Blastomere uniformity and number 105

Blood group and Rh status 451
Breast and ovarian cancer 78
Buffer system 169
Buserelin 85, 86

C

Calcium free media 288
Carbon
   dioxide and oxygen concentration in incubator 179
   filters 3
Cause of
   high volume 45
   increased viscosity 45
   low volume 44
   poor endometrial response 362t
Centrifuge 14
Cervical mucus removal 108
Changing room 7
Charges of semen banking 454
Choice
   and dose of gonadotropin 71t
   of catheter and outcome of embryo transfer 105
   of dosage 70
Choline 288
Clean air work station 11
Cleaning cervical mucus 120
Clinical significance of positive test 64
Clomiphene
   challenge test 27
   citrate 362t
   in mild stimulation protocol 76
Closed pulled straws 358
Coagulation 41t, 42
Coiled tails 58
Coitus interruptus 40

Combined oral contraceptive pill 34
Common indications for autologous semen banking 304
Commonly used GnRH agonists 86
Complications of pregnancy reduction 412
Computer
   aided sperm analysis 51
   assisted semen analyzer 14
   automated semen analysis 178
Conference room 7
Congenital absence of Vas 46t, 49
Connecting tubing 135
Consanguinity and limiting donor 454
Constituents of
   culture media 168t
   media 290t, 311t
Container for collection 40
Controlled ovarian stimulation in PCOS 32
Cooling and warming rates 309
Critical OHSS 398
Cross-infection in semen banks 313
Cryofreezing 119
Cryopreservation 453
   of embryo and subsequent replacement 394
   of epididymal sperms 314
   of immature oocytes 288
   of testicular sperms 315
Cryoprotectant dimethylosulfoxide 306
Cryoprotective media 306
C-terminal peptide 79
Culture media 15
   in IVF and embryo culture 167

Cumulative embryo score 153
Cumulus
   expansion 232
   oocyte complexes 232*t*
Cusco's speculum 120
Cytoplasmic droplets 58

D

Damage to endometrium 106
Death of donor 455
Debris laden or viscous sample and for CASA analysis 55
Decreasing dose of hCG 393
Degradation of deoxyribonucleic acid 312
Dehydrogesterone 379
Delaying hCG 393
Density gradient centrifugation method 214
Denudation 238
Deposition of embryo transfer into uterine cavity 121
Disadvantages of
   antagonists 98
   GnRH agonists 90
   long protocol 89
   short protocol 90
Disposable
   in ART 191
   polysterene pipettes 199
Disruption of meiotic spindle 287
Diuretics 397
DNA fingerprinting 451
Donor
   rights 451
   sperm banking 304
Dopamine 397
Drainage of hydrosalpinx 374

E

Echogenic tip 131
Echogenicity 368
Ejaculatory duct obstruction 44, 46*t*
Electronic thermometer 15
Embryo
   assessment 153
   glue 109
   grading 160*f*, 251*t*
   metabolics 105
   reduction needle 16*t*
   respiratory rate 105
   selection 151
   transfer 152, 422
      and troubleshooting 103
      catheter 16t, 114*f*
      media 114*f*
      step by step 112
   vitrification 329
Embryology pertaining to embryo transfer 112
Embryonic fragmentation 105
Embryos for
   cryopreservation 252, 253
   transfer 253
Embryos respiratory rate 105
Empty follicle syndrome 146
Endometrial
   culture and histopathology for infections 367
   histology 366
   histopathology 366
   preparation for frozen embryo transfer 370
   thickness 368
   vascular changes 366
   vascularity 368

Endometriosis 29
Endotoxin level 177
Epididymal
   and testicular sperm 220
   sperm 220
Equilibration media 296
Essential
   of sperm preparation 208
   prerequisites for embryo growth 167f
   principles of
      controlled rate cooling 284
      thawing 286
Estradiol supplementation in luteal phase 380
Estrogens 370
Ethical and legal aspectsin ART 441
Evaluation of
   embryo quality 155
   oocyte quality 286
   ovarian reserve 24
Exogenous FSH ovarian reserve test 25t, 27
External quality control 18
Extrinsic buffer system 168t

F

Factors affecting
   clinical efficiency of oocyte cryopreservation 287
   embryo transfer 103, 104
Failed emission 44
Falcon polystyrene IVF test tubes 198f
Fertilization assessment 154
Fibroids and polyps 28
Fixed
   protocol 93
   versus flexible antagonist administration 95
Flexible protocol 93
Floor plan of ART center 9f
Follicle
   aspiration 394
   flushing 136
Follicular maturation 432f
Food and Drug Administration 194
Foot control of rocket suction pump 132f
Fornax test tube warmer 140f
Four well plate polystyrene plate 200f
Fragmentation index 65
Freezing 309
French protocol 93, 94f
Frequent ejaculation 46
Fructose 42t
Fyrite kit 15

G

Gamete cryopreservation 283
Gastrointestinal complications 390
Genital tract infection 53
Gentle and atraumatic technique 107
Germinal vesicle breakdown 230
Glass
   marking pencil 16t
   micropipettes 331
Glucocorticoids 33
Glucose consumption 105
Glucosidase 42t
Glycerol egg-yolk citrate 307
GnRH
   agonist 85
      for ovulation trigger 91
   antagonists 92

Golan's classification of OHSS2 386*t*
Gonadotropin 69
  releasing hormone 99
Good Manufacturing Practice 176
Goserelin 85, 86
Gradient double density 229*f*
Grading of
  cumulus–oocyte complexes 232*t*
  motility 53
Graduated conical tubes 16*t*
Grouping of scored zygotes 241

H

Hamster egg human sperm penetration assay 61
Head with small acrosomal area 57
Heat sealing machines 14
Heating
  appliances 13
    ventilation and air conditioning 3
Hemizona assay 42*t*, 61
HEPA filters 3
Hepatic dysfunction 93
Hepatitis 19
High security vitrification kit 332*t*, 358
Highly purified
  HMG 69
  urinary FSH 69
HIV positive
  donor 445
  husband 445
  status 445
  women 445
Human
  chorionic gonadotropin 69, 80, 379
  immunodeficiency virus 18
  menopausal gonadotropins 69
  pituitary gonadotropin 69
  sperm
    motility bioassay testing 194
    preserving medium 307
Huntington's chorea 305
Husband's sperm 448
Hydrosalpinx 29
Hyperandrogenemia 362*t*
Hyperprolactinemia 362*t*
Hyperstimulation syndrome 77
Hypogonadism 44
Hypo-osmotic swelling test 41*t*, 60, 225
Hysteroscopy 369

I

ICSI micropipettes 16t
Ideal sperm separation technique 225
Immature germ cells 59
Immotile cilia syndrome 53
Immunobead test 43*t*, 63
Immunocytochemical assay 60
Immunological
  aspects of endometrial implantation 365
  infertility 22t
Implantation potential point 111
Improvement of motility and sperm function 223
Improving uterine receptivity 372*t*
In vitro fertilization 151, 421
Increased vascular permeability of mesothelial surfaces 388
Incubation 236, 240
Incubator handling 179

Indications for
  donor semen banking 305
  ICSI 34*t*
  IVF 22*t*
  semen cryopreservation 304
Initial
  basic microscopic examination 47
  microscopic examination 46
Insemination 235, 236, 240
  protocols in ART 233
Insertion of outer sheath 120
Inspection for retained embryos 122
Instruction to couple before IVF 35*t*
Insulin sensitizer 32
Intracytoplasmic sperm injection 283
Intramuscular depot injections 86
Intrauterine
  adhesions 29
  insemination 315
  synechiae 362*t*
Intrinsic testicular disease 49
Invasive hemodynamic monitoring 395
IVF conical test tubes 198*f*

K

Kremer test 42*t*

L

Laboratory purification system 12
Laminar
  air flow 181
  flow hoods 11
Laparotomy 398
Large granular lymphocytes 365

L-arginine 371
Laser system 14
Learning curve 146
Leukocytes 59
Leuprolide 86
Level of estradiol 392
Liquefaction 41, 43
Live spermatozoa 210
Liver dysfunction 390
Loading embryos in inner catheter 121
Location of laboratory 1
Lubeck protocol 93, 94*f*
Lupreolide 85
Lysis of uterine synechia 374

M

Management of
  ascitis 397
  failure to aspirate follicular fluid 145
  OHSS 390
MAR test 43*t*, 209
Masturbation 40
Matrix metalloproteinases 410
Measurement of VOC 3
Media for
  sperm preparation and insemination 233
  vitrification of cleavage stage embryos 342
Medical treatment of endometritis 374
Medication after embryo transfer 111
Metformin 394
Method of
  assessment of sperm concentration 50

collection 40
preparation 54
endometrial evaluation 367*t*
insemination 235
semen freezing 310*t*
Micro-droplet method 237
Micromanipulator 8, 12
Microscopes 12
Mild
OHSS 396
stimulation protocol 74
Minimum drops size 332
Miscarriage 78
Mixed antiglobulin reaction test 63
Modes of ovulation induction in PCOS 33
Modified Tyrode's medium containing glycerol, sucrose, glucose, glycine as cryoprotective agents, human serum albumin 307
Morphological
features of normal embryos and blastocyst 255*t*
parameters 105
Mouse embryo assay test 193
Multidose protocol 93
Multifetal pregnancy reduction 401, 402
Multiple pregnancy 77

N

Naferelin 85
Nasal spray 86
National ART registry of India 401
Navot's classification 387
Neck and midpiece defects 58
Needle
handle 134
sharpness 131

Neisseria gonorrhoea 450
Nitric oxide levels 105
Nitroglycerine 371
Nonpyrogenicity 193
Nonsteroidal anti-inflammatory drugs 112
Nontoxic
condom 40
gloves 16*t*
Normal values for semen analysis 43*t*
Nuclear chromatin decondensation test 41*t*
Number of
follicles on ultrasonography 393
sperms 52

O

Obstruction in male genital tract 44
Obstructive azoospermia 220
Oocyte
and embryo quality 430
aspiration 131*f*
cryopreservation 283
denudation 286
donation 456
freezing 283
protocol 289*t*
in equilibration media 297*f*
maturity 231*t*
pick-up 370
retrieval set 16*t*
vitrification and thawing 292
Open pulled straw 331
Operation theater 8
OPU step by step 137
Outline of cryoprotectants in semen cryopreservation 306

Ovarian
  cyst 30, 91
  function 283
  hyperstimulation syndrome 91, 385, 387t
  reserve tests 25t
  stimulation with GnRH antagonists 96
  volume 26
Ovum
  aspiration pump 12
  donation cycles 421
  pickup 127
    and troubleshooting 127
    needle 130, 134f
    procedure 132f

P

Packaging of semen sample 308t
Paracentesis of hydrothorax 398
Parameters for semen analysis 41t
Partial obstruction of ejaculatory duct 53
Pasteur's pipette 16t
Pathophysiology of OHSS 388, 389
Peak systolic velocity 433
Pelvic inflammatory disease 22t
Pentoxifylline 223
Peroxidase-positive leukocytes 209
Petri dish warmer 13
pH values 46t
Phosphate buffer 171
Physiology of
  blastocyst media 175
  IVF fertilization medium 172
  sequential culture media 171
Pipette stands 16t
Piroxicam 374

Place of embryo deposition in uterine cavity 110
Plastic
  Pipettes 200f
  test tube stand 16t
Platelet-activating factor 223, 224
Polybutadiethylene 192
Polycystic ovary patients 31
Polyethylene 192
Polypropylene 192
Polystyrene 192
Poor sperm
  function 63
  motility 63
Position of patient during embryo transfer 107
Postejaculatory urine sample 40
Premature
  endogenous luteinizing hormone 85
  release of cortical granules 287
Preparation of
  embryo transfer media plate 113, 113f
  flushing syringes 115
  needle and tubing 143
  styrofoam box with liquid nitrogen 335
  transfer plates 112
  vagina 128
Pressure gradient 3
Pretreatment hormone assessment to optimize IVF outcomes 24
Prevention of thrombosis 397
Previous pelvic surgery 22t
Primary testicular failure 49
Principles of
  vitrification 329
  warming 330

Procedure of
  oocyte
    slow freezing 289
    thawing 290
  sperm preparation 216
Progressive motility 53, 209, 210
Pronuclei
  scoring 155
  stage scoring 156*f*
Prostatic specific antigen 42*t*
Protocol
  for examination of sperm morphology 51
  for insemination and embryo culture 234
  for retained embryos 122
  of ovarian stimulation 392
Purified urinary FSH 69

Q

Quality
  checks 4
  control 17
    testing for culture media 176
  of consumables used in laboratory 15
  of water 171

R

Reactive oxygen species 62
Recent advances in cryopreservation media 288
Recombinant
  FSH 69, 78, 79
  hCG 69
  LH 69, 80
Record room 7
Recovery room 7
Recurrent intrauterine insemination failure 22*t*
Reducing
  insulin 31
  uterine contractility 374
Relaxing patient during procedure 106
Relevance of embryo selection and grading 104
Relieve financial burden on infertile couple 211
Renal dysfunction 93
Requirements for sperm donor 450
Retained embryos and repeat embryo transfer 111
Retrograde ejaculation 22*t*, 221
Rights of
  child born by donor gamete 448
  homosexuals and lesbians 447
  single woman to ART 447
Risk factors for OHSS 391*t*
Ritodrine 374
Rocket suction pump 131*f*
Role of
  GnRH
    agonists and antagonists in ART 85
    antagonist in mild stimulation 75
  oil overlay 237
  oral contraceptive pill 96
    before ART cycle 34
  ultrasound and mock embryo-transfer before procedure 106
  uterine contractility in success of embryo transfer 108
Room for intrauterine insemination 7

S

Sample
  collection and delivery 39
  with low sperm count 54
Scoring of agglutinates 48*t*
Scrub station 8
Secretion of seminal vesicles and prostate 44
Semen
  analysis 41, 43, 451
    and assessment of male partner 39
  banks 449
  collecting containers 16*t*
  cryopreservation 303
  culture 42*t*
  preparation for IVF 207
  processing laboratory 7
  volume 209
Seminal
  fructose 43*t*, 210
  neutral glucosidase 43*t*, 210
  zinc 43*t*, 209
Sequential media 173*f*
Serum estradiol 391
Setting up of ART center 1
Severe
  endometriosis 22*t*
  infection 49
  intrauterine adhesions 22*t*
  OHSS 396
  oligoasthenoteratospermia 22*t*
Sex hormone binding globulin 31, 32
Sexual intercourse post-transfer 111
Short
  abstinence interval 44
  denudation method 239
Sildenafil 371

Single
  dose protocol 93
  embryo transfer 113*f*
  versus multiple dose GnRH antagonist protocol 93
Size and number of follicles 391
Social impact of donor insemination 442
Sodium bicarbonate 170
Speed of smear 54
Sperm
  agglutination 63
  concentration 43*t*, 48, 209, 210, 233
  count/ejaculate 210
  counting chamber 14
  cryopreservation 303
  fertilizing capability 41*t*
  immobilization test 178
  injection 231
  longevity test 61
  membrane binding 61
  morphology 53, 209
  motility 50
  penetration assay 42*t*
  preparation 235
  survival test 178
Spermatogenesis 49
Spermatozoa 52*t*
Spindle imaging system 14
Squamous metaplasia 362*t*
Stage warmer 13
Step
  down protocol 73
  of oocyte warming 302
  up high dose protocol 71
  up low dose protocol 72
Stereomicroscope 8
Stereozoom microscope 12

Sterility test 178
Steroids 394
Storage
 and handling of gametes 445
 of media 189*t*
Store room 7
Study of hyperactivated motility 41*t*
Subcutaneous injections 86
Suboptimal
 estrogens 362
 progesterones 362
Subseptate uterus 29
Sucrose concentration 288
Superiority of various vitrification methods 333
Surgical sperm retrieval techniques 305
Swemed glass pipettes and handle 201*f*

T

Tails of irregular width 58
Techniques of semen preparation 212
Teratospermic index 56
Termination of pregnancy 398
Test tube warmer 133*f*
Testicular
 dysfunction 53
 or epididymal sperms 34*t*
 sperm extraction-open method 220
Testing for HIV in couple 445
Tests for sperm membrane integrity 60
Thawing 313

Time
 interval between embryo loading and transfer 110
 of insemination 233
Tip of ovum pickup needle 135*f*
Tissue culture grade plastic test tubes 16*t*
Total
 motility 53, 209, 210
 progressive motility 53
 sperm number 43*t*, 209
Transabdominal reduction 404
Transcervic alaspiration 403
Transportation of semen 40
Transvaginal
 fetal reduction 405
 sonogram of ovary 434*f*
Treatment of
 luteal phase defect 377
 poor uterine receptivity 370
Triptorelin 85, 86
Tubal and pelvic adhesions 22*t*
Tuberculosis 21, 22*t*
Two step gradient 229
Types of
 disposables 195
 embryo transfer medium used durin gembryo transfer 109
 grades 157*f*

U

Ultrapure water system 15
Ultrasonographic examination 395
Ultrasonography 77
Ultrasound
 and color Doppler 368
 assessment of endometrial receptivity and oocyte and embryo quality 419

for bladder status 119
machine 14
  with TVS probe 129f
  to visualize cervical canal and uterine cavity 120
Ultraviolet light 4
Unexplained infertility 22t
Unique vitrification devices 331
Use of
  GnRH agonist in COH protocols 87
  oil overlay in ART 176
  ultrasound-guidance during embryo transfer 109
USP class VI and elution test 193
Uterine septum 362t

V

Vacuolated heads 57
Vaginal administration 379
Varicocele 53
Vascularization flow index 427
Vigorous curettage 362
Virtual organ computer aided analysis 424
Viscosity 41t, 45
  of semen 45
Visualization of embryos and grading 118

Vitamins 168
Vitrification
  devices 331t
  media 296
  simplified 292
  step by step 334
  technique for ultrarapid freezing 315
Volatile organic compounds 2

W

Warming
  blocks 13
  rate 309
  steps 347
Wash and swim-up method 228f
Washing
  denuded oocytes 240, 242
  of OCC 240
Water supply 2
WHO criterion for sperm morphology 56
Withholding hCG 392

Z

Z score 242t
Zona
  pellucida 230, 252, 342f, 356f
  hardening 287